M. Lemmerling · S. S. Kollias (Eds.)

Radiology of the Petrous Bone

With Contributions by

C. Bartolozzi · A. Behin · S. Berrettini · C. Cappelli · D. Caramella · J. Chiras · C. Czerny
B. De Foer · I. Dhooge · A. Dirisamer · R. Hermans · H. Imhof · S. S. Kollias · M. Lemmerling
N. Martin-Duverneuil · E. Neri · E. Oschatz · S. Sunaert · H. Tanghe · L. van den Hauwe

Foreword by

A. L. Baert

With 271 Figures in 633 Separate Illustrations, 19 in Color and 16 Tables

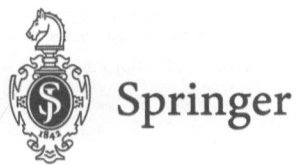 Springer

MARC LEMMERLING, MD
Medische Beeldvorming
A. Z. St. Lucas
Groenebril, 1
9000 Gent
Belgium

SPYROS S. KOLLIAS, MD
Institute of Neuroradiology
University Hospital of Zurich
Frauenklinikstrasse 10
8091 Zürich
Switzerland

MEDICAL RADIOLOGY · Diagnostic Imaging and Radiation Oncology
Series Editors: A. L. Baert · L. W. Brady · H.-P. Heilmann · M. Molls · K. Sartor

Continuation of Handbuch der medizinischen Radiologie
Encyclopedia of Medical Radiology

ISBN 978-3-642-62315-8

Radiology of the petrous bone / M. Lemmerling, S. S. Kollias (eds.) ;
with contributions by B. DeFoer ... [et al.] ; foreword by A. L. Baert.
    p. ; cm. -- (Medical radiology)
    Includes bibliographical references and index.
    ISBN 978-3-642-62315-8   ISBN 978-3-642-18836-7 (eBook)
    DOI 10.1007/978-3-642-18836-7
    1. Ear--Diseases--Diagnosis. 2. Ear--Radiography. 3. Temporal
bone--Tumors--Diagnosis. 4. Diagnostic imaging. I. Lemmerling, M. (Marc) 1964- II.
Kollias, S. S. (Spyros S.) III Series.
    [DNLM: 1. Diagnostic Imaging--methods. 2. Ear Diseases--diagnosis. 3.
Ear--pathology. 4. Skull Neoplasms-pathology. 5. Temporal Bone--pathology. WV 210
R129 2003]
    RF123.5.I4 R336 2003
    617.8'0757--dc21   2002042649

http//www. springer.de

© Springer-Verlag Berlin Heidelberg 2004

Originally published by Springer-Verlag Berlin Heidelberg New York in 2004
Softcover reprint of the hardcover 1st edition 2004

Cover-Design and Typesetting: Verlagsservice Teichmann, 69256 Mauer

21/3150xq – 5 4 3 2 1 0 – Printed on acid-free paper

Foreword

The petrous bone is a organ with a very complex anatomy and a very limited accessibility by conventional radiology.

With the introduction of CT and MRI, detailed and spectacular display of the very small osseous and non-osseous structures of the middle and inner ear became possible. Consequently, a new era opened in clinical radiology of this organ.

This volume covers comprehensively the imaging techniques, radiological anatomy and congenital and acquired pathological conditions of the petrous bone as visualized by the new cross-sectional methods. The eminently readable text is enriched by numerous superb illustrations.

The book has been prepared and edited by two outstanding head and neck radiologists: M. Lemmerling and S.S. Kollias are both well known for their excellent contributions to the scientific literature on petrous bone imaging. The other authors of individual chapters were invited to contribute because of their expertise and long experience in the field. I would like to congratulate the editors and the authors most sincerely for their efforts.

I am confident that this outstanding text will meet with great interest from general radiologists , neuroradiologists, and head and neck radiologists, and also from neurosurgeons and ENT specialists. I am sure that it will enjoy the same success with the readers as many previous volumes published in this series.

Leuven   ALBERT L. BAERT

Preface

When I tried to analyse the temporal bone during my studies, I had to restudy its anatomy over and over again, even before beginning to understand which diseases could be radiologically diagnosed. Honestly, the latter only became clear to me after many more years of communication with the referring physicians. Bearing these personal experiences in mind while compiling the present volume, I decided from the outset to include a chapter on temporal bone anatomy and a section on the opinion of the otologist.

The continued improvement in the ability to define the many minute structures present in the petrous bone, and to visualise exceedingly small disease processes, created an increased interest in our subspecialty from otologists and neurotologists. I am very grateful to all contributing authors who made it possible to provide a complete and up-to-date volume in this subject area. Without their expertise and work this publication would never have been accomplished. The book aims to provide a guide to many aspects of temporal bone imaging, including those that are not yet performed by all of us in this field, such as functional MRI and virtual endoscopy. Most of the information in this volume, however, should offer the radiologist a practical answer to most questions about the petrous bone.

The initiative for writing this book came from Prof. A.L. Baert. I consider his request to write this book as a sign of his appreciation for my contributions in the field of temporal bone imaging. I am very grateful for being given the chance and hope that I have fulfilled his expectations.

Last but not least, I would like to thank my family for their understanding and patience. Although this project seemed endless, they supported me all the way. A special thanks goes to Nancy Verpoort, who spent a considerable amount of time editing the figures and texts.

Gent   MARC LEMMERLING

Contents

1 Technique and Radiologic Anatomy

M. Lemmerling

CONTENTS

1.1
Technique

Computed tomography and MR imaging are the most commonly used techniques to image the temporal bone. Through this book the indications for both techniques will become clear. In this first chapter the radiologic anatomy of the temporal bone is shown for both techniques. On consecutive images made in daily practice the different visualized structures are indicated. First of all, the currently used imaging protocols are described.

1.1.1
CT Technique for Temporal Bone Imaging

The images are acquired in a single imaging plane using a multislice detector scanner, but without using the spiral mode technique. The patient lies on his/her back and the gantry of the scanner is not tilted. The following imaging parameters are used: (a) 120 kV; (b) 250 mAs; (c) collimation 0.5 mm; (d) scan time 1.0 s; and (e) cycle time 2.0 s.

After acquiring this raw data set, 20 images are reconstructed with a slice thickness of 1 mm and by using an ultra-high-resolution reconstruction mode.

M. Lemmerling, MD, PhD
Medische Beeldvorming, A.Z. St. Lucas, Groenebriel 1, 9000 Gent, Belgium

The technicians are taught to make this reconstruction in a plane parallel to the lateral semicircular canal. This is the axial imaging set. The coronal imaging set is reconstructed exactly perpendicular to this axial set of images. On the most cranial axial image the superior semicircular canal is shown. The most anterior coronal image is made just anterior to the geniculate ganglion of the facial nerve. This procedure is repeated for both the right and left temporal bones separately, which means that four films with 20 images are made and printed using a window width of 4000 HU and a window level of 200 HU. These parameters for windowing only have an indicative value, and each radiologist has to make his/her own choice. Systematic visualization of both, stapes crura and of the suspensory ligaments in the middle ear cavity, can be a helpful indicator when choosing the windowing parameters.

1.1.2
MR Technique for Temporal Bone Imaging

A lot of discussion exists as to which MR imaging protocol should be used for the temporal bone. Controversy exists regarding which sequences should be used, what the exact slice thickness of the images should be, and even on the eventual use of contrast agents. The following imaging protocol can be considered as an example of how a good protocol can appear, but each radiologist can omit or add sequences or make changes to it according to personal experiences or according to different indications. These sequences are standard in my department:
1. Axial 5-mm-thick turbo-spin-echo (TSE) T2-weighted images through the brain, brain stem, and posterior fossa, performed to study the brain for cerebral anomalies causing hearing loss, tinnitus, vertigo, etc. (e.g., cerebral arteriovenous malformations and tinnitus, brain stem ischemia, and vertigo)
2. Axial 3-mm-thick T1-weighted SE images through the temporal bone

3. Axial 0.7-mm-thick 3D T2-weighted TSE images through the inner ear structures
4. Gadolinium-enhanced axial 3-mm-thick T1-weighted SE images through the temporal bone, and if an enhancing lesion is seen on this sequence, the following is added
5. Gadolinium-enhanced coronal 3-mm-thick T1-weighted SE images

The following changes are currently made:
- Performing T1-weighted images in 3D technique with the use of thinner slices (e.g., 1 mm). This technique is especially interesting in studying the relationship between small tumors and the cranial nerves in the internal auditory meatus.
- Performing reconstructions of the 3D T2-weighted TSE sequence in planes other than the axial one. This is most often done to study the relationship between different small structures in the cerebellopontine angle and internal audi-tory meatus, such as cranial nerves, vessels, and small tumors.
- Performing additional MR angiographic sequences, which is especially interesting if vascular lesions are detected.

1.2
Radiologic Anatomy

1.2.1
Axial CT Images (Figs. 1–22)

The images are shown from a left temporal bone, from cranially to caudally. The last image is not part of the previous series. The last image is an enlarged view at oval window level in another person, showing the anterior and posterior stapes crus. All images have a 1-mm slice thickness.

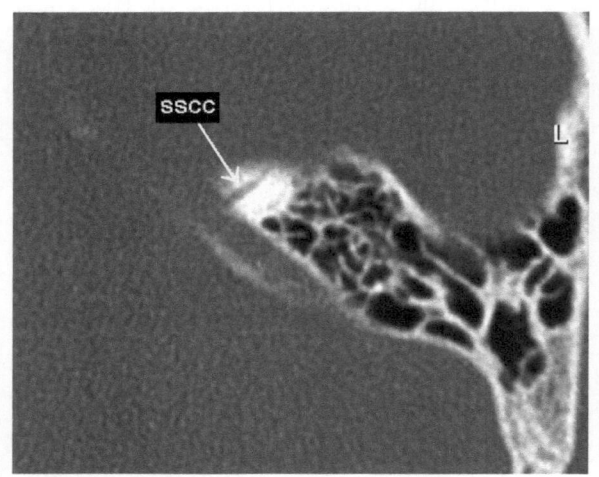

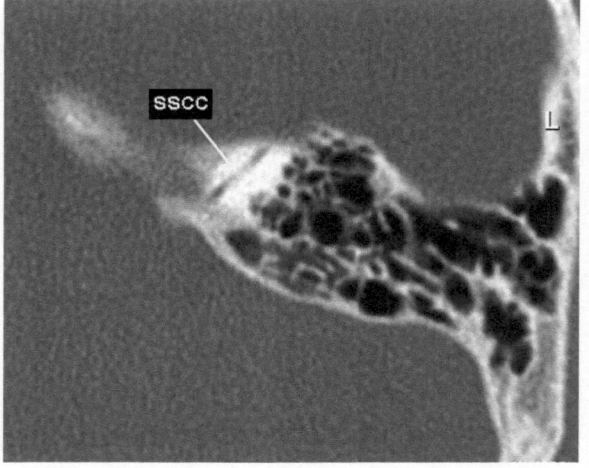

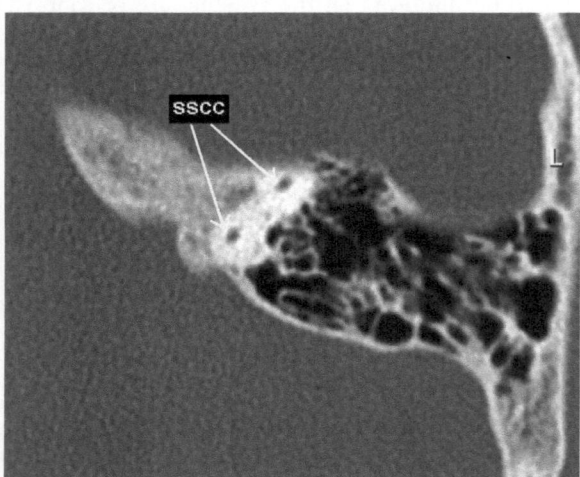

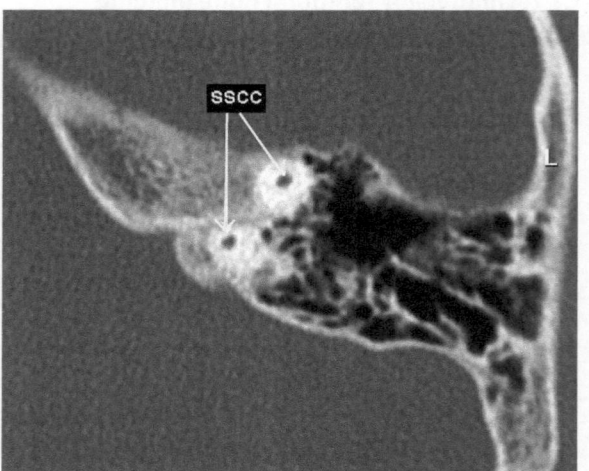

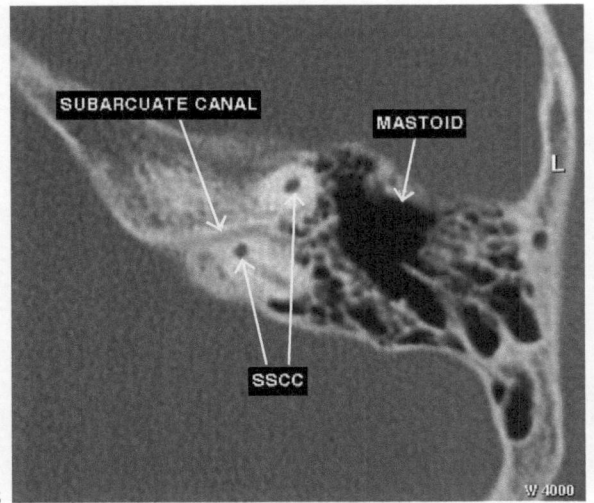

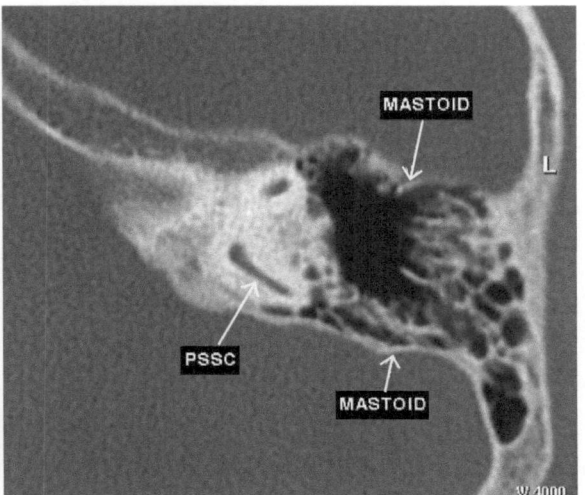

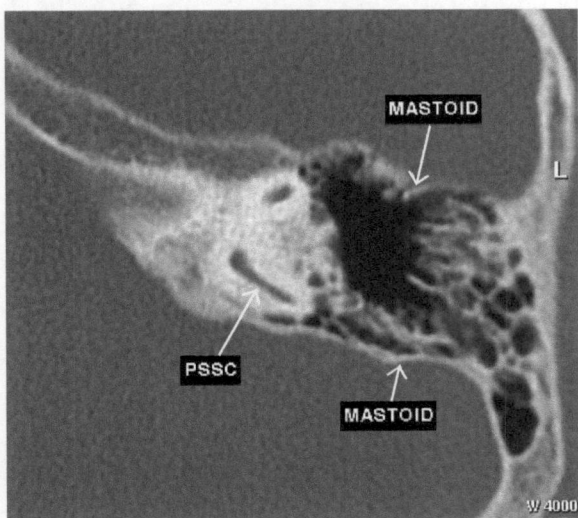

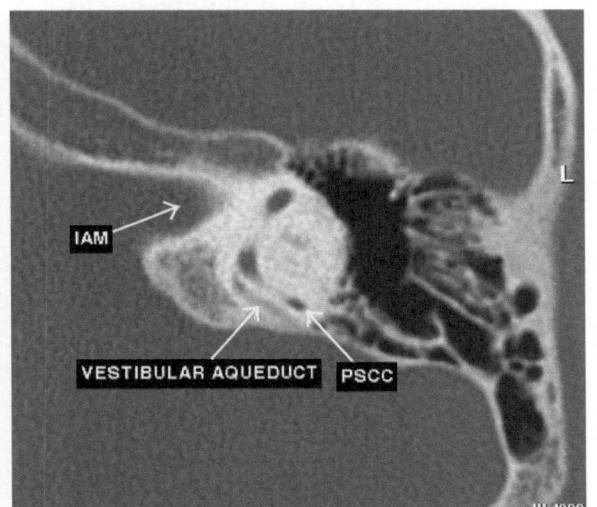

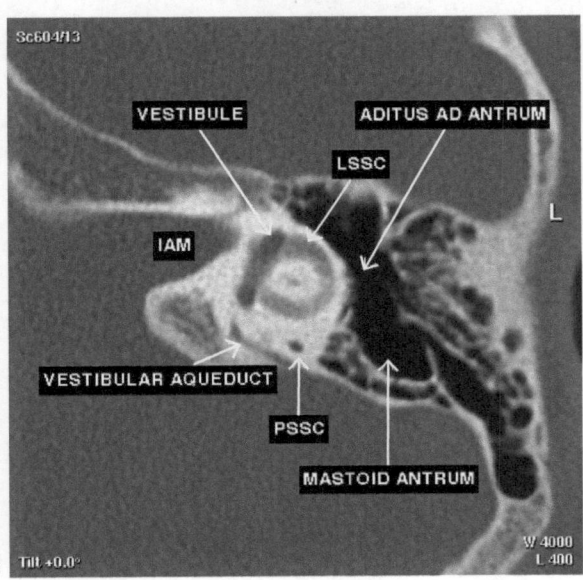

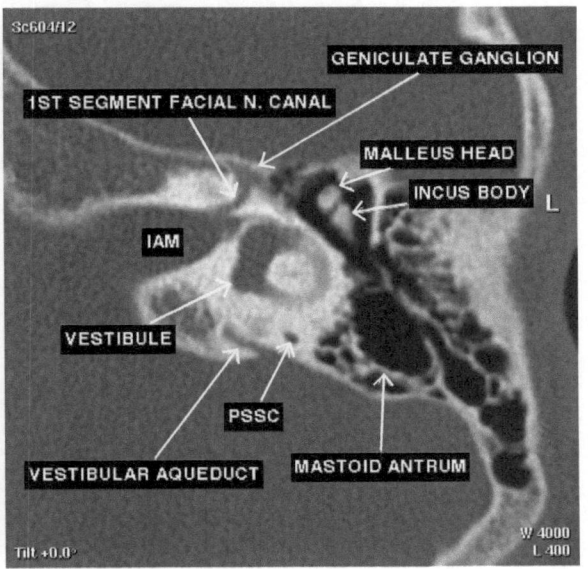

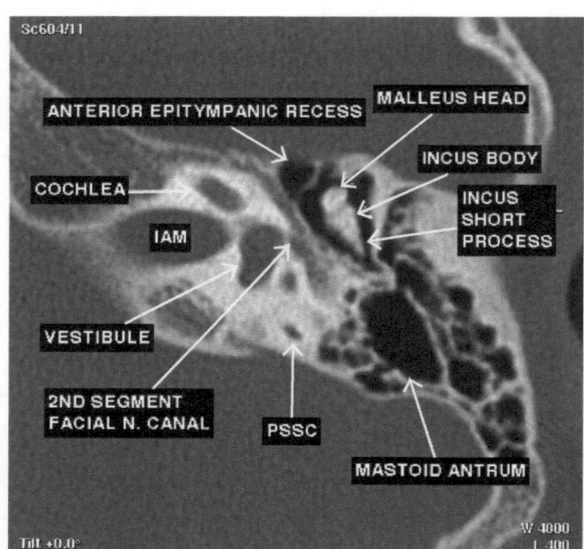

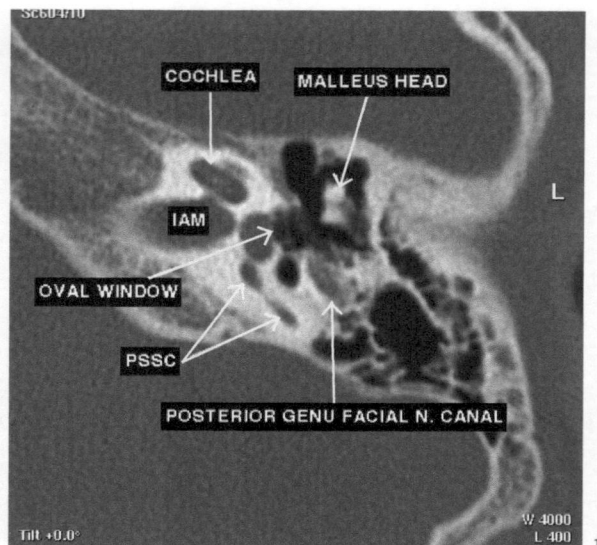

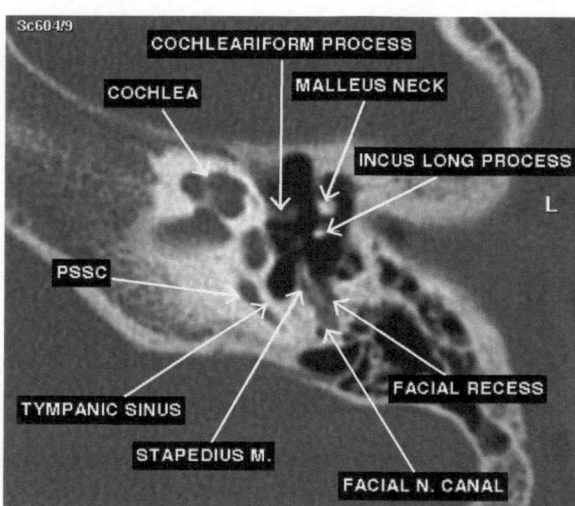

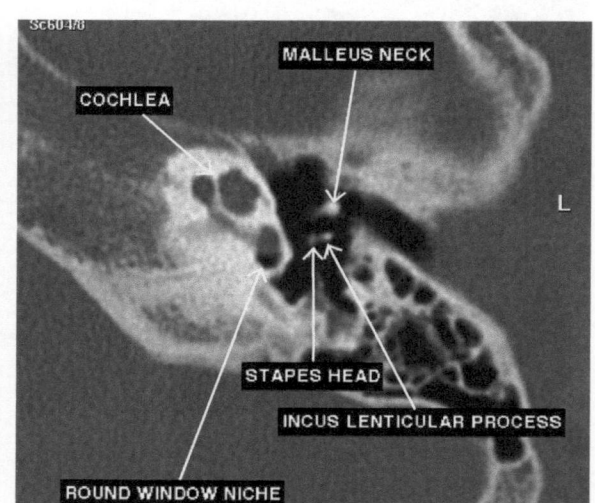

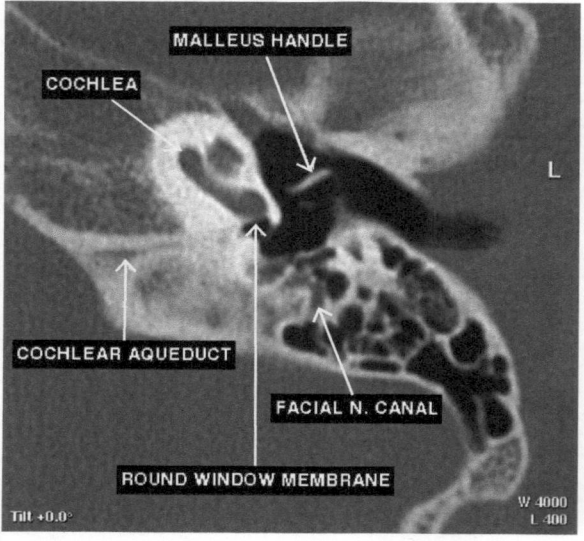

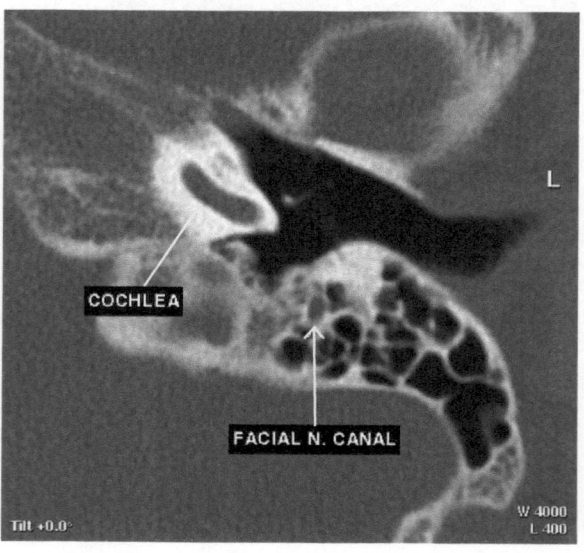

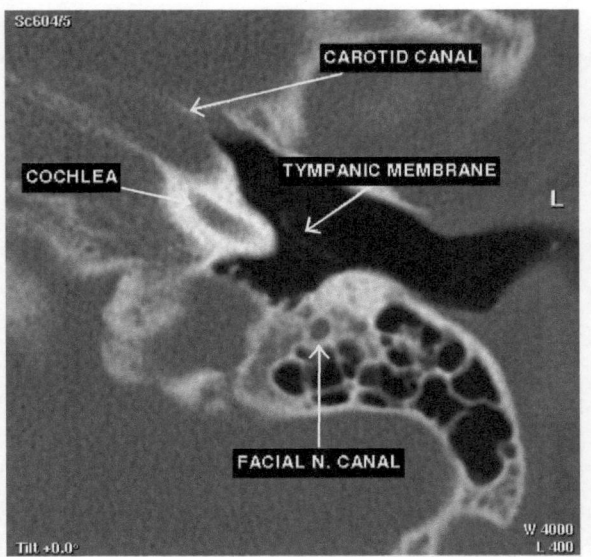

17

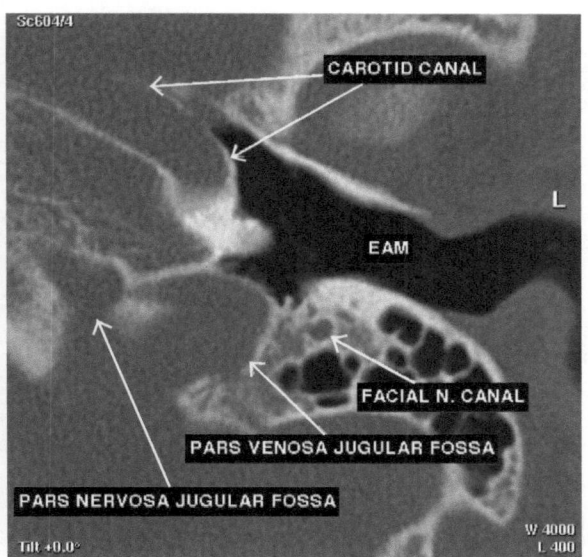

18

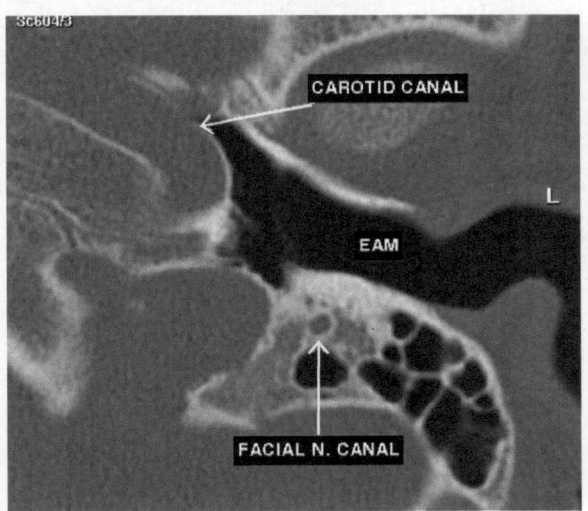

19

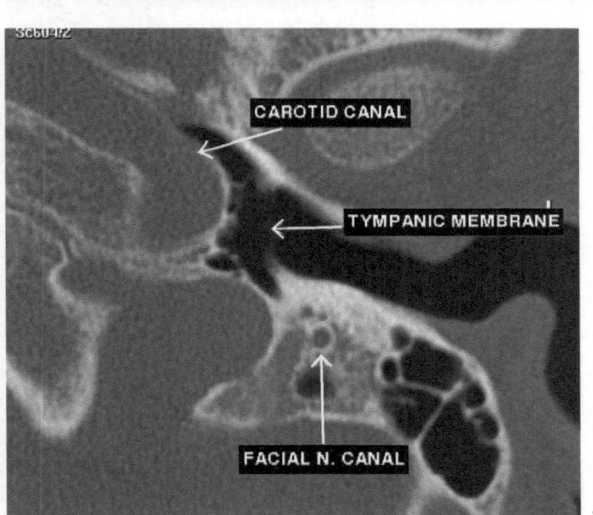

20

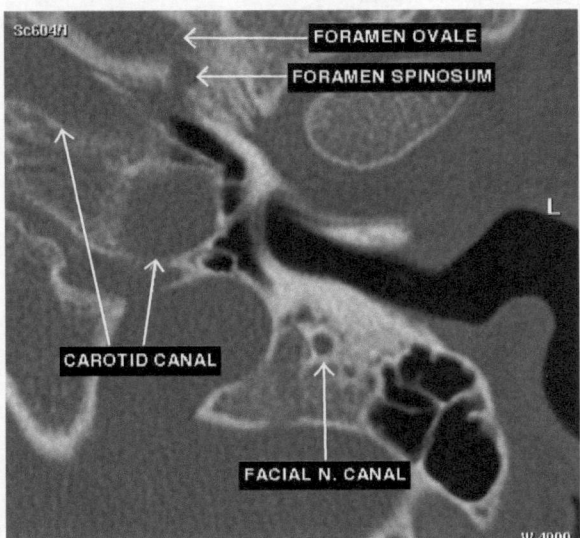

21

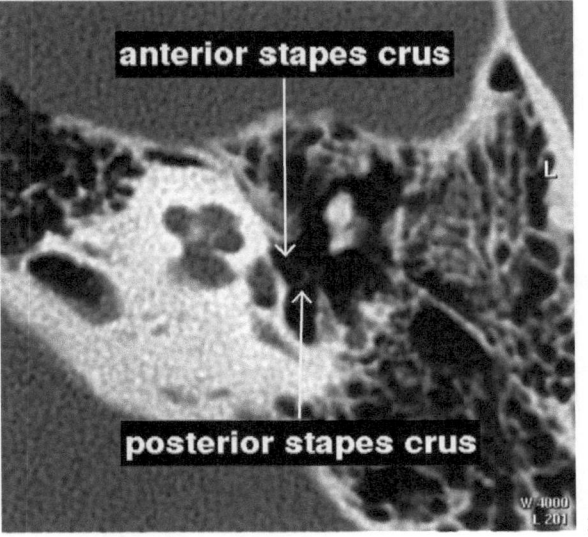

22

1.2.2
Coronal CT Images (Figs. 23–41)

The images are shown from a left temporal bone, from anteriorly to posteriorly. All images have a 1-mm slice thickness.

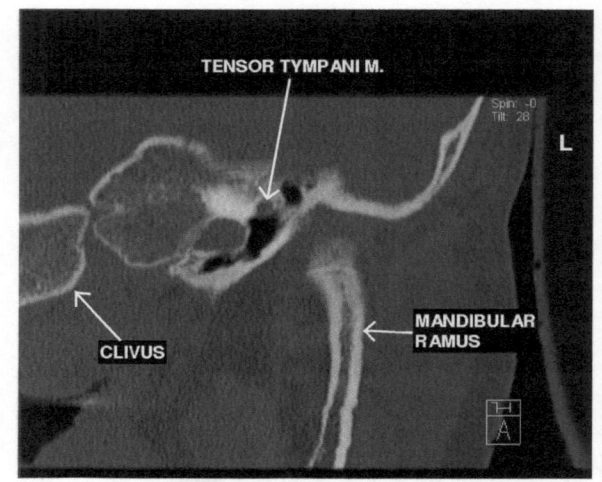

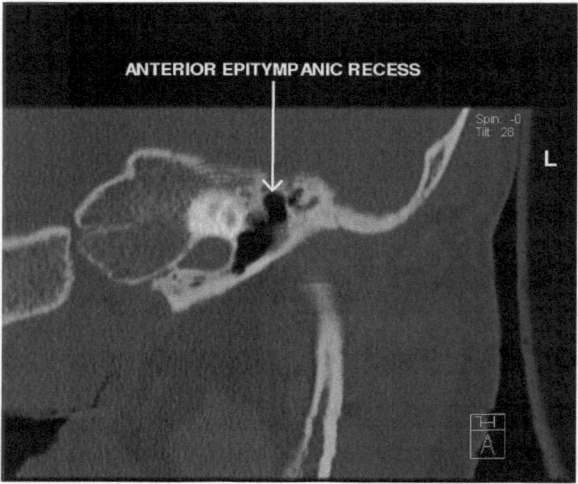

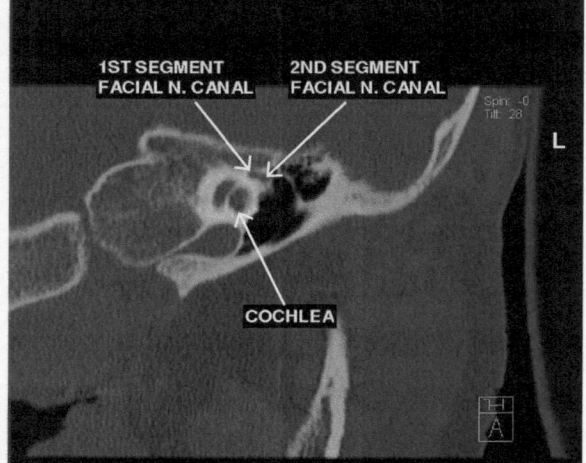

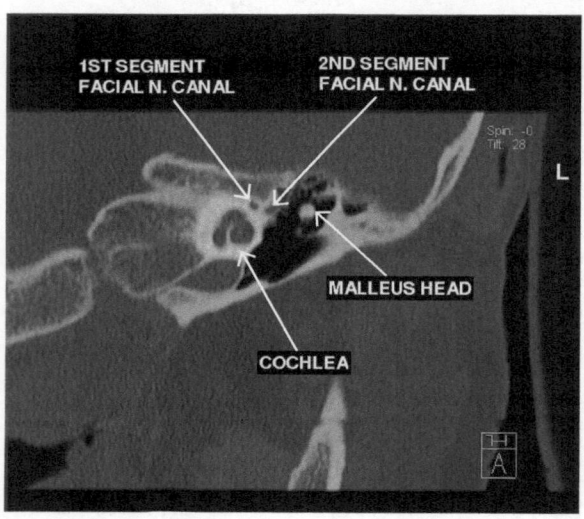

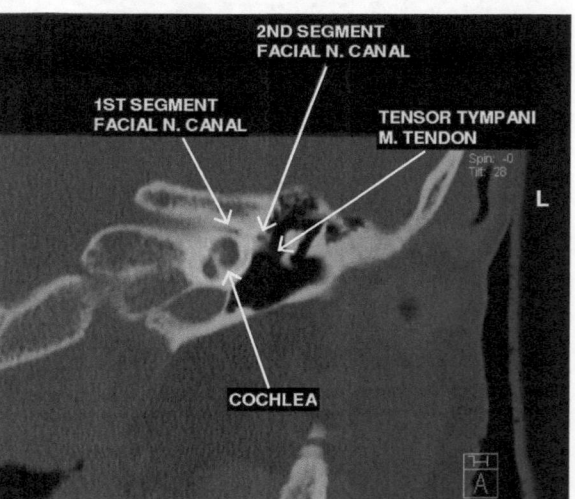

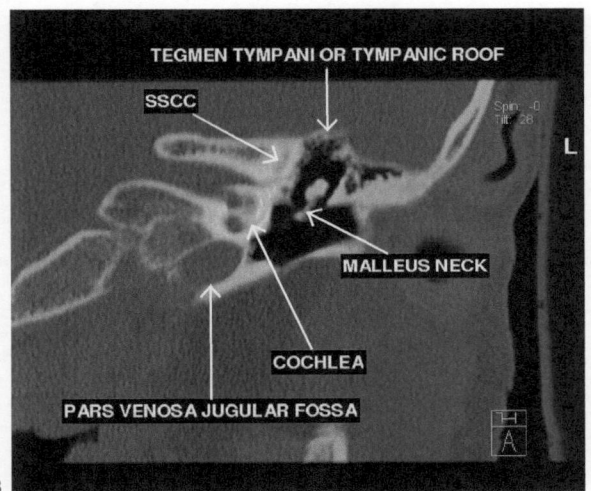

28

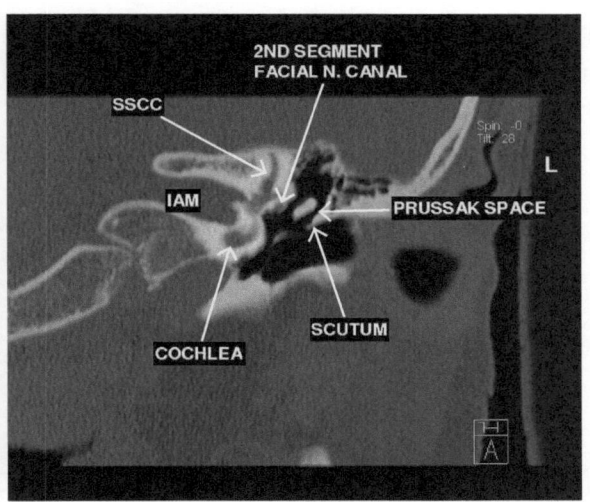

29

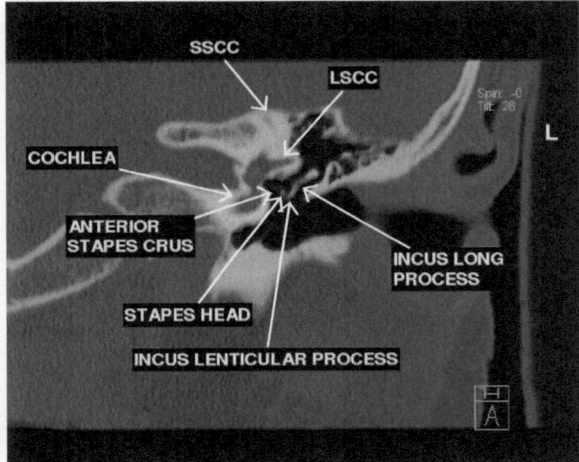

30

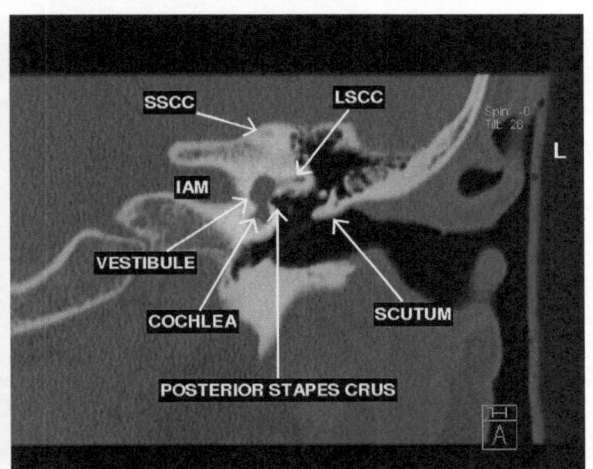

31

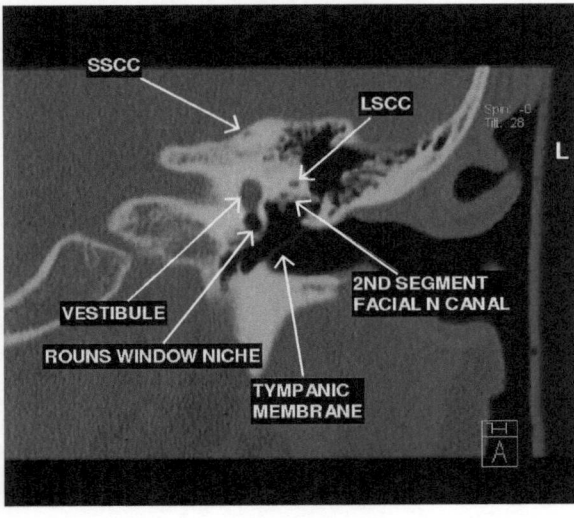

32

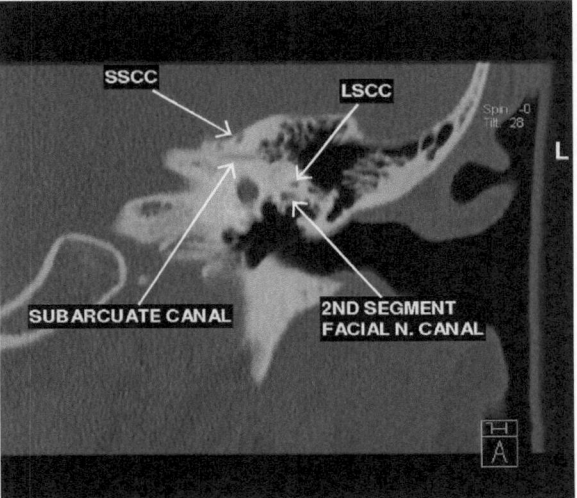

33

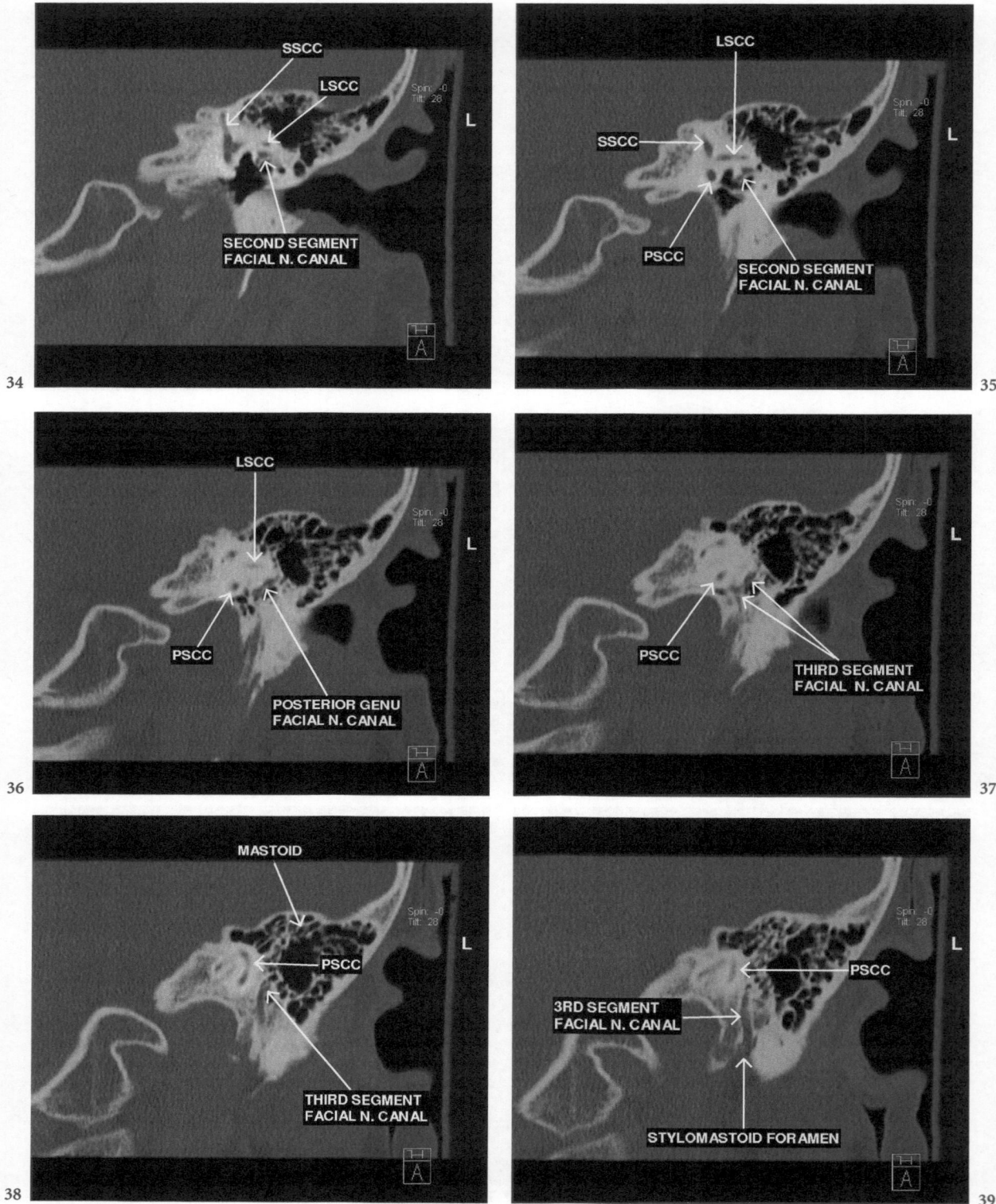

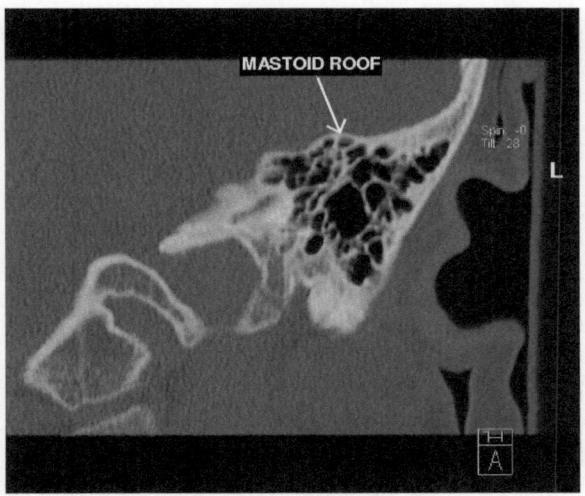

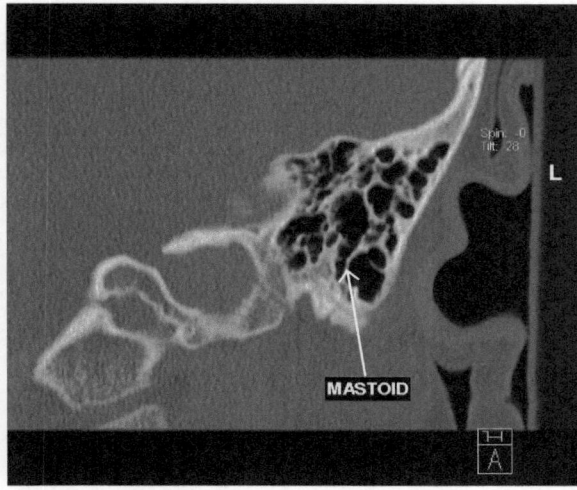

40

41

1.2.3
Axial T2-weighted MR Images (Figs. 42–59)

The images are shown from a left temporal bone, from cranially to caudally. All images have a 0.7-mm slice thickness.

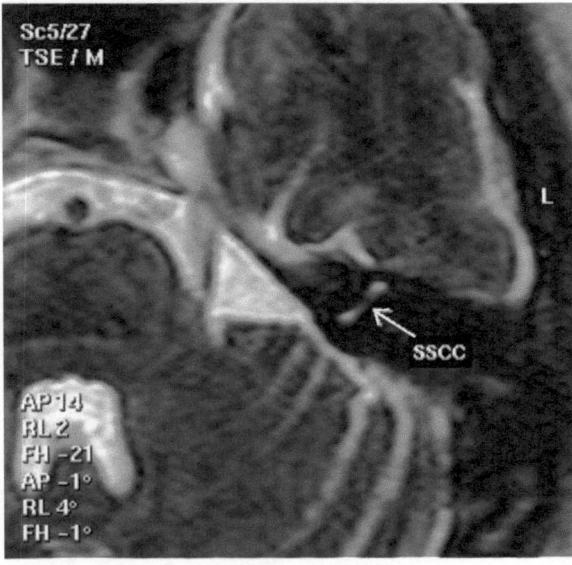

42

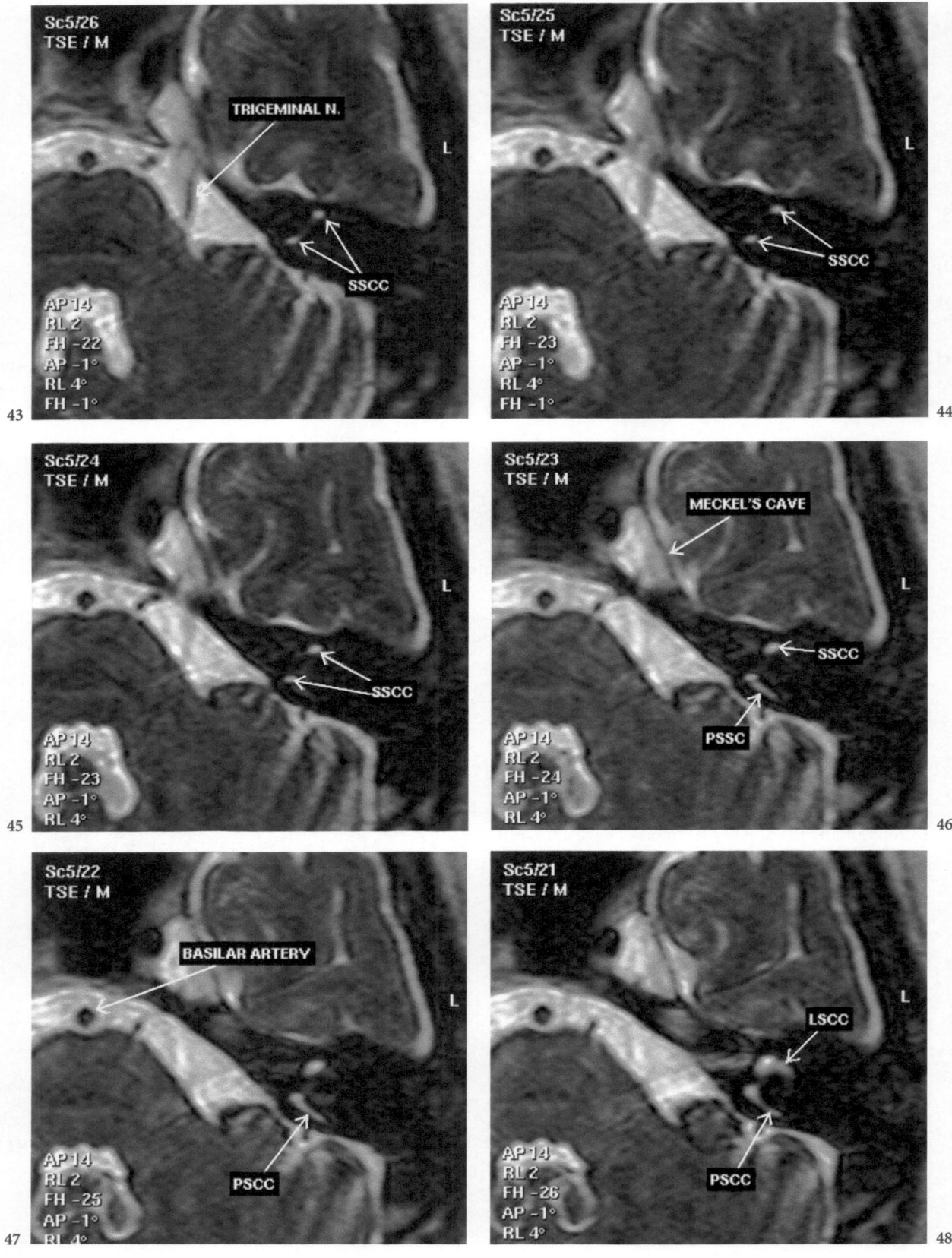

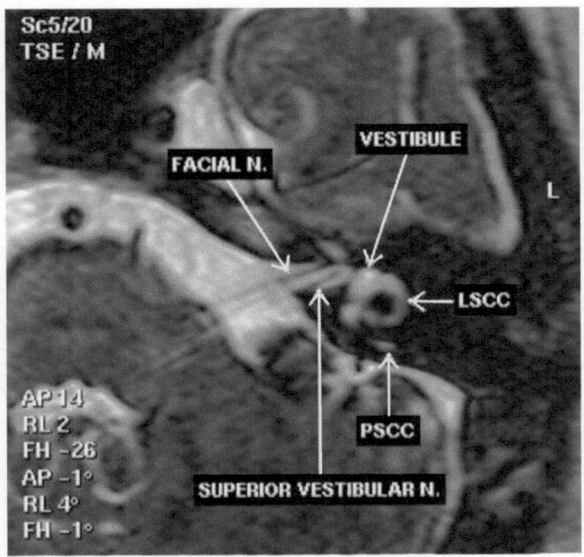

Sc5/20
TSE / M

FACIAL N.
VESTIBULE
L
LSCC
PSCC
SUPERIOR VESTIBULAR N.

AP 14
RL 2
FH −26
AP −1°
RL 4°
FH −1°

49

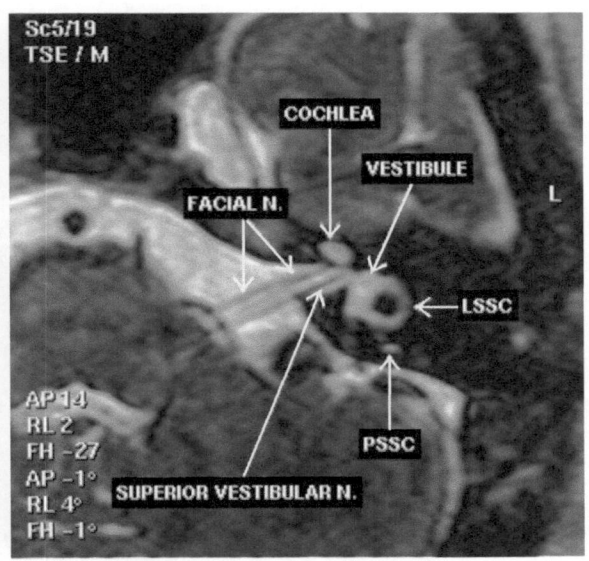

Sc5/19
TSE / M

COCHLEA
VESTIBULE
FACIAL N.
L
LSSC
PSSC
SUPERIOR VESTIBULAR N.

AP 14
RL 2
FH −27
AP −1°
RL 4°
FH −1°

50

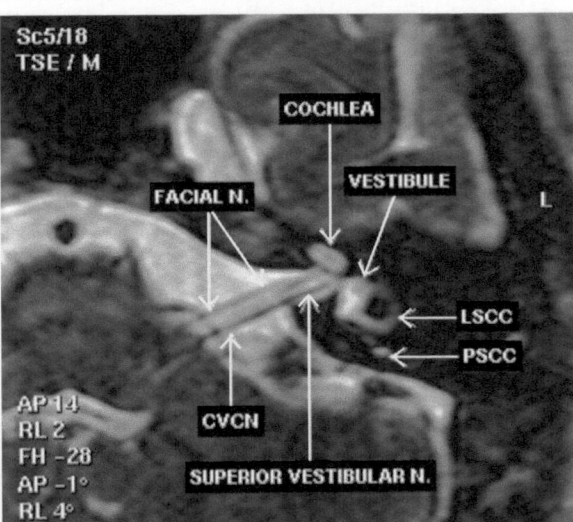

Sc5/18
TSE / M

COCHLEA
FACIAL N.
VESTIBULE
L
LSCC
PSCC
CVCN
SUPERIOR VESTIBULAR N.

AP 14
RL 2
FH −28
AP −1°
RL 4°

51

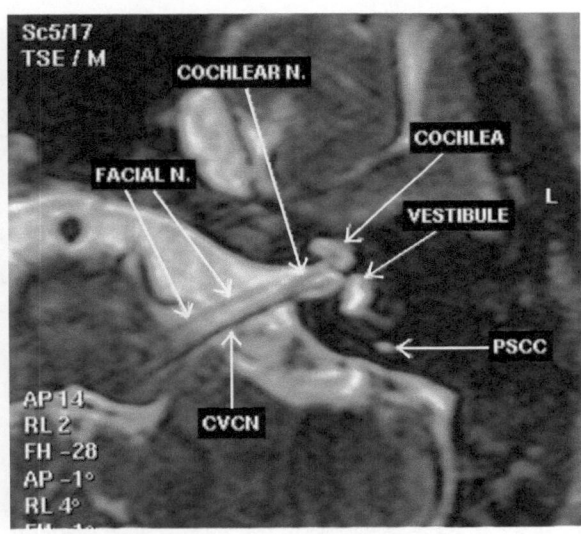

Sc5/17
TSE / M

COCHLEAR N.
FACIAL N.
COCHLEA
VESTIBULE
L
PSCC
CVCN

AP 14
RL 2
FH −28
AP −1°
RL 4°

52

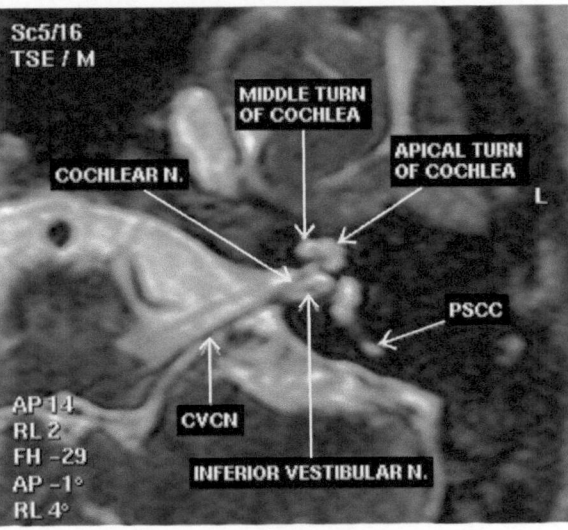

Sc5/16
TSE / M

MIDDLE TURN
OF COCHLEA
APICAL TURN
OF COCHLEA
COCHLEAR N.
L
PSCC
CVCN
INFERIOR VESTIBULAR N.

AP 14
RL 2
FH −29
AP −1°
RL 4°

53

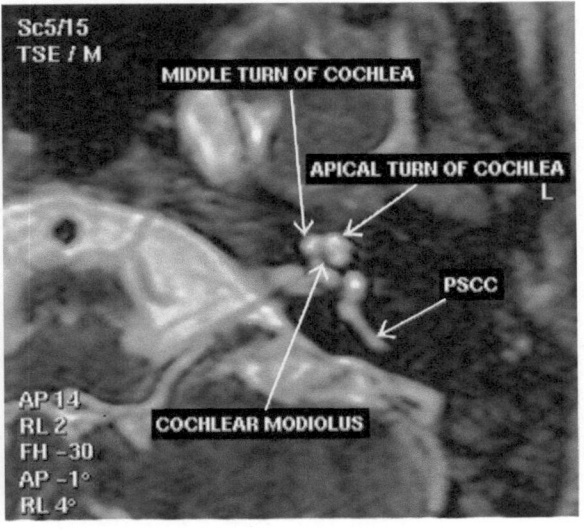

Sc5/15
TSE / M

MIDDLE TURN OF COCHLEA
APICAL TURN OF COCHLEA
L
PSCC
COCHLEAR MODIOLUS

AP 14
RL 2
FH −30
AP −1°
RL 4°

54

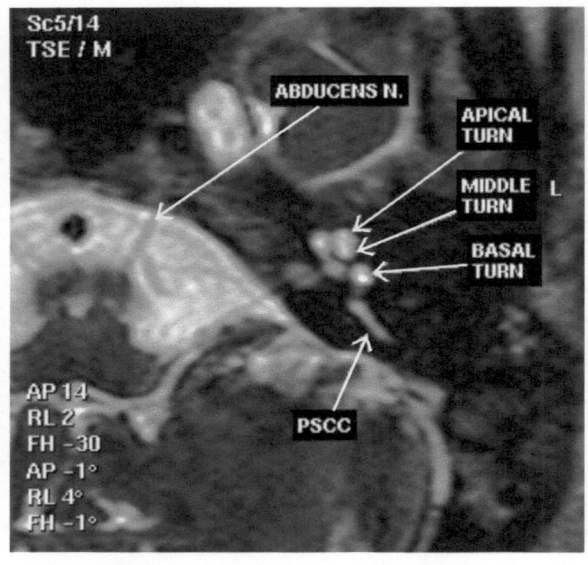

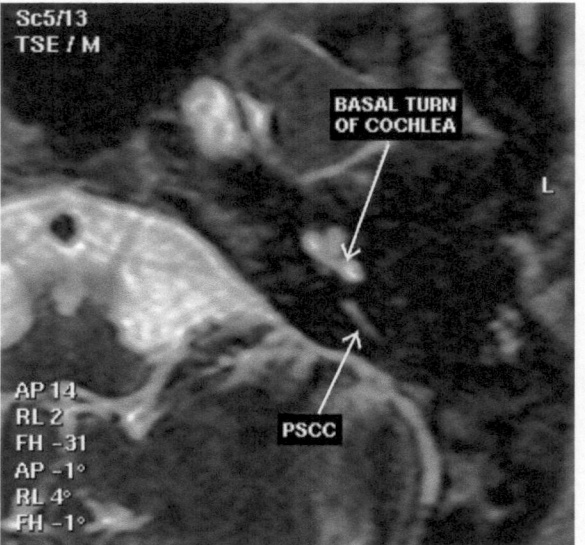

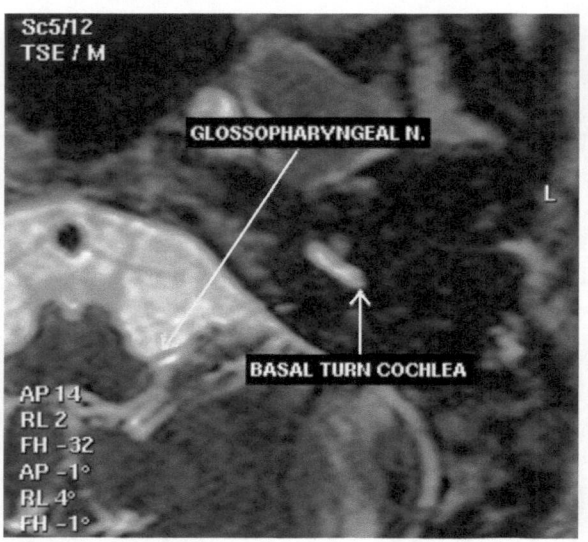

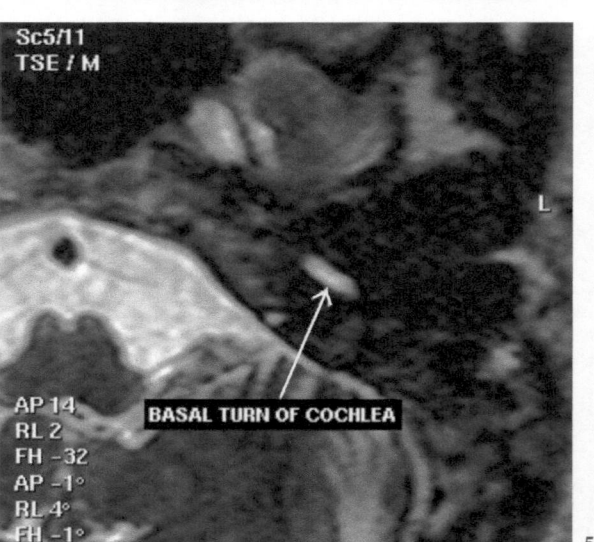

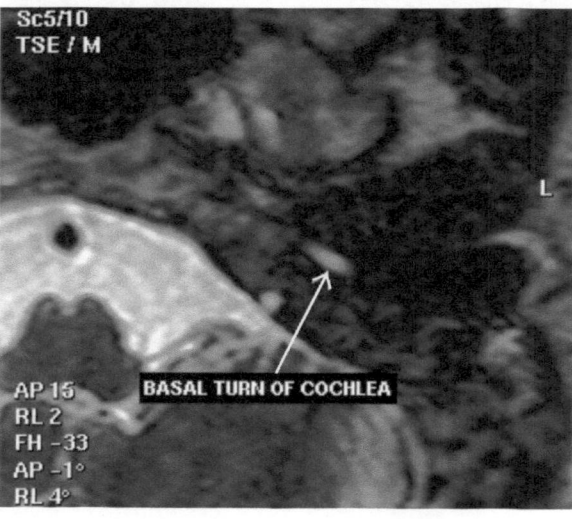

1.2.4
Axial T1-weighted MR Images (Figs. 60–68)

The images are shown from a right temporal bone, from cranially to caudally. All images have a 3.0-mm slice thickness.

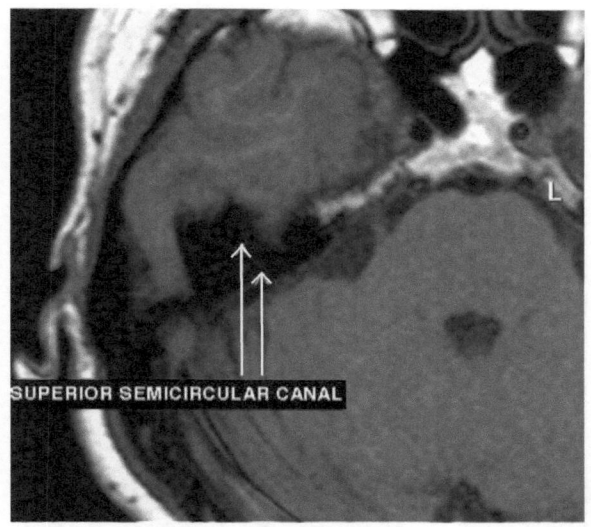

60

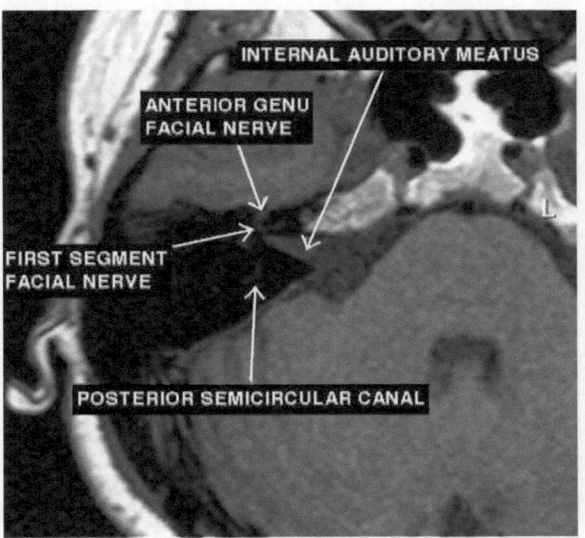

61

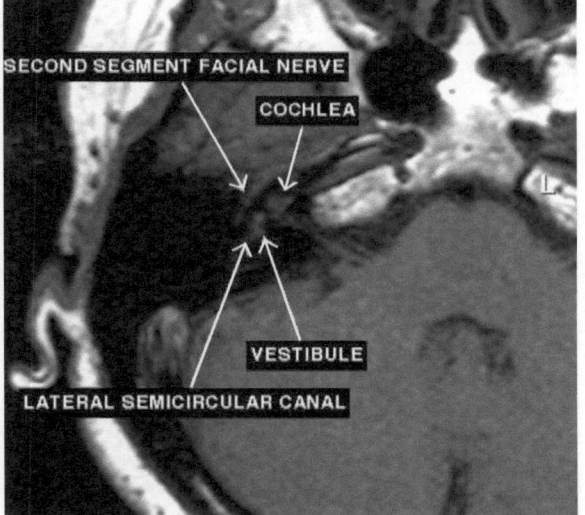

62

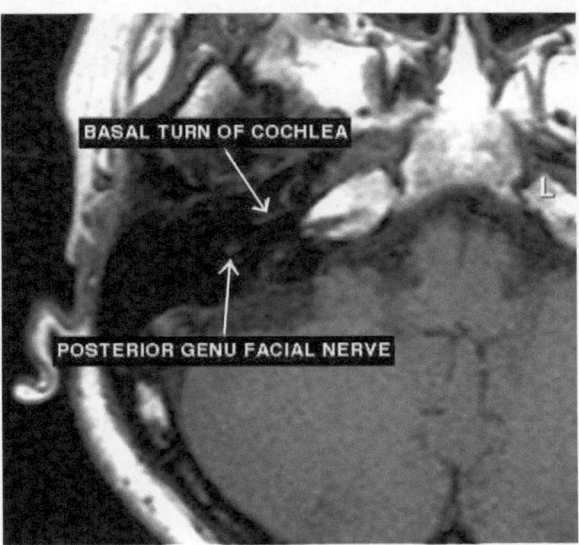

63

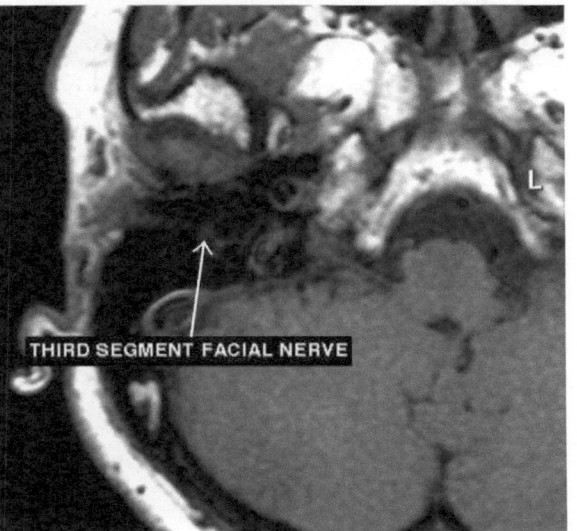

64

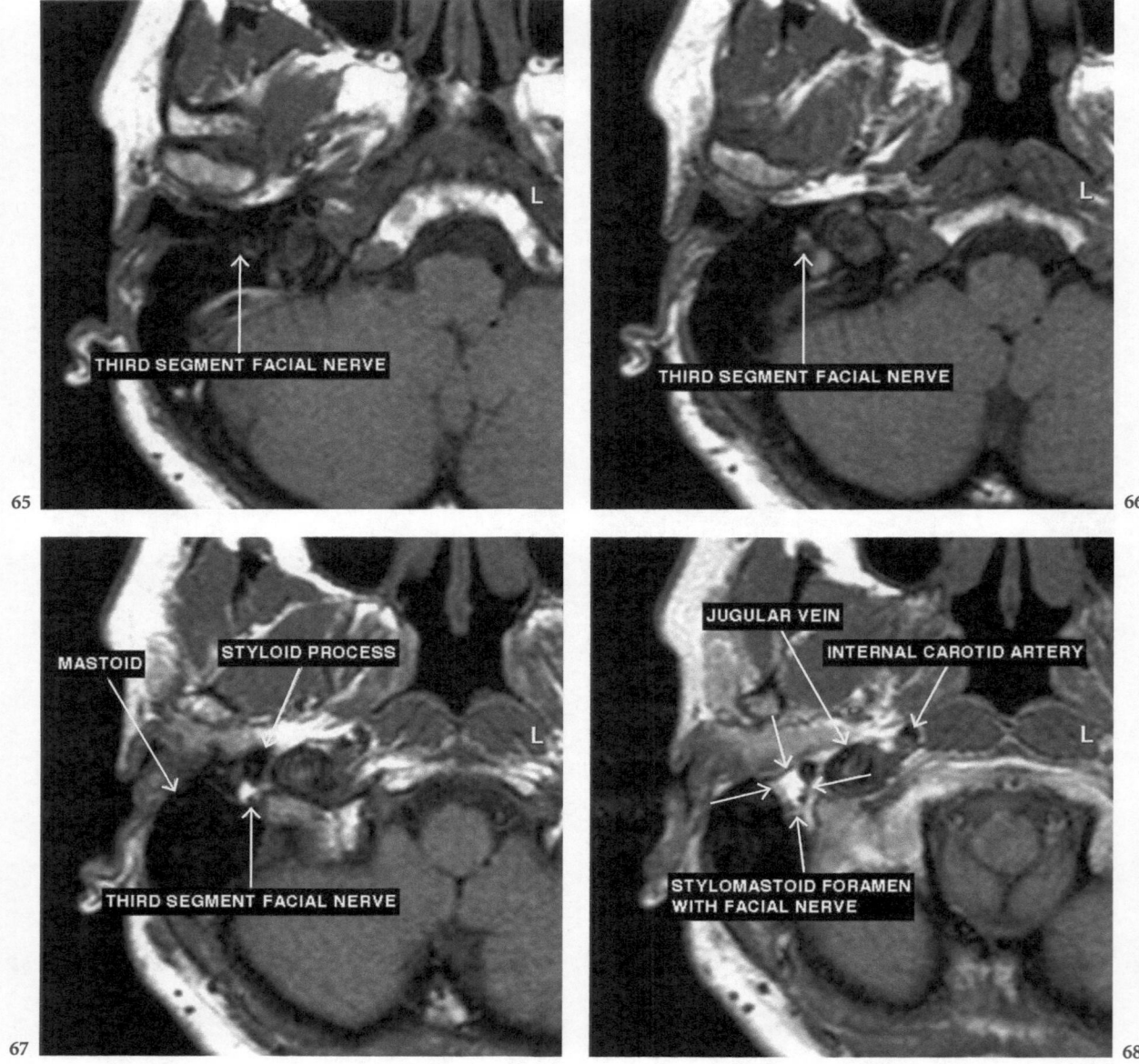

65

66

67

68

2 External Ear Imaging

R. Hermans

CONTENTS

2.1 Introduction

The external ear is easily examined clinically; therefore, in most cases, imaging has no or only a minor role to play. However, when the external auditory canal is severely deformed or obstructed, clinical inspection is hampered or impossible, making the imaging studies of much greater importance in patient management.

2.2 Congenital Malformations

2.2.1 Aural Dysplasia

The incidence of aural dysplasia is between 1/3300 and 1/10,000 births. Failure of the first branchial cleft

R. Hermans, MD, PhD
Department of Radiology, University Hospitals Leuven, Herestraat 49, 3000 Leuven, Belgium

to canalize causes stenosis or atresia of the external auditory canal. Very often, these patients have an abnormal auricle. The degree of deformity of the auricle is attributed to the severity of the external canal deformation. In cases of minor microtia, stenosis of the external auditory canal is most common, whereas in patients with major microtia, atresia is predominant (Mayer et al. 1998).

Aural dysplasia is usually unilateral and not associated with other deformities; however, it may be associated with numerous syndromes (Table 2.1). Commonly, abnormalities of the middle ear and mastoid are associated with aural dysplasia. The inner ear structures are usually normal.

A narrow and/or short external auditory meatus is associated with dysplasia of the tympanic bone. The canal often runs in an abnormal direction, sloping more upwards than usual. Sometimes, in such cases the medial portion of the canal may be in a more horizontal position. Apart from narrowing of the bony portion of the external canal, associated fibrosis may further narrow or completely obstruct the external ear canal. The tympanic membrane may be present or absent. Imaging shows the narrow external auditory canal, which may lack a bony floor.

When no external auditory canal is formed, the tympanic bone is not present (aplasia). A bony plate is present where the tympanic membrane is usually

Table 2.1. Syndromes associated with aural dysplasia. (Adapted from Swartz and Harnsberger 1998)

Treacher Collins syndrome
Crouzon syndrome
Nager syndrome
Hemifacial microsomia/Goldenhar syndrome
Klippel-Feil syndrome
Pierre Robin syndrome
Möbius syndrome
Duane retraction syndrome
Craniometaphyseal dysplasia
Osteopetrosis
Chromosome 18 deletion syndrome
Thalidomide embryopathy

located. This "atresia plate" may correspond to a "frust" tympanic bone or to downward extension of the squamous part of the temporal bone, meeting the floor of the middle ear.

The size of the tympanic cavity is often diminished, making surgery more difficult. The tegmen may have a low position, which also may complicate the surgical approach. The air content of the mastoid is often reduced, correlating with the degree of abnormality of the external ear.

The size of the bony eustachian tube may be reduced, but sometimes this structure appears enlarged (MAYER et al. 1998).

Ossicular chain abnormalities are very frequently associated with aural dysplasia. Aplasia of the tympanic bone is associated with fusion of the neck of the malleus to the atresia plate (Fig. 2.1). Also other ossicular anomalies may be present: fusion of the malleus and incus, with absence of the normal malleo-incudal joint, is common, and the long process of the incus may have an abnormal orientation or be hypoplastic or absent. The most important ossicular structure to look for on CT is the stapes. Absence of the stapes makes surgical reconstruction more complex. Furthermore, the presence and width of the oval window should be checked. On coronal images, it should have a diameter of approximately 2 mm (YEAKLEY and JAHRSDOERFER 1996).

The tympanic segment of the facial nerve canal is often displaced caudally, sometimes reaching as low as the round window (MAYER et al. 1998). The second genu and mastoid portion of the facial nerve typically have a more anteriorly position than normal, which is important for the surgeon to know, as they may appear in the surgical pathway. The mastoid portion of the facial nerve may curve anteriorly towards the area of the temporomandibular joint, or leave the temporal bone in a more lateral direction. Determining the exact course of the facial nerve is of utmost importance to avoid postoperative facial paralysis (Fig. 2.2).

When the tympanic bone is aplastic, the position of the temporomandibular joint is frequently more posterior than normal, due to lack of posterior bony support. Confluence of the temporomandibular joint soft tissue with the middle ear is regarded unfavorable for surgery, as this makes maintaining support for the surgically created hearing apparatus difficult (YEAKLEY and JAHRSDOERFER 1996).

The CT study should also exclude the presence of a (congenital or acquired) cholesteatoma.

Although rare, abnormalities of the inner ear should be sought. Usually, when associated with aural dysplasia, these inner ear malformations are minor. The labyrinthine function is not necessarily abnormal. The internal auditory canal may appear widened and more angled than normal.

2.2.2
Branchiogenic Anomalies

Although aural dysplasia can be regarded as a branchiogenic anomaly (see above), other anomalies arising from the branchiogenic apparatus may occur around the external ear.

Defects of the branchial apparatus manifest as cysts, sinuses, fistulas, and ectopic glands. Anomalies of the branchial complex are vestigial remnants, resulting from incomplete obliteration of the branchial apparatus or buried epithelial cell rests.

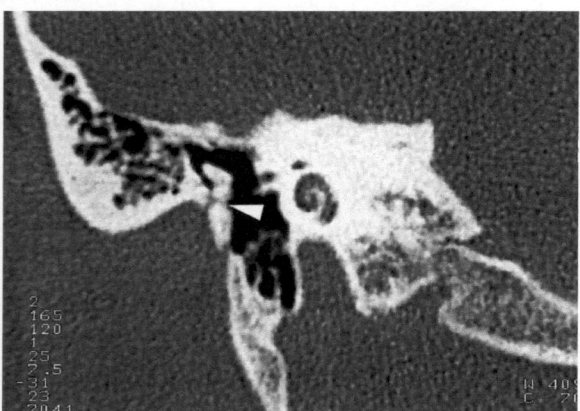

Fig. 2.1. Coronal CT image through right temporal bone. Atresia of the external auditory canal. The neck of the malleus is fused with the atresia plate (*arrowhead*). (Reprinted from HERMANS 2000)

Fig. 2.2a–i. Right-sided Goldenhar syndrome. **a–d** Axial CT images through right temporal bone. The facial nerve canal shows a relatively long labyrinthine segment (**a**, *arrowhead*); note the associated hypoplastic appearance of the ossicular chain (**a**, *arrow*). Short tympanic segment of facial nerve (**b**, *arrowheads*). A second genu cannot be clearly identified, but the mastoid segment of the facial canal is running posterolaterally to the tympanic cavity (**c**, *arrowhead*). At a lower level, the mastoid segment of the facial nerve is seen running

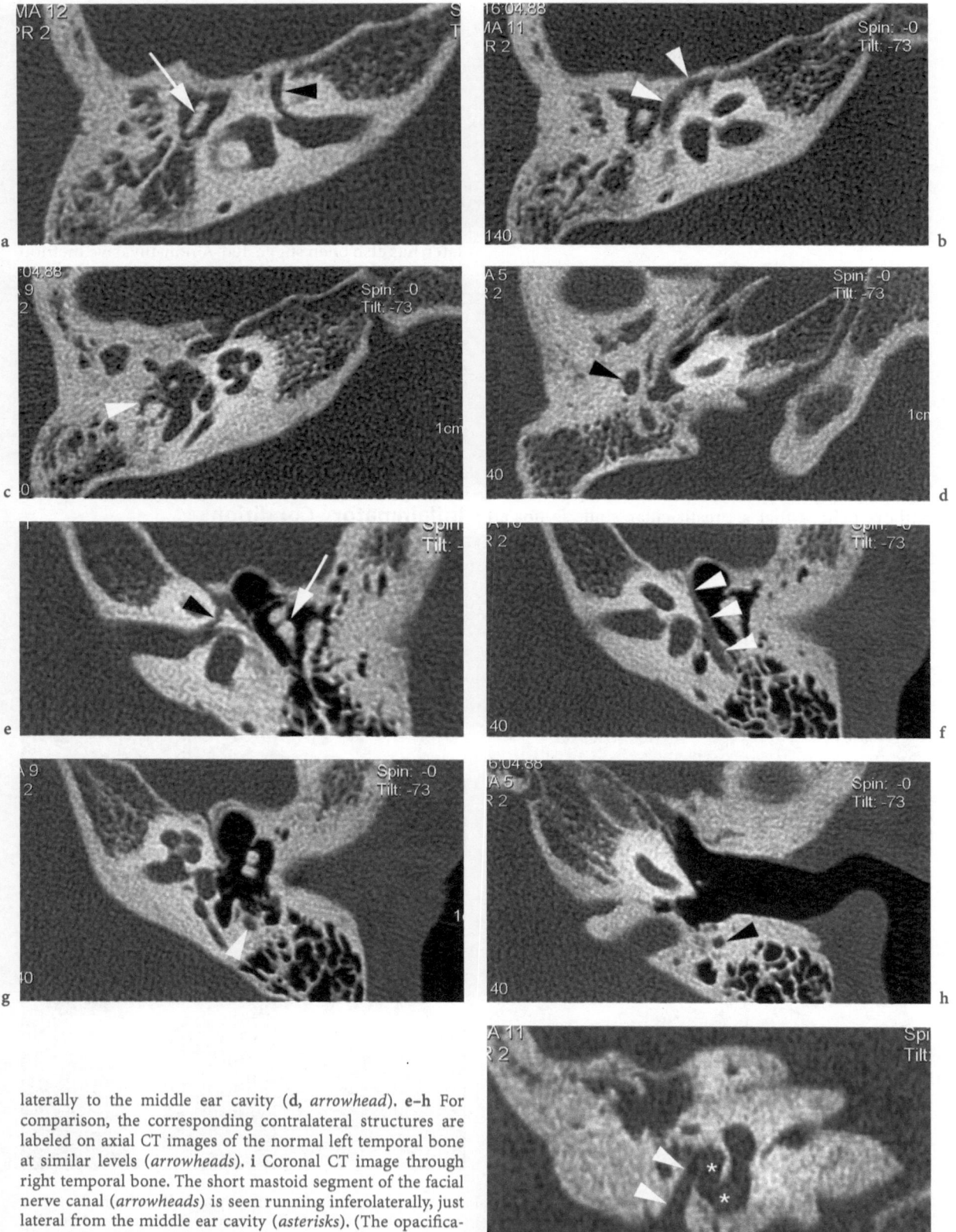

laterally to the middle ear cavity (**d**, *arrowhead*). **e–h** For comparison, the corresponding contralateral structures are labeled on axial CT images of the normal left temporal bone at similar levels (*arrowheads*). **i** Coronal CT image through right temporal bone. The short mastoid segment of the facial nerve canal (*arrowheads*) is seen running inferolaterally, just lateral from the middle ear cavity (*asterisks*). (The opacification of the right middle ear cavity is presumably caused by chronic dysfunction of the Eustachian tube.)

First branchial cleft anomalies may originate anywhere along the nasopharynx, middle ear cavity, or external auditory canal (Fig. 2.3). These sinuses, fistulas, or cysts may extend downwards below the angle of the mandible, where they can present as an inflammatory mass lesion. As the first branchial cleft persists as the epithelium of the external auditory canal, such cleft anomalies may communicate with this anatomic structure (Fig. 2.4).

2.2.3
Preauricular Sinus

The auricle develops from six mesenchymal proliferations surrounding the first pharyngeal cleft. These swellings fuse and gradually form the definitive auricle. As this fusion is a complicated process, developmental abnormalities may arise (LANGMAN 1981). A sinus results when one of the sulci between the auricular hillocks incompletely disappears. Most authors believe that a preauricular sinus is not an anomaly of the first branchial apparatus

A preauricular sinus is a relatively common congenital abnormality. It consists of a blind-ending opening in the external ear, often located at or near the anterior crus of the helix. The diagnosis is made clinically. Most of these sinuses remain asymptomatic, but repeat infection may cause chronic discharge, repeated abscess formation, and scarring, making surgical excision of the sinus and its possible ramifications necessary. Recurrences may follow incomplete resection (CURRIE et al. 1996).

Preoperative visualization of the extent of the lesion may be helpful to prevent incomplete resection. Usually, injection of the sinus tract with contrast medium is not successful, as the lumen is often blocked by epithelial debris (LAU 1983). Forced injection of methylene blue, followed by surgery a few days later, has also been suggested. A non-invasive method is high-resolution ultrasound, allowing visualization of the sinus, its branches, and any associated cystic component in the subcutaneous tissues. Also the relationship of the lesion to the auricular cartilage and parotid gland can be demonstrated (AHUJA et al. 2000).

2.3
Inflammatory Conditions

2.3.1
External Otitis

In most cases of external otitis, imaging studies are not required as the disease can be well inspected and followed-up by clinical examination.

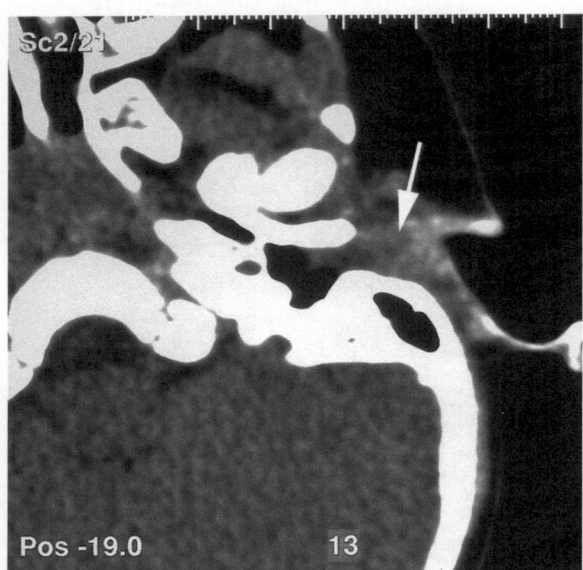
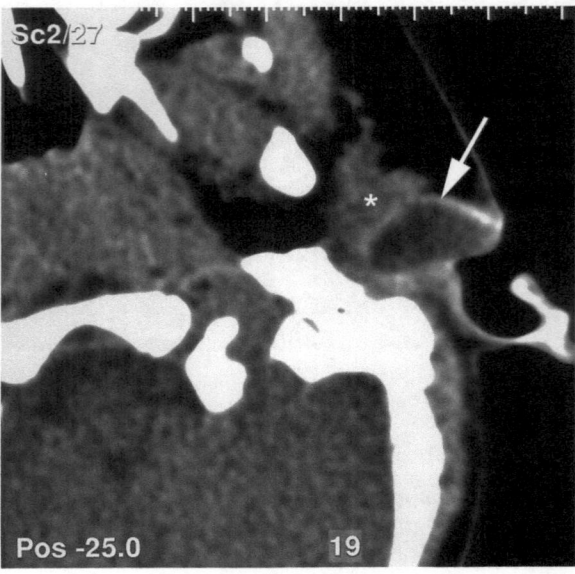

Fig. 2.3a, b. Newborn child with obliteration of the left external auditory canal, clinically caused by a swelling from its antero-inferior wall. Axial CT shows soft tissue obliteration of the canal (**a**, *arrow*), by a cystic structure, antero-inferior to and running parallel to the canal (**b**, *arrow*). The cyst has a close relationship with the upper-posterior part of the parotid gland (**b**, *asterisk*). First branchial cleft cyst

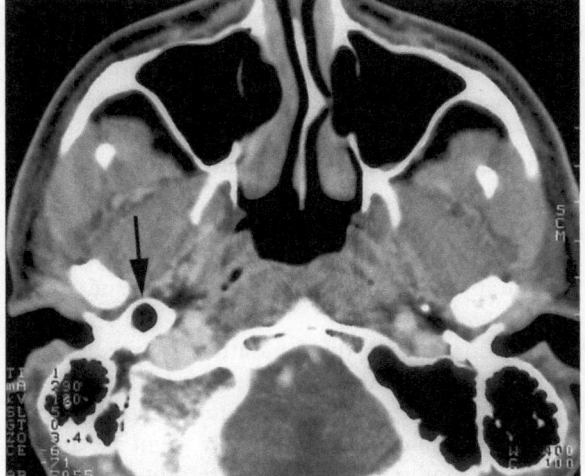
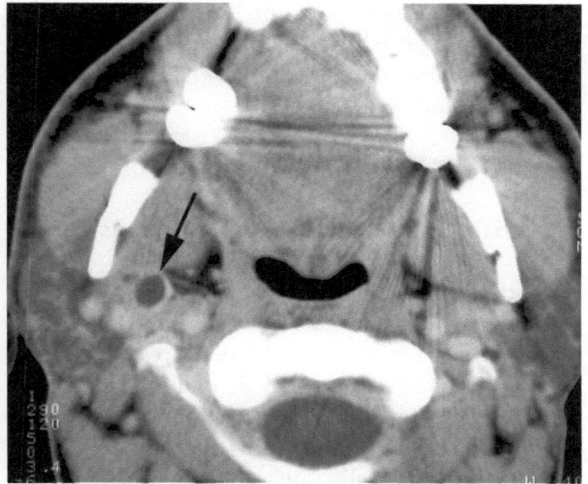
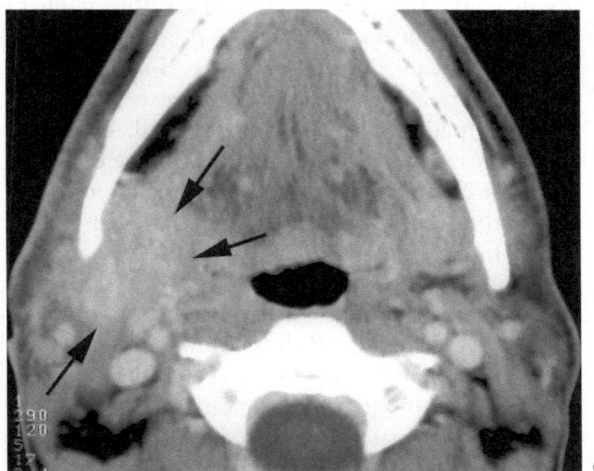

Fig. 2.4a–c. Axial contrast-enhanced CT images. Right-sided tubular anomaly communicating with the malformed tympanic bone (**a**, *arrow*), extending inferiorly just deep to the parotid gland (**b**, *arrow*), ending in an inflammatory mass in the submandibular space (**c**, *arrows*). First branchial cleft anomaly. (From HERMANS 2000)

External otitis, also known as swimmer's ear, is a common condition. Maceration by water or trauma are often the etiologic factors. Also dermatologic and endocrinologic conditions may give rise to external otitis. External otitis presents with itching, sometimes severe pain, and a cheesy discharge. The ear canal is diffusely swollen and tender. Most cases are controlled with topical treatment. In severe cases, cellulitis of the surrounding structures may be present, requiring systemic antibiotic treatment.

External ear furuncles are also common; they appear as localized, tender, and possibly fluctuant swellings. Treatment is by drainage of fluctuant areas and topical antibiotics. Systemic antibiotics are needed when there is cellulitis or systemic symptoms.

Chronic external otitis may lead to acquired atresia of the external auditory canal (KEOHANE et al. 1993). Recurrent inflammation with formation of granulation tissue may eventually lead to fibrosis and stenosis.

Treatment is either by surgical correction or by a hearing aid.

Ramsay-Hunt syndrome (also known as herpes zoster oticus) corresponds to acute facial neuritis, causing facial paralysis, otalgia, and vesicles in the external ear. It is thought to be a cranial polyneuropathy caused by the herpes zoster virus (DE and PFLEIDERER 1999). Sometimes also hearing loss, tinnitus, or vertigo may be present. Magnetic resonance imaging shows enhancement of the facial nerve, similar to that in Bell's palsy. Enhancement of the intracanalicular portion of the vestibulocochlear nerve and the labyrinth may sometimes be seen.

Relapsing polychondritis is a rare inflammatory disease of cartilage of unknown origin, producing a bizarre form of arthritis. It may involve the cartilages of the ear, nose, and respiratory tract. Involvement of the auricle and cartilaginous portion of the external auditory canal is clinically apparent. Imaging is not required for evaluation of the external ear. Also the inner ear may be involved in this condition. Enhancement of the labyrinthine structures has been reported (VOURTSI et al. 1998).

2.3.2
Necrotizing ("Malignant") External Otitis

Necrotizing external otitis is a severe infection of the external ear, almost exclusively caused by *Pseudomonas aeruginosa*. Because of the aggressive clinical course, it has also been called "malignant external otitis" (CHANDLER 1968); however, the disease is not neoplastic, and it also does not remain limited to the external ear. Generally, "necrotizing external otitis" is considered the most accurate descriptive name of this disease process.

Most patients suffer from diabetes or are otherwise immunocompromised. The disease also occurs in elderly patients. It usually occurs unilaterally, but bilateral cases have been described. Severe otalgia is the most common symptom. The patients may also suffer from purulent otorrhea. Clinical examination shows inflammatory changes and the presence of granulation tissue at the junction of the bony and cartilaginous part of the external auditory canal.

The exact pathogenesis is unknown. *Pseudomonas* is not a commensal of the external auditory canal but may colonize this structure. Colonization may occur after indiscriminate use of broad-spectrum antibiotics for ear infection or after irrigation of the ears with non-sterile tap water containing *Pseudomonas* (RUBIN and YU 1988). Ischemic conditions, related to diabetic microangiopathy or the effect of aging, result in hypoperfusion and may increase susceptibility to infection. Also decreased activity of white blood cells may be a contributing factor.

The infection rapidly spreads to involve surrounding bone and soft tissues. The disease may erode into the bone of the mastoid. Anterior spread causes extension into the temporomandibular joint, possibly causing destructive osteomyelitis (MIDWINTER et al. 1999). Anterior spread may also cause involvement of the parotid gland.

Anteromedial extension into the infratemporal space may occur. Facial nerve palsy develops in 24–43% of cases (RUBIN and YU 1988). The facial nerve usually becomes affected by infratemporal spread of the infection towards the stylomastoid foramen. Other cranial neuropathies can result as the infection spreads below the skull base. Intracranial extension may occur in advanced cases.

Both CT and MRI are excellent techniques to visualize the disease extent (Figs. 2.5, 2.6). Magnetic resonance imaging is the preferred modality if intracranial spread is suspected. Abnormalities of the external auditory canal, with or without bone destruction, can be seen. In many patients also soft tissue thickening or fluid is seen in the middle ear and mastoid. Infiltration of the parapharyngeal space is commonly present. Serial imaging during successful therapy shows improvement of soft tissue disease (RUBIN et al. 1990).

The radiographic differentiation from true malignant neoplasia may be difficult; occasionally, both conditions are present at the same time (RUBIN et al. 1990). In cancer, the bone involvement is expected to display a more contiguous pattern of destruction, whereas in necrotizing otitis media "skip" areas may be present. The clinical picture in external ear cancer is different, without or with only minimal pain; however, cancer may occasionally mimic necrotizing otitis media in its clinical appearance (MATTUCI et al. 1986; AL-SHIHABI 1992).

The treatment consists of surgical débridement of the external auditory canal, drainage of collections, and intravenous antibiotics. Malignant otitis externa used to have a grave prognosis, but with the advent of more effective antibiotics, the infection can be controlled in the majority of cases. Cranial nerve involvement is often quoted as a bad prognostic sign. It does reflect more extensive disease, and the mortality rate is higher in these patients; however, recovery of facial nerve function after successful treatment has been observed.

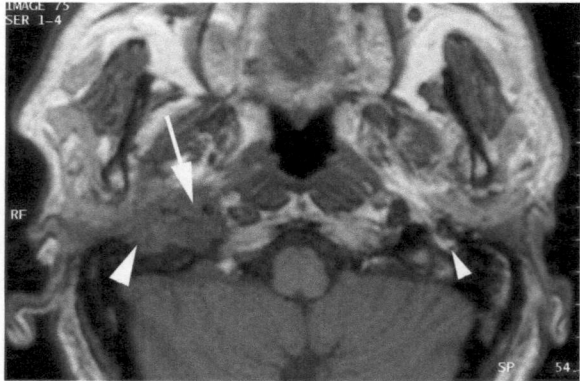

Fig. 2.5. Axial T1-weighted MR image. Diabetic patient suffering from right-sided external otitis and facial palsy. In continuity with the external auditory canal, infratemporal soft tissue infiltration is seen, extending in the fat pad below the stylomastoid foramen (*large arrowhead*), and into the carotid space (*arrow*). On the left, note normal facial nerve just below the stylomastoid foramen (*small arrowhead*). Necrotizing external otitis

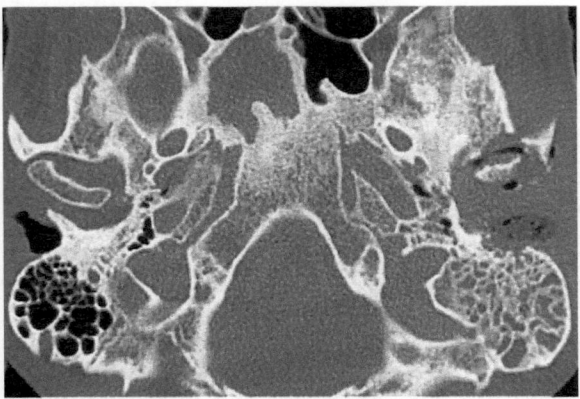
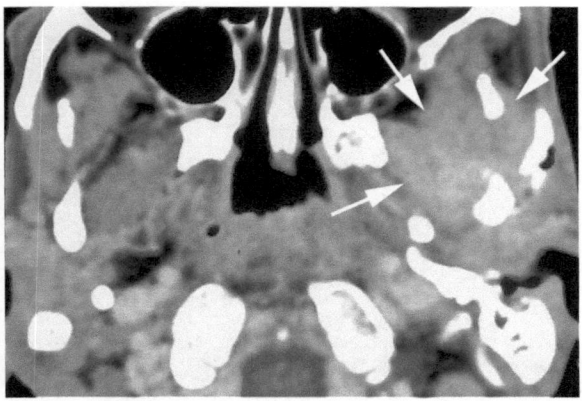

a   b

Fig. 2.6. Axial CT images through skull base show destruction of the bony external auditory canal, erosion of the mastoid bone, and invasion of the temporomandibular joint (**a**). The contrast-enhanced image reveals extension of the infection into the soft tissues of the infratemporal fossa (**b**, *arrows*). (From HERMANS 2000)

2.4
Trauma

Trauma to the external canal is most commonly caused by instrumentation, either by the patient himself, or by a physician. Most of these smaller lacerations or canal hematomas can be handled with antibiotic drops, but more complex lacerations need temporary packing of the ear canal in order to avoid fibrotic stenosis.

Fractures of the tympanic bone are quite frequent. They are usually caused by the impact of a posteriorly displaced mandibular condyle, itself resulting from a blow to the chin region. Care should be taken not to misinterpret the normal petrotympanic suture as a fracture line (Fig. 2.7).

Longitudinal fractures of the temporal bone run more or less along the long axis of the temporal bone. Such a fracture typically originates from a blow to the temporoparietal portion of the skull, with inferior propagation of the fracture line through the mastoid into the lateral wall of the middle ear, passing behind, through, or in front of the external auditory canal (Fig. 2.8).

Fractures through the external auditory canal are treated by temporary packing of the canal to prevent canal stenosis.

Soft tissue trauma to the external ear canal, without recognizable fracture, may lead to fibrosis and stenosis of the external auditory canal (Fig. 2.9).

Posttraumatic canal stenosis may lead to accumulation of debris deep to the stenosis, and formation of a cholesteatoma (MCKENNAN and CHOLE 1992). Posttraumatic cholesteatoma may also develop as a result of implantation of ear canal squamous epithelium into the fracture line (MCKENNAN and CHOLE 1989).

Entrapment of epithelium may occur due to complex displacement of bony fragments or diastasis of suture lines. A tear of the tympanic membrane is also believed to be a possible origin for cholesteatoma formation (FREEMAN 1983). Posttraumatic cholesteatoma of the external ear may only become symptomatic after a delay of several years. Imaging shows the presence of a soft tissue mass, possibly associated with surrounding bone erosion. A close topographic relationship to a fracture line usually exists (Fig. 2.10; FRANSSENS et al. 1993). As these patients have no prior history of ear

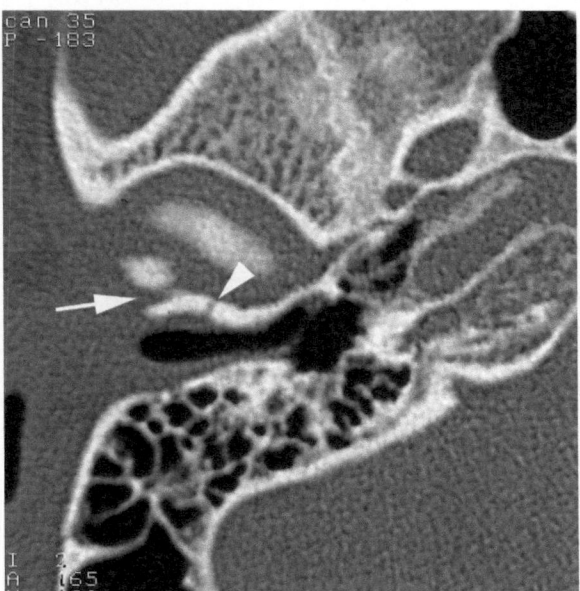

Fig. 2.7. Axial CT image in a patient with posttraumatic ear bleeding. A non-displaced fracture of the right tympanic bone is seen (*arrowhead*). No other temporal bone fractures were apparent. Note (normal) petrotympanic suture (*arrow*)

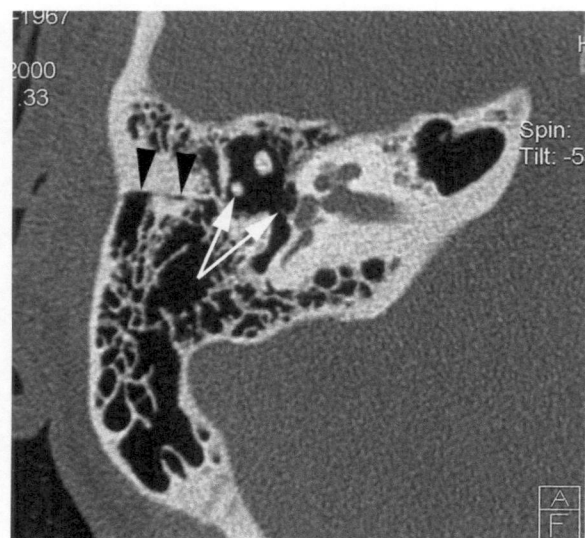

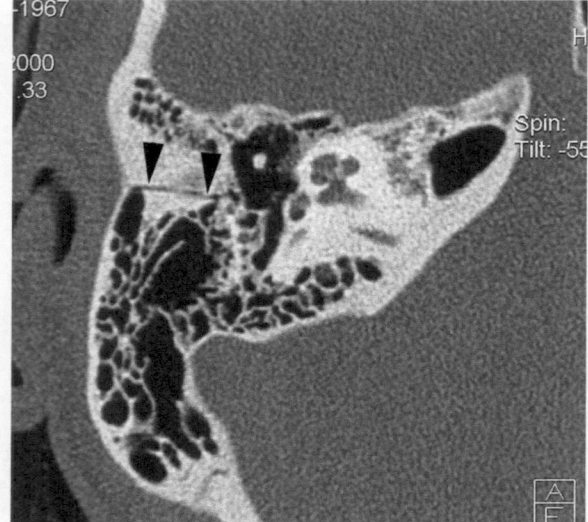

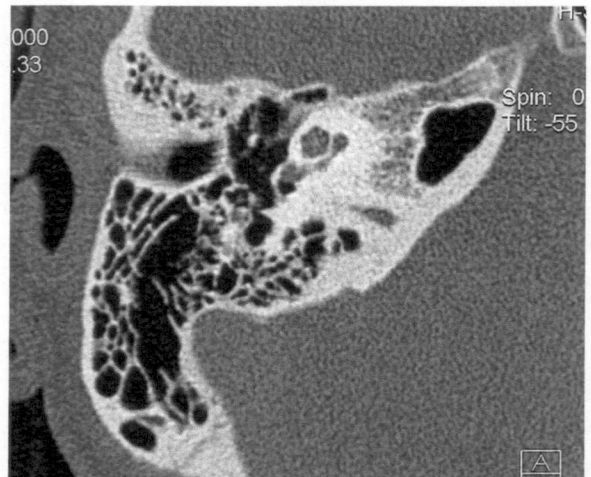

Fig. 2.8a–c. Axial adjacent CT images in a patient with posttraumatic conductive hearing loss. A longitudinal temporal bone fracture (*arrowheads*) is extending in the lateral wall of the middle ear, as well as in the superior wall of the external auditory canal. The incus is luxated. Dissociation is seen between long process of incus and stapedial superstructure (**a**, *arrows*)

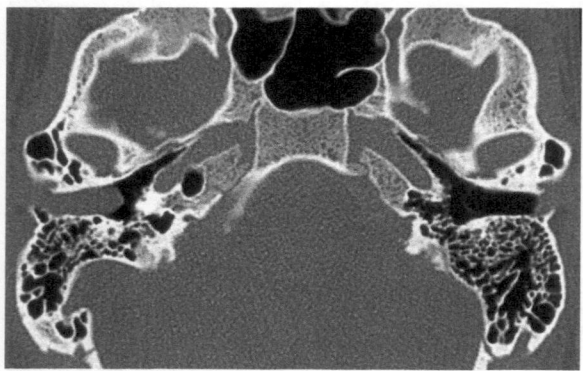

Fig. 2.9. Right-sided conductive hearing loss after cranial trauma. Clinical examination shows complete soft tissue obliteration of the right external ear canal. Axial CT image confirms soft tissue obliteration of this structure; normal aeration of the middle ear cavity. Posttraumatic fibrosis and stenosis

disease, a well-pneumatized mastoid air-cell complex usually is present, allowing extensive growth of the lesion. Histologically, there is no difference with the non-traumatic type of cholesteatoma. Treatment consists of removal of the cholesteatoma and restoration of a wide patent ear canal (FREEMAN 1983).

2.5
Fibrous Dysplasia

Fibrous dysplasia is a condition in which normal medullary bone is replaced by an abnormal proliferation of fibrous tissue, resulting in asymmetric distortion and expansion of bone. It may be confined to a single bone (monostotic fibrous dysplasia) or involve

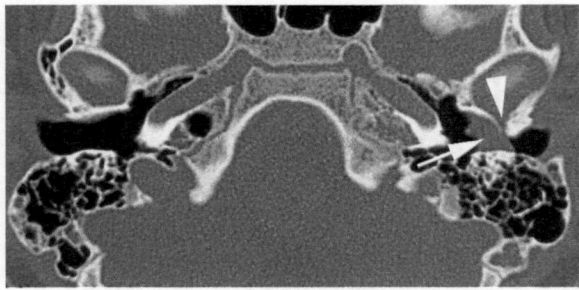

Fig. 2.10. Left-sided conductive hearing loss 1 year after craniocerebral trauma with left temporal bone fracture. Otoscopy revealed presence of a cyst-like lesion. Axial CT image shows a bone defect in the anterior wall of the external auditory canal (*arrowhead*), extending into the temporomandibular joint, with adjacent soft tissue mass deep in the ear canal (*arrow*). Explorative surgery was done and a (posttraumatic) cholesteatoma was found in the ear canal

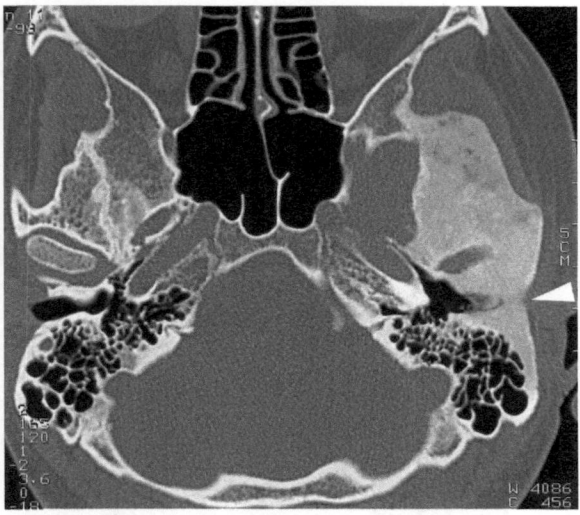

Fig. 2.11. Axial CT image. Enlargement of the squamous part of the left temporal bone, showing the typical ground-glass appearance of fibrous dysplasia; the enlargement of the bone causes stenosis of the external ear canal (*arrowhead*). (Courtesy of B. De Foer)

multiple bones (polyostotic fibrous dysplasia). The monostotic form may involve any of the facial bones but is most commonly seen in the maxilla. The association of the polyostotic form with sexual precocity and cutaneous pigmentation in women is known as McCune-Albright syndrome.

Fibrous dysplasia is a disease of young patients. It may be an incidental finding. In the temporal bone, fibrous dysplasia most commonly involves the squamous portion. The most common symptom in temporal bone involvement is stenosis of the external auditory canal, resulting in conductive hearing loss. As in any stenosis of the external canal, a secondary cholesteatoma may develop deep to the stenosis (Vrabec and Chaljub 2000). Occasionally, other parts of the temporal bone may be involved by fibrous dysplasia.

Usually no new lesions appear after the cessation of skeletal growth. The lesions become more sclerotic with time but may continue to grow slowly into adulthood. Occasionally, reactivation of the lesions occurs during pregnancy. Secondary malignant degeneration into a sarcoma (approximately 0.5% of cases) should be considered when stable or recurrent fibrous dysplasia produces pain or soft tissue extension (Schwartz and Alpert 1964).

Radiologically, fibrous dysplasia usually appears as enlarged bone with a dense "ground-glass" aspect (Fig. 2.11). Sometimes, the lesions have a more osteolytic aspect with regions of dense calcification within them (Fig. 2.12; Brown et al. 1995).

On CT, the bone remodeling associated with a middle fossa meningioma may roughly mimic fibrous dysplasia; however, in meningioma the thickened

and sclerotic bone appears irregularly delineated. The bone delineation in fibrous dysplasia usually is sharply defined. In case of doubt, a complementary MRI study should be performed.

On MRI, the lesions usually have a low signal intensity on T1-weighted images and either high or low signal intensity on T2-weighted images. The signal intensity on T1- and T2-weighted images and the degree of contrast enhancement on T1-weighted images depends on the amount of bony trabeculae, degree of cellularity, and presence of cystic and hemorrhagic changes (Jee et al. 1996). Incidentally found fibrous dysplasia may be confused with a neoplastic lesion on an MR study.

The treatment of fibrous dysplasia affecting the external ear has traditionally been conservative, directed toward the management of the external canal stenosis (Megerian et al. 1995).

2.6
Benign Neoplasms

2.6.1
Cholesteatoma

Cholesteatoma is a tumor-like mass of exfoliated keratin within a sac of stratified squamous epithelium,

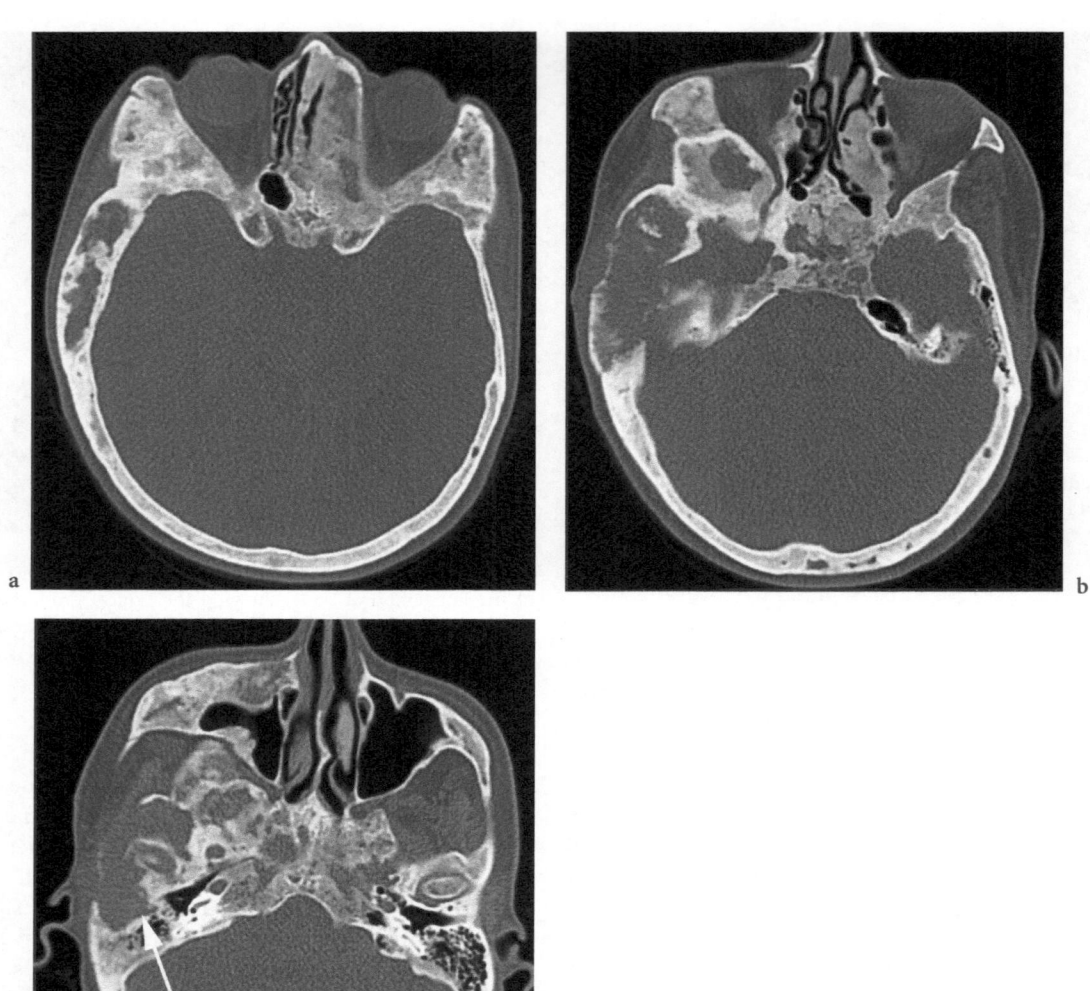

Fig. 2.12a–c. McCune-Albright syndrome. Both sides of the sphenoid bone, left ethmoid bone, and squamous part of the right temporal bone show expansion of the bone, with a mixed osteolytic appearance, areas of dense calcifications, and partly a ground-glass appearance (**a, b**). Stenosis of the left external ear canal by the bone expansion (**c,** *arrow*)

most often occurring in the middle ear. Cholesteatoma is usually an acquired disease ("secondary cholesteatoma") but may be congenital ("primary cholesteatoma"). Congenital cholesteatoma is an ectoblastic derived tumor, originating from epithelial rests. As they have been found everywhere in the temporal bone, they may also occur in the external auditory canal.

Cholesteatoma most commonly occurs within the middle ear. External auditory canal cholesteatoma is uncommon.

A patient with external canal cholesteatoma may present with itching, pain, and foul-smelling otorrhea. In a review of 39 external canal cholesteatomas,

VRABEC and CHALJUB (2000) identified several possible causes. In their practice, most cases were seen after tympanomastoid surgery and therefore classified as "iatrogenic." These cases present as invagination of skin through a defect in the posterior canal wall or as a subepithelial mass lesion. Imaging revealed destruction of the canal wall lateral to the scutum. The second more common cause was described as "spontaneous" external canal cholesteatomas, and was believed to be related to focal osteitis, minor trauma to the external canal skin, or retention of hard cerumen. Presumably, they may also arise from ectopic epithelium. Imaging studies show a

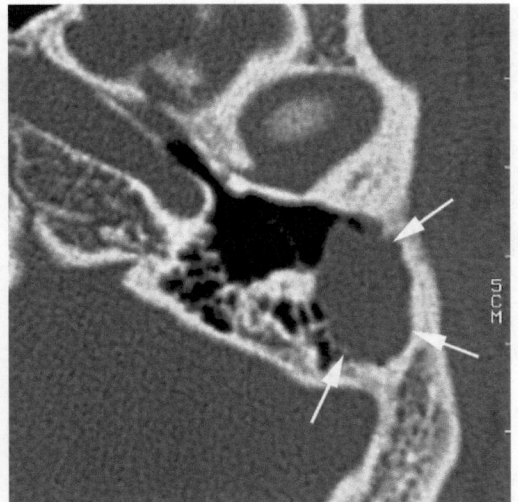

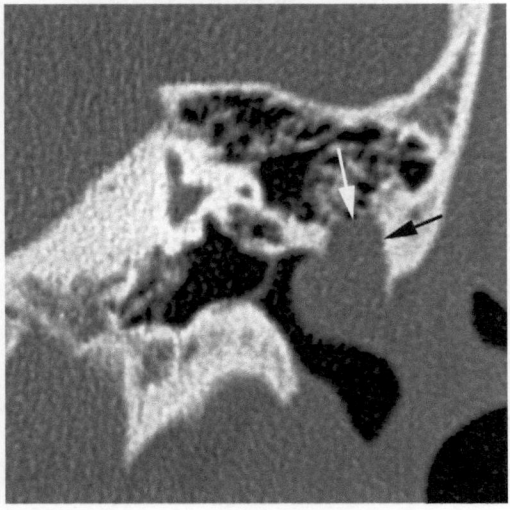

Fig. 2.13. Axial (**a**) and coronal (**b**) CT image of left temporal bone. Soft tissue mass eroding through the posterocranial wall of the external auditory canal into the mastoid (*arrows*). External auditory canal cholesteatoma. (From HERMANS 2000)

in Paget's disease and with external canal osteoma. It may also occur with acquired stenosis due to external otitis, if such stenosis is located laterally in the canal.

In patients with external canal cholesteatoma, the middle ear and mastoid may be extensively pneumatized. Once such a cholesteatoma has gained access to these cavities, it may become quite large. Reported complications include facial nerve paralysis, ossicular erosions, and labyrinthine fistula (BROOKES and GRAHAM 1984; VRABEC and CHALJUB 2000).

2.6.2
Keratosis Obturans

Keratosis obturans is a condition in which an epidermal keratin plug is found in the external auditory canal, often bilaterally. The presenting symptoms are pain and conductive hearing loss. These symptoms may be acute, caused by swelling of the plug when moistened (e.g., after swimming).

There is evidence that keratosis obturans is caused by abnormal epithelial migration across the tympanic membrane and out of the external ear canal (CORBRIDGE et al. 1996).

The accumulation of large plugs of desquamated epithelium may lead to a greatly widened bony canal; however, the tympanic membrane is usually spared. In young patients, an association with sinusitis and/or bronchiectasis has been noted in up to 77% of cases, but this concurrence is less often found in adult patients (approximately 20%). Also, bilateral involvement is more frequently seen in juvenile cases than in adults.

On CT, soft tissue thickening is seen in the external auditory canal, possibly with ballooning and erosion of its bony borders.

The differential diagnosis is external auditory canal cholesteatoma, which is usually a unilateral disease, presenting as otorrhea and a more chronic, dull pain (PIEPERGERDES et al. 1980); CT shows a more localized erosion of the canal wall in cholesteatoma.

well-localized bone erosion, often in the anterior–inferior part of the canal, just lateral to the annulus (Fig. 2.13). Trauma was believed to be the third most common cause; posttraumatic cholesteatoma is described more extensively above.

In some of the patients described by VRABEC and CHALJUB (2000), stenosis of the external auditory canal caused cholesteatoma (two patients had congenital stenosis, the other patient suffered from acquired stenosis due to fibrous dysplasia). Any process causing occlusion or narrowing of the external canal may result in retention of squamous debris medial to the stenosis. This has also been described

2.6.3
Exostoses and Osteoma

Exostoses are multinodular bony masses developing due to prolonged irritation of the external auditory canal, most commonly secondary to excessive contact with cold sea water ("surfer's ear"). They commonly are bilateral lesions, although the patient may have unilateral symptoms. On CT, they appear as broad-based bony excrescences, usually multiple, narrowing the bony external auditory canal. (Fig. 2.14).

Osteomas are less common than exostoses. Typically, an osteoma is a solitary, unilateral, and pedunculated bony growth (Fig. 2.15).

2.6.4
Other Tumors

Other kinds of benign tumors may be encountered within the external auditory canal. All of these lesions are rare.

Chronic external otitis may be associated with the formation of a (non-neoplastic) aural polyp. Several types of tumors arising from the ceruminous glands may be seen. Vascular malformations, hemangiomas, smooth muscle tumors, and tumors of neural origin have been described. Very rarely, the external auditory canal may become invaded by a meningioma originating from the middle cranial fossa (Fig. 2.16; TSUNODA and FUKAYA 1997).

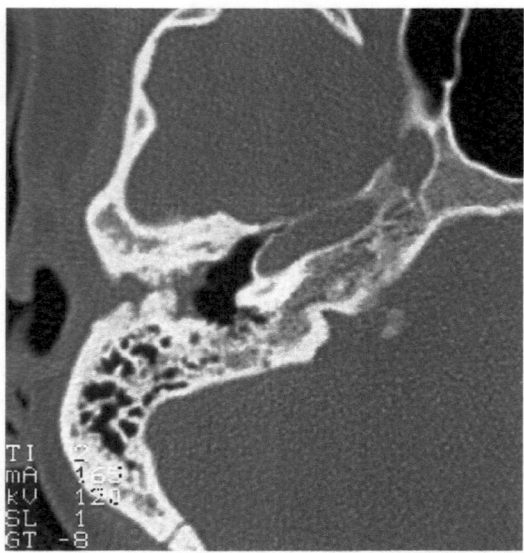

Fig. 2.14. Axial CT image through right temporal bone. Multinodular bone masses, associated with soft tissue inflammation in the external auditory canal: exostoses. (From HERMANS 2000)

2.7
Malignant Neoplasms

Primary external ear malignant neoplasms are uncommon. External ear cancer initially appears as a painless lesion. Enlarging lesions cause minor bleeding, itching, pain, and intermittent drainage of serous fluid. Often, these symptoms are attributed to external otitis. Eventually, as the clinical situation progressively becomes worse, further exploration will reveal the true nature of the lesion. More advanced cancer may cause stenosis of the external auditory canal, trismus, conchal and preauricular swelling, and facial nerve palsy (MILLION et al. 1994). Spread toward the middle ear, and more rarely inner ear, may occur.

Histologically, external ear malignancies usually correspond to squamous cell carcinoma or basocellular carcinoma. On rare occasions, adenocarcinoma (developing from the ceruminous glands), lymphoma, or malignant melanoma are encountered in the external canal.

As assessment of bone detail is critical to treatment planning, CT is normally the first study (Fig. 2.17). Surrounding structures are likely to become involved with further tumor growth, such as the parotid gland and temporomandibular joint. Perineural tumor spread along the facial or auriculotemporal nerve may be seen. Also intracranial

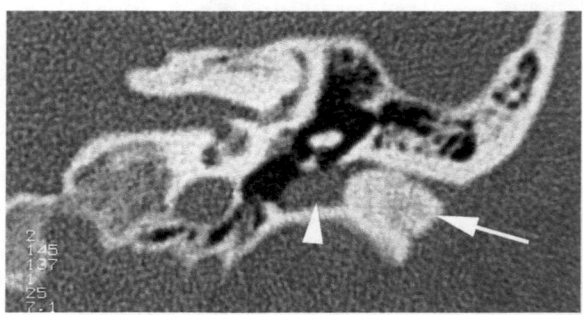

Fig. 2.15. Coronal CT image through left temporal bone. Solitary bony outgrowth, attached to the tympanic bone: osteoma (*arrow*). Some retro-obstructive debris or inflammation is present between the osteoma and the tympanic membrane (*arrowhead*)

spread is possible. Magnetic resonance imaging is frequently used as an adjunct in such cases (Fig. 2.17). Tumor spread to the neck lymph nodes is possible. The parotid and higher parajugular lymph nodes are at risk and an imaging study of the neck is therefore desirable.

Treatment is by radiotherapy, surgery, or a combination of both. After radical treatment of extensive neoplasms, it is useful to obtain a baseline imaging study (optimal timing probably approximately 4 months after completion of treatment), and to perform periodic follow-up imaging studies, in order to

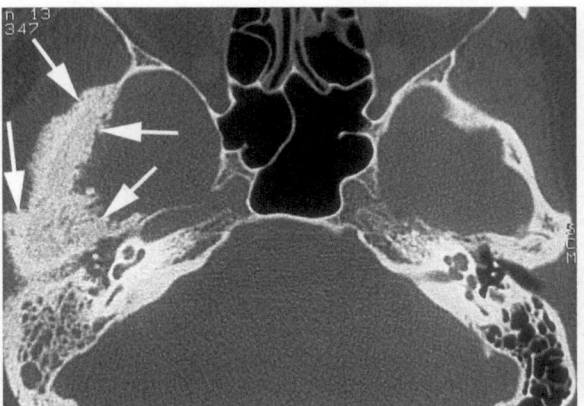

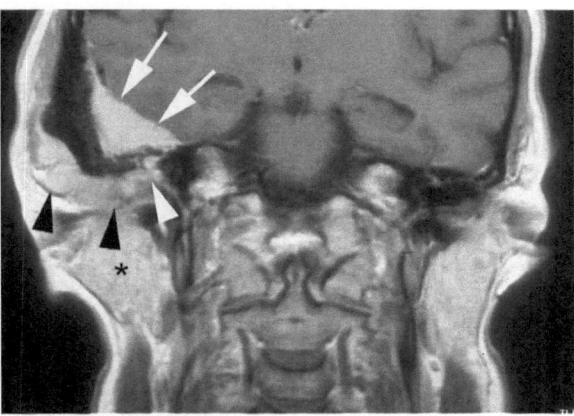

a   b

Fig. 2.16a, b. Patient with acquired soft tissue stenosis of the right external ear canal. Axial CT image (**a**) shows extensive sclerotic bone remodeling of the squamous part of the right temporal bone (*arrows*). Although somewhat reminiscent of the ground-glass aspect seen in fibrous dysplasia (see Fig. 2.11), the appearance of the surface should arouse the suspicion of hyperostosis induced by a meningioma. Opacification of the right middle ear cavity is seen. Coronal enhanced T1-weighted spin-echo image (**b**). A strongly enhancing mass lesion is seen in the middle cranial fossa (*arrows*), with transosseous extension into the middle ear, external ear canal, and along the outside of the squamous bone (*arrowheads*). Biopsy of the external ear mass revealed meningioma. Parotid gland is indicated by *asterisk*

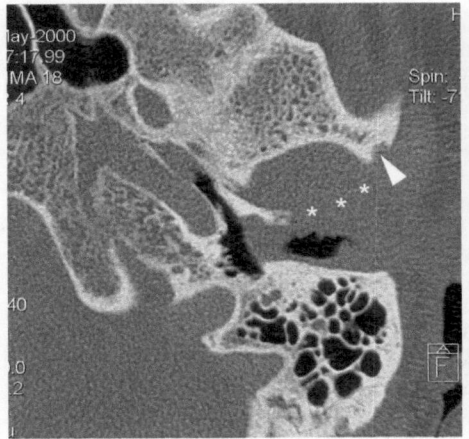

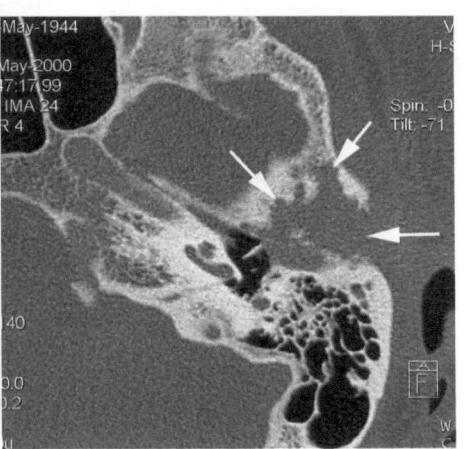

a   b

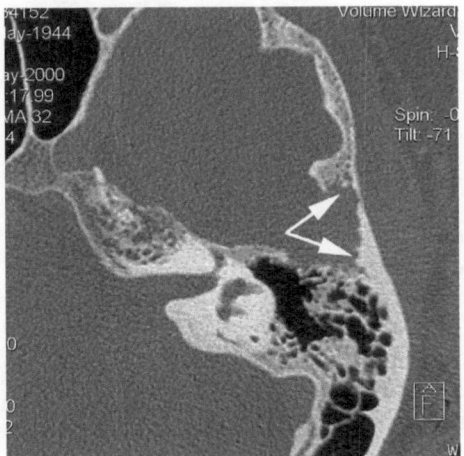

c

Fig. 2.17a–h. Patient known with squamous cell carcinoma of the left external ear canal. Axial CT images (bone window) show soft tissue thickening in the external ear canal, with erosion of its anterior bony wall (tympanic bone: **a**, expected position indicated by *asterisks*). Some osteolysis at the origin of the zygomatic process is seen (*arrowhead*). More superiorly, erosion of the roof of the ear canal and adjacent part of the squamous portion (**b**, *arrows*). Several millimeters more cranially, slight erosion of the inner table of the squamous portion is seen, indicating intracranial tumor extension (**c**, *arrows*). Coronal (**d**) and sagittal (**e**) reformation confirm extensive osteolysis of the tympanic bone and superior extension in the squamous portion of the temporal bone (*arrows*). The mandibular condyle (**e**) appears intact. Axial contrast-enhanced CT ▷

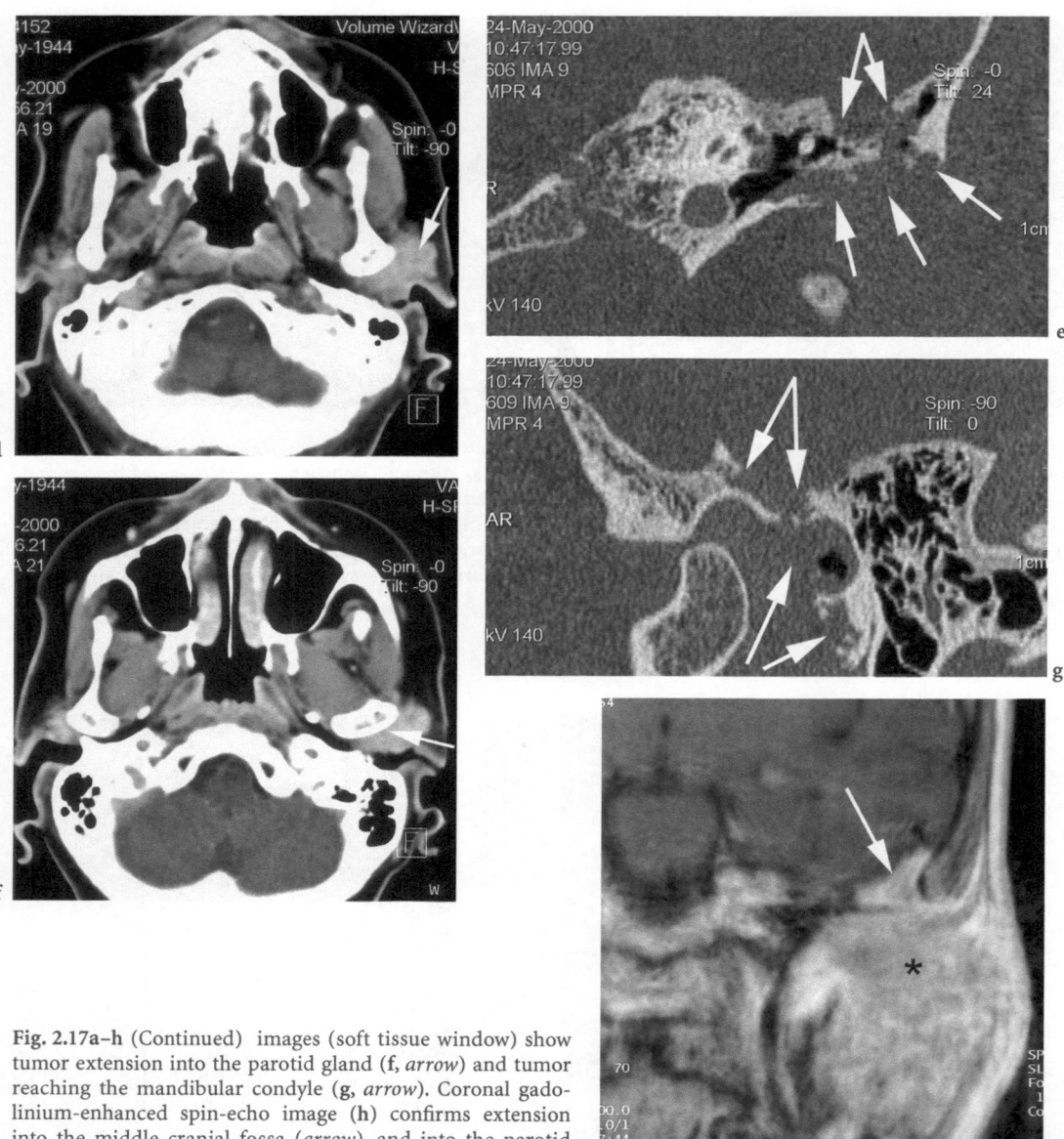

Fig. 2.17a–h (Continued) images (soft tissue window) show tumor extension into the parotid gland (**f**, *arrow*) and tumor reaching the mandibular condyle (**g**, *arrow*). Coronal gadolinium-enhanced spin-echo image (**h**) confirms extension into the middle cranial fossa (*arrow*), and into the parotid gland (*asterisk*)

detect recurrent tumor as early as possible (MILLION et al. 1994).

Malignant neoplasms secondarily invading the external auditory canal may arise from neighboring structures, such as the periauricular skin or parotid gland. Occasionally, hematogenous spread to the external auditory canal from a distant site is encountered. It may be seen with breast cancer, but also metastatic lung or urogenital cancer has been reported at this site.

References

Ahuja AT, Marshall JN, Roebuck DJ, King AD, Metreweli C (2000) Sonographic appearances of preauricular sinus. Clin Radiol 55:528–532

al-Shihabi BA (1992) Carcinoma of temporal bone presenting as malignant otitis externa. J Laryngol Otol 106:908–910

Brookes GB, Graham MD (1984) Post-traumatic cholesteatoma of the external auditory canal. Laryngoscope 94:667–670

Brown EW, Megerian CA, McKenna MJ, Weber A (1995) Fibrous dysplasia of the temporal bone: imaging findings. Am J Roentgenol 164:679–682

Chandler JR (1968) Malignant external otitis. Laryngoscope 78:1257–1294

Corbridge RJ, Michaels L, Wright T (1996) Epithelial migration in keratosis obturans. Am J Otolaryngol 17:411–414

Currie AR, King WW, Vlantis AC, Li AK (1996) Pitfalls in the management of preaurciular sinuses. Br J Surg 83:1722–1724

De S, Pfleiderer AG (1999) An extreme and unusual variant of Ramsay Hunt syndrome. J Laryngol Otol 113:670–671

Franssens Y, Hermans R, Feenstra L, Baert AL (1993) Posttraumatic external auditory canal cholesteatoma. J Belge Radiol 76:320–321

Freeman J (1983) Temporal bone fractures and cholesteatoma. Ann Otol Rhinol Laryngol 92:558–560

Hermans R (2000) Head and neck imaging. In: Pettersson H, Allison D (eds) The encyclopedia of medical imaging. The NICER Institute, Oslo, part VI

Jee WH, Choi KH, Choe BY, Park JM, Shinn KS (1996) Fibrous dysplasia: MR imaging characteristics with radiopathologic correlation. Am J Roentgenol 167:1523–1527

Keohane JD, Ruby RR, Janzen VD, MacRae DL, Parnes LS (1993) Medial meatal fibrosis: the University of Western Ontario experience. Am J Otol 14:172–175

Langman J (ed) (1981) Ear. In: Medical embryology, 4th edn. Williams and Wilkins, Baltimore, pp 303–304

Lau JT (1983) Towards better delineation and complete excision of preauricular sinus. Aust NZ J Surg 53:267–269

Mattuci KF, Setzen M, Galantich P (1986) Necrotizing otitis externa occurring concurrently with epidermoid carcinoma. Laryngoscope 96:264–266

Mayer TE, Brueckmann H, Siegert R et al. (1998) High-resolution CT of the temporal bone in dysplasia of the auricle and external auditory canal. Am J Neuroradiol 18:53–65

McKennan KX, Chole RA (1989) Posttraumatic cholesteatoma. Laryngoscope 99:779–782

McKennan KX, Chole RA (1992) Traumatic external auditory canal atresia. Am J Otol 13:80–81

Megerian CA, Sofferman RA, McKenna MJ, Eavey RD, Nadol JB Jr (1995) Fibrous dysplasia of the temporal bone: ten new cases demonstrating the spectrum of otologic sequelae. Am J Otol 16:408–419

Midwinter KI, Gill KS, Spencer JA, Fraser ID (1999) Osteomyelitis of the temporomandibular joint in patients with malignant otitis externa. J Laryngol Otol 113:451–453

Million RR, Cassisi NJ, Mancuso AA, Stringer SP (1994) Temporal bone. In: Million RR, Cassisi NJ (eds) Management of head and neck cancer: a multidisciplinary approach, 2nd edn. Lippincott, Philadelphia, pp 751–764

Piepergerdes JC, Kramer BM, Behnke EE (1980) Keratosis obturans and external auditory canal cholesteatoma. Laryngoscope 90:383–391

Rubin J, Yu VL (1988) Malignant external otitis: insights into pathogenesis, clinical manifestations, diagnosis and therapy. Am J Med 85:391–398

Rubin J, Curtin HD, Yu VL, Kamerer DB (1990) Malignant external otitis: utility of CT in diagnosis and follow-up. Radiology 174:391–394

Schwartz DT, Alpert M (1964) The malignant transformation of fibrous dysplasia. Am J Med Sci 247:35–54

Swartz JD, Harnsberger HR (eds) (1998) Imaging of the temporal bone, 3rd edn. Thieme, New York

Tsunoda R, Fukaya T (1997) Extracranial meningioma presenting as a tumour of the external auditory meatus: a case report. J Laryngol Otol 111:148–151

Vourtsi A, Papadopoulos A, Golfinopoulos S et al. (1998) Abnormal enhancement of the membranous labyrinth in a case of relapsing polychondritis. Ann Otol Rhinol Laryngol 107:81–82

Vrabec JT, Chaljub G (2000) External canal cholesteatoma. Am J Otol 21:608–614

Yeakley JW, Jahrsdoerfer RA (1996) CT evaluation of congenital aural atresia: what the radiologist and surgeon need to know. J Comput Assist Tomogr 20:724–731

The Clinician's View

I. Dhooge

The external ear is composed of the auricle and the external auditory canal. It has great functional (protective and acoustic) and cosmetic significance. It may be involved in numerous dermatoses and general systemic disorders. It is also the site of injuries, tumors, and infections. When deformed, it can be the source of considerable psychological distress. Because of the accessibility of the external ear, most of the diagnoses are made by history and clinical examination. Imaging becomes important in selected problems.

Necrotizing "malignant" external otitis, for example, is a life-threatening disease where the infection of the external auditory canal is complicated by progressive osteitis and osteomyelitis of the temporal bone. Complete radiologic evaluation is helpful in determining the extent of disease, the involvement of middle ear or mastoid, the occurrence of lateral sinus thrombosis, etc. Imaging is also important in monitoring the response to therapy. The radiographic extent of disease correlates closely with the intensity and duration of therapy required and is therefore of prognostic value.

Imaging of the external ear can also help in determining the extent of a cholesteatoma of the external auditory canal. The extent of the disease will determine the surgical approach which may vary from transcanal debridement and curettage to canalplasty to full tympanomastoidectomy.

Radiology can help in differentiating between numerous benign tumors that can arise in or around the ear (benign osseous neoplasms, chondroma, eosinophilic granuloma, vascular neoplasms, mesen-chymal neoplasms, glandular neoplasms).

Malignant tumors of the external ear canal are rare. Since the therapeutic approach and the progno-sis merely depend on the extent of the tumor, imaging is of the utmost importance in evaluating the extent of the lesion and its relation with adjacent structures such as the parotid gland, postauricular area, upper jugular digastric area, and all cranial nerves. Using primarily the CT scan, the lesion is staged according to the TNM system described by ARRIAGA (1990).

Magnetic resonance imaging scans are helpful if middle or posterior fossa involvement is suspected.

Reference

Arriaga M, Curtin H, Takahashi H et al. (1990) Staging pro-posal for external auditory meatus carcinoma based on preoperative clinical examination and computed tomogra-phy findings. Ann Otol Rhinol Laryngol 99:714–721

3 Imaging of Cholesteatomatous and Non-Cholesteatomatous Middle Ear Disease

M. Lemmerling and B. De Foer

CONTENTS

3.1
Introduction

The natural history of chronic middle ear disease is different from that of acute middle ear disease. For a well understanding of both entities it is important to consider them as two completely different diseases. In contrast to acute otomastoid diseases that usually develop in the well-pneumatized mastoid of a child, chronic otitis media is most often seen in the more sclerotic mastoid and on the basis of dysfunction of the eustachian tube. The treatment of non-cholesteatomatous chronic otitis media consists of tympanoplastic reconstruction. Debate exists on the usefulness

M. Lemmerling, MD, PhD
Medische Beeldvorming, A.Z. St. Lucas, Groenebriel 1,
9000 Gent, Belgium
B. De Foer, MD
Department of Radiology, A.Z. Sint Augustinus,
Oosterveldlaan 24, 2610 Antwerp (Wilrijk), Belgium

of performing a combined aerating mastoidectomy (Ruhl and Pensak 1999; Mishiro et al. 2001).

There is no general agreement about the usefulness of performing preoperative CT evaluations in patients with chronic otitis media. A literature search of English language clinical and basic science publications was performed, reviewing major otolaryngology texts on the clinical experience and recommendations of experienced otologic surgeons and radiologists regarding the use of radiologic studies in case of chronic otitis media. The conclusion was that no single accepted standard exists on this matter (Blevins and Carter 1998). Often otoscopy allows to obtain enough information. In cases of simple otitis media CT is not useful. In cases of suspected cholesteatoma imaging studies provide information that allows for better planning of the surgical procedure, and offers the otologist the possibility to inform the patient more accurately on what result can be expected from the surgical intervention. Good indications for preoperative CT imaging in cases of chronic middle ear disease are the following: difficult otoscopy or doubtful diagnosis; suspicion that a malformation is present; single functional ear; temporal bones after mastoidectomy; and suspicion for the presence of intracranial complications (Garber and Dort 1994; Rocher et al. 1995; Falcioni et al. 2002). Each clinician must assess the benefits derived from these studies in his or her daily practice (Blevins and Carter 1998).

3.2
Chronic Otitis Media
Without Cholesteatoma

3.2.1
Middle Ear Effusion

Middle ear effusion is commonly present and in non-complicated cases a CT examination adds no information to what has been otoscopically noted. Middle ear effusions are easily seen with CT and have an intermediate density, like all other fluids in the body.

Performing density measurements in unnecessary and will not result in reliable interpretations of the type of effusion, serous or mucoid.

3.2.2
Tympanic Membrane Changes

Almost all tympanic membrane changes are better appreciated otoscopically than with CT, but the CT finding of such changes has to alert the radiologist to perform a detailed analysis of the associated middle ear changes. Prior to tympanic membrane surgery, the otologist wants to be informed in detail about the ossicular status and about the status of the middle ear cavity in general.

3.2.2.1
Tympanic Membrane Thickening and/or Perforation

Tympanic membrane thickening and perforation are easily observed otoscopically. Both conditions are of course also easily seen with CT, but the otologist will be more interested in what can be visualized behind the membrane (Figs. 3.1, 3.2).

3.2.2.2
Tympanic Membrane Retraction

Tympanic membrane retraction is easy to identify otoscopically as well as with CT. In extended cases the tympanic membrane can become adherent to the stapes head. In such cases the term "nature's myringostapediopexy" (SWARTZ et al. 1986) or "spontaneous type-III myringostapediopexy" is used, referring to the similar finding that is seen after a surgical type-III myringostapediopexy procedure (Fig. 3.3). In such cases hearing will be preserved (SCHUKNECHT 1993).

3.2.3
Ossicular Erosion

3.2.3.1
Etiology and Location

Since many years it is known that chronic otitis media can lead to the development of erosions of the ossicular chain. Many theories have been proposed to believe that mononuclear inflammatory cells and osteocytes (GANTZ and MAYNARD 1982) or osteoclasts (CHOLE

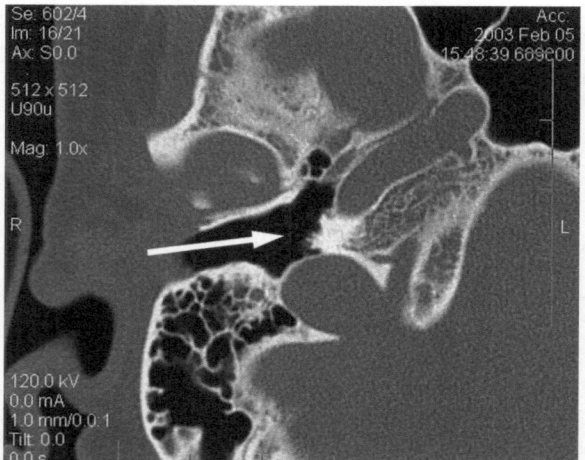
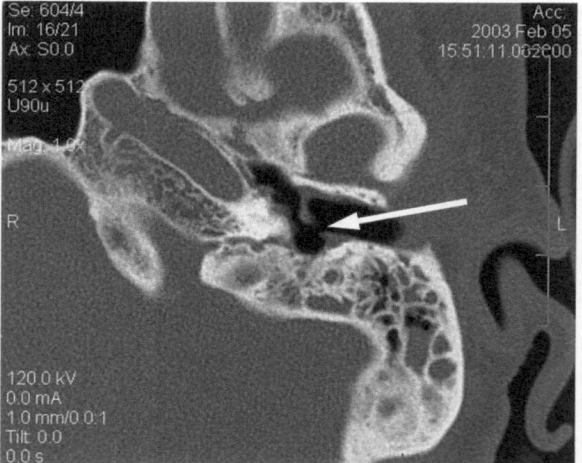
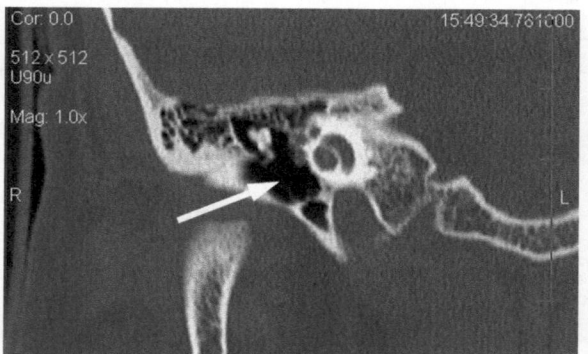
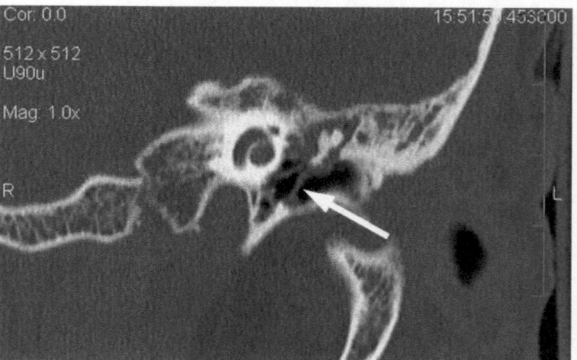

Fig. 3.1. In this patient with non-cholesteatomatous middle ear disease on the left side the normal tympanic membrane (*arrow*) on the right side (**a** axial, **c** coronal) is in obvious contrast with the thickened membrane (*arrow*) contralaterally (**b** axial, **d** coronal)

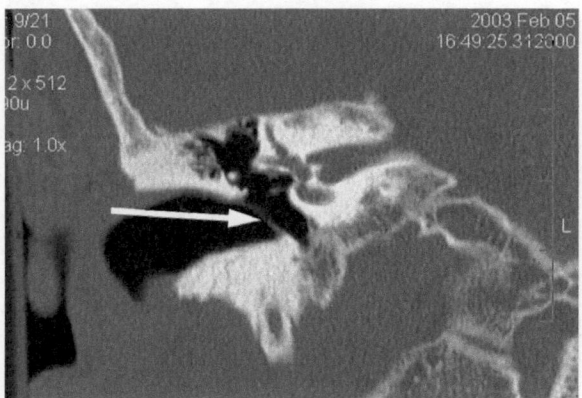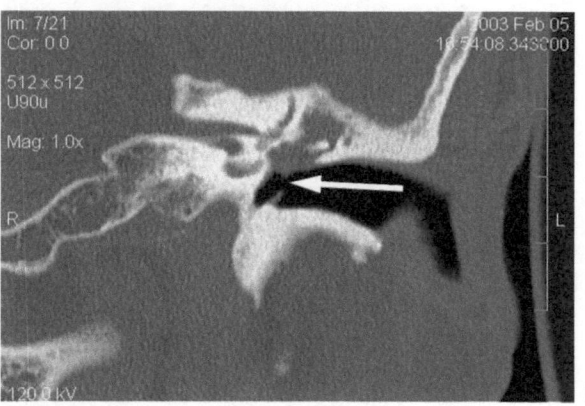

a   b

Fig. 3.2. In this patient with moderate chronic otitis media on the right side a moderate tympanic membrane thickening (*arrow*) is noted **a** on the coronal CT images. **b** In the contralateral temporal bone severe chronic middle ear disease is present, with cholesteatoma formation. Tympanic membrane perforation (*arrow*) is seen

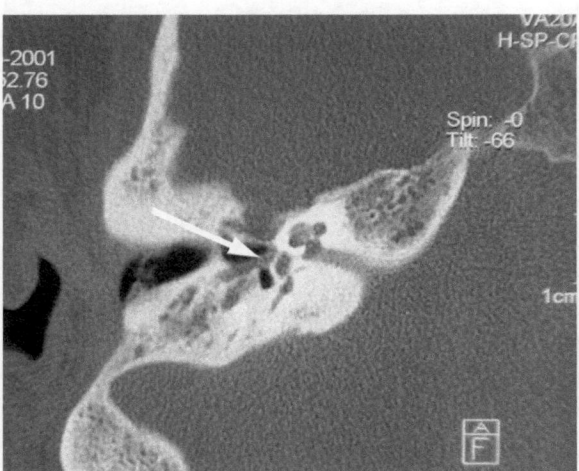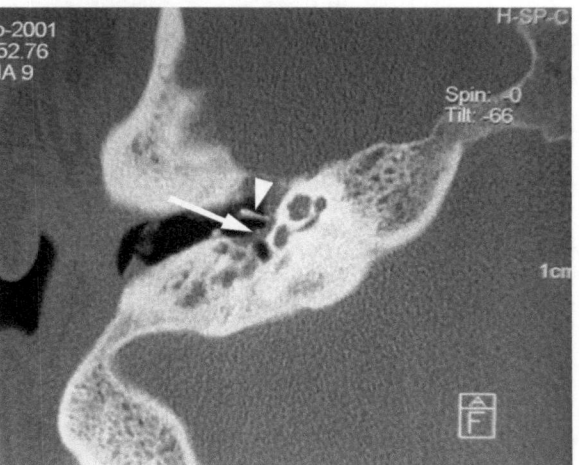

a   b

Fig. 3.3. Two axial CT images are shown in a patient with tympanic membrane retraction, in a way that the membrane is now positioned immediately on the stapes (*arrow*): spontaneous type-III myringostapediopexy or nature's type-III myringostapediopexy. Note that the malleus (*arrowhead*) is excluded from conduction

1988) release substances that erode the ossicles. The incus long process and incus lenticular process are the most vulnerable ossicular structures in the whole chain, followed by the stapes head. The malleus and incus body are more resistant to the process of ossicular erosion (SWARTZ 1984).

3.2.3.2
Reliability of CT

In the early 1990s studies were performed to assess the usefulness and limitations of high-resolution CT for evaluating the condition of the ossicular chain in the opacified middle ear. It was clear that the malleus head and incus body were more easily studied with success than were the more minute structures of the chain, such as the stapes superstructure and the incudostapedial joint (FUSE et al. 1992). With an

improving quality of the images made by recently built scanners, this has changed a lot. In the late 1990s a new study was conducted to establish the computed visibility of the incudostapedial joint and of the stapes superstructure in normal and opacified middle ears. In normal ears, both the stapes crura and the continuity between the incus and stapes were seen in almost 100% of cases, whereas the actual incudostapedial joint was identified in 86 and 67% of cases in the axial and coronal planes, respectively. The position of the incudostapedial joint was just below footplate level on the axial images and mostly at or anterior to the midportion of the foot plate on the coronal images. In clinically confirmed diseased middle ears, the status of the stapes superstructure in all cases and that of the incus in 11 cases was correctly predicted with CT. The findings make clear that it is now possible to

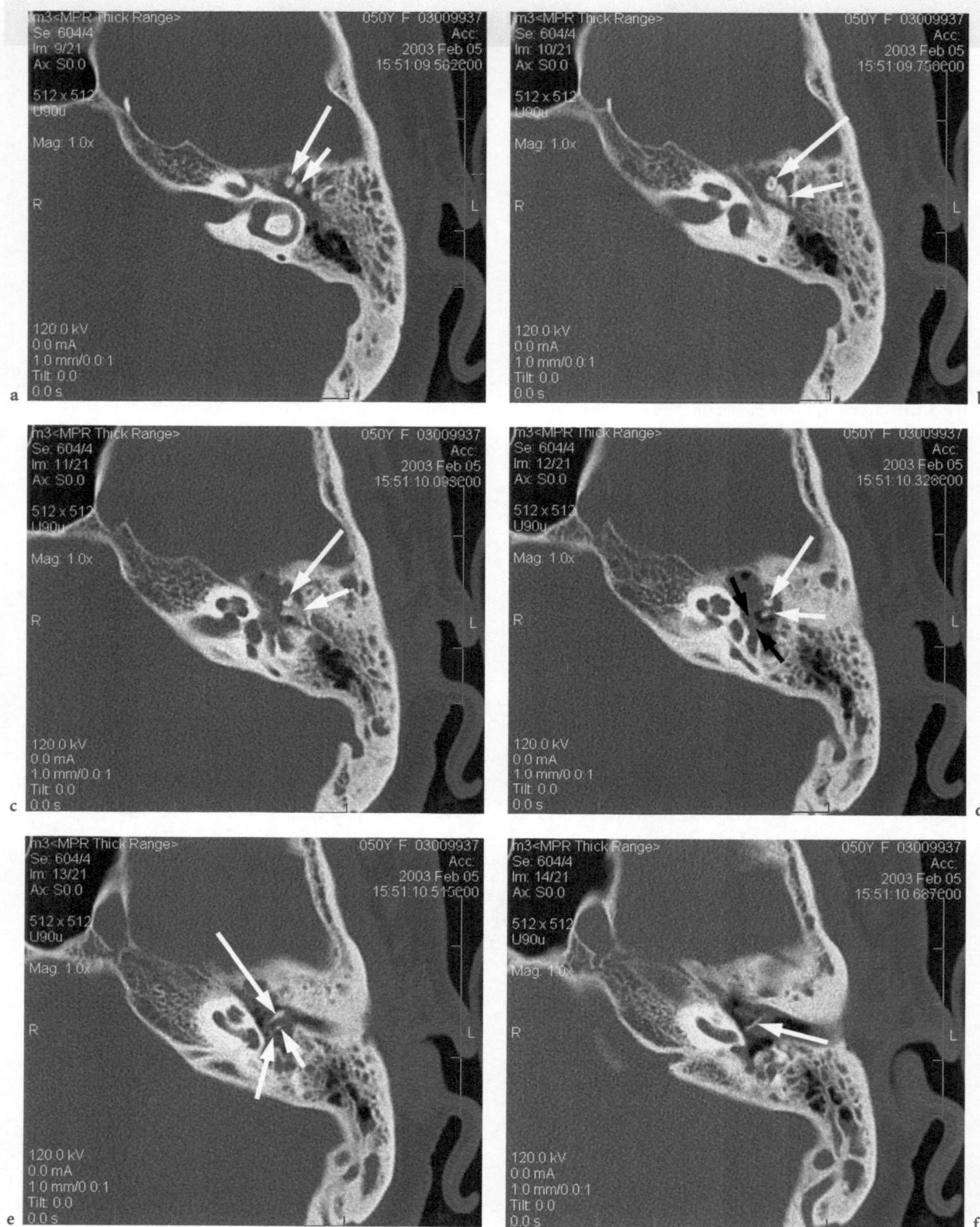

Fig. 3.4a–f. In a patient with non-cholesteatomatous chronic otitis media without ossicular erosion on the left side six consecutive axial CT images are shown. A good knowledge of the ossicular CT anatomy is important in order to identify all normal ossicular elements from the chain. **a** Malleus head (*large arrow*), incus body (*small arrow*). **b** Malleus head (*large arrow*), incus short process (*small arrow*). **c** Malleus head (*large arrow*), incus body, and short process (*small arrow*). **d** Anterior and posterior stapes crus (*black arrows*), malleus neck (*large white arrow*), and incus long process (*small white arrow*). **e** Malleus handle (*large arrow*), incus lenticular process (*small arrow*), and capitulum stapedis (*middle arrow*). **f** Malleus handle

visualize routinely the incudostapedial joint and stapes superstructure at CT, even in an opacified middle ear (Fig. 3.4). Absence of these structures in an opacified middle ear strongly indicates abnormality (LEMMERLING et al. 1997a).

3.2.4
Postinflammatory Ossicular Fixation

The term "postinflammatory ossicular fixation" refers to a group of phenomena taking place in temporal bones with chronic inflammatory disease, in which granulation tissue formation takes place.

3.2.4.1
Fibrous Tissue Fixation

Fibrous tissue formation appears on CT as non-bony non-calcific soft tissue debris encasing some or all of the ossicular chain (Fig. 3.5).

3.2.4.2
Tympanosclerosis

Typically the ear with tympanosclerosis is free of suppuration. Otoscopy reveals tympanosclerosis as whitish plaques in the tympanic membrane and nodular deposits in the submucosal layers of the middle ear.

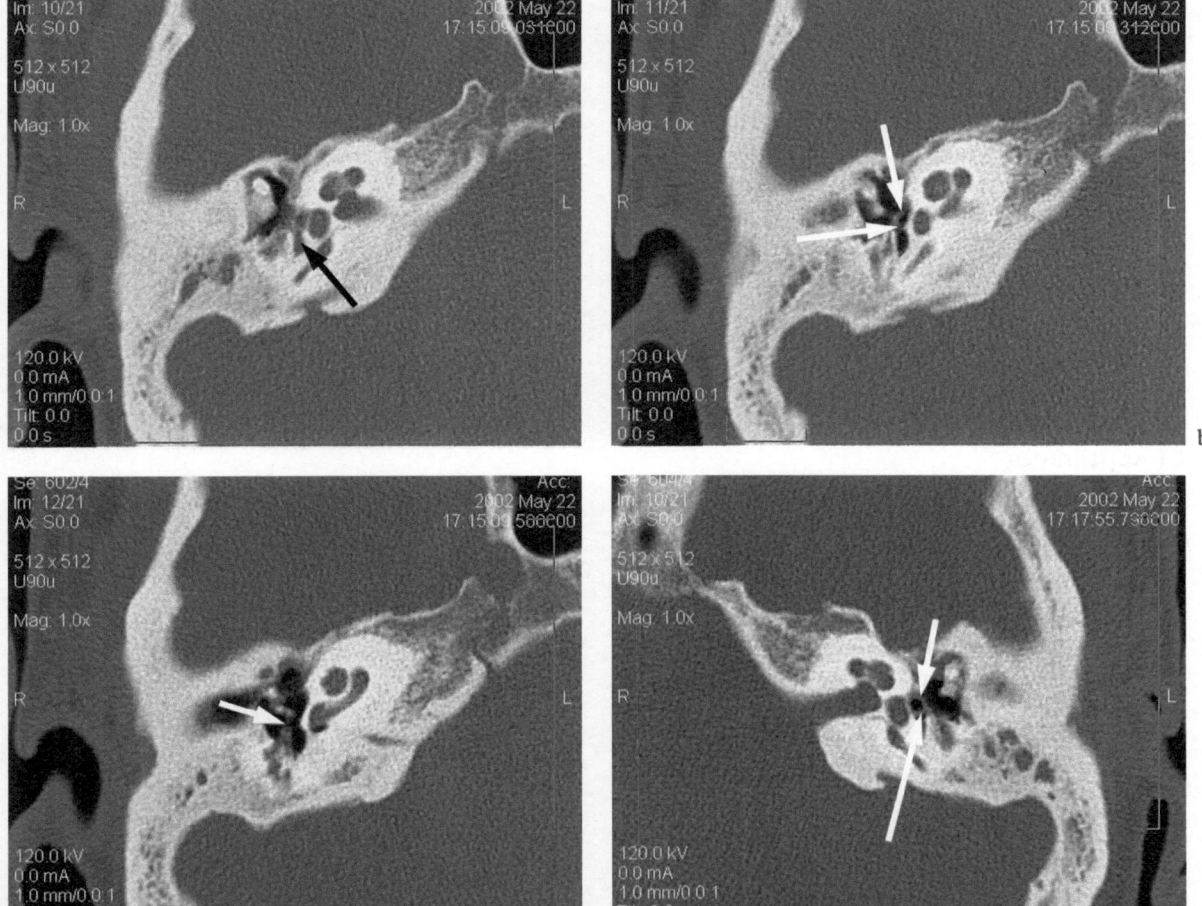

Fig. 3.5. In the right temporal bone of a patient with non-cholesteatomatous chronic middle ear disease fibrous tissue formation with opacification (*arrow*) is seen **a** in the sinus tympani, and fibrous tissue formation is also present on **b** both stapes crura (*arrows*). This latter phenomenon is referred to as "peristapedial tenting." **c** Fibrous tissue formation is seen along the stapedius muscle tendon (*arrow*). **d** In this same patient chronic otitis media without cholesteatoma is also present on the left side, and tympanosclerosis is demonstrated here, with calcific debris on both stapes crura which have become much more dense than in normal conditions (*arrows*)

The latter localization often causes ossicular fixation (SCHUKNECHT 1993). Tympanosclerosis appears on CT as unifocal or multifocal punctate or web-like calcifications in the middle ear cavity or on the tympanic membrane. It may be in direct apposition to the ossicular chain or the suspensory ligaments of the ossicles (SWARTZ et al. 1985). All these ligaments are actually almost constantly visualized (LEMMER-LING et al. 1997b), and a good knowledge of their presence and course makes it possible to provide a detailed description of the tympanosclerotic foci (Figs. 3.5, 3.6).

3.2.4.3
New Bone Formation

New bone formation is the least common of the three forms of postinflammatory ossicular fixation. It appears on CT as thick bony webs or general bony encasement (Fig. 3.7; SWARTZ et al. 1985). In cases of osteoneogenesis osteoid tissue is deposited on existing bone by osteoblastic activity, which leads to the formation of lamellar new bone, progressively obliterating the intervening spaces (SCHUKNECHT 1993).

3.3
Cholesteatoma

3.3.1
CT Appearance

Acquired cholesteatomas, which account for almost all cholesteatomas, result from ingrowth of keratinizing stratified squamous epithelium through the eardrum into the middle ear cavity, and can simply be considered as the presence of skin in the wrong place. For this good reason some authors call them "keratoma," although the term "cholesteatoma" is in general use. This epithelized pocket will grow slowly in a dry ear, but exfoliation is hastened in the presence of infection. The created mass will erode the ossicles and bony walls of the tympanic cavity and mastoid (SCHUKNECHT 1993). This latter phenomenon is generally believed to occur on the basis of pressure erosion, although some say that the activity of collagenase is partially responsible (ABRAMSON et al. 1988).

Two types of acquired cholesteatoma have been described: pars flaccida cholesteatoma (also referred to as primary acquired cholesteatoma, attic cholesteatoma, or Prussak's cholesteatoma) and pars

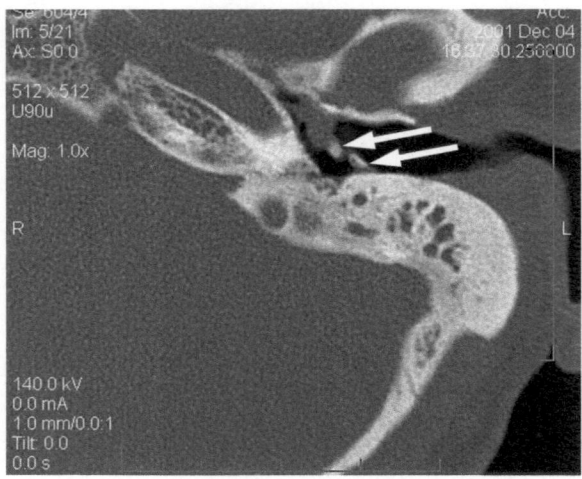

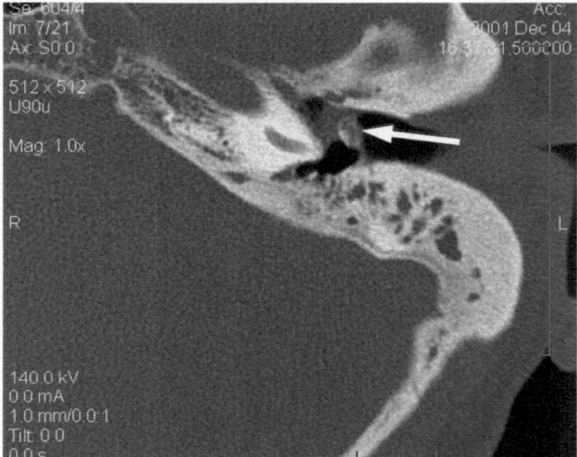

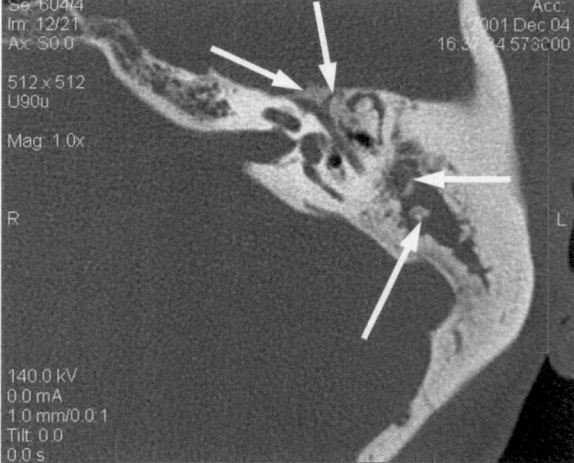

Fig. 3.6. In this patient with chronic middle ear disease and tympanosclerosis large calcified debris (*arrows*) are seen **a, b** on the thickened tympanic membrane. **c** On the axial CT image performed through the epitympanum more calcifications are visible in the anterior epitympanic recess (*both anterior arrows*) and even in the mastoid cavity (*both posterior arrows*)

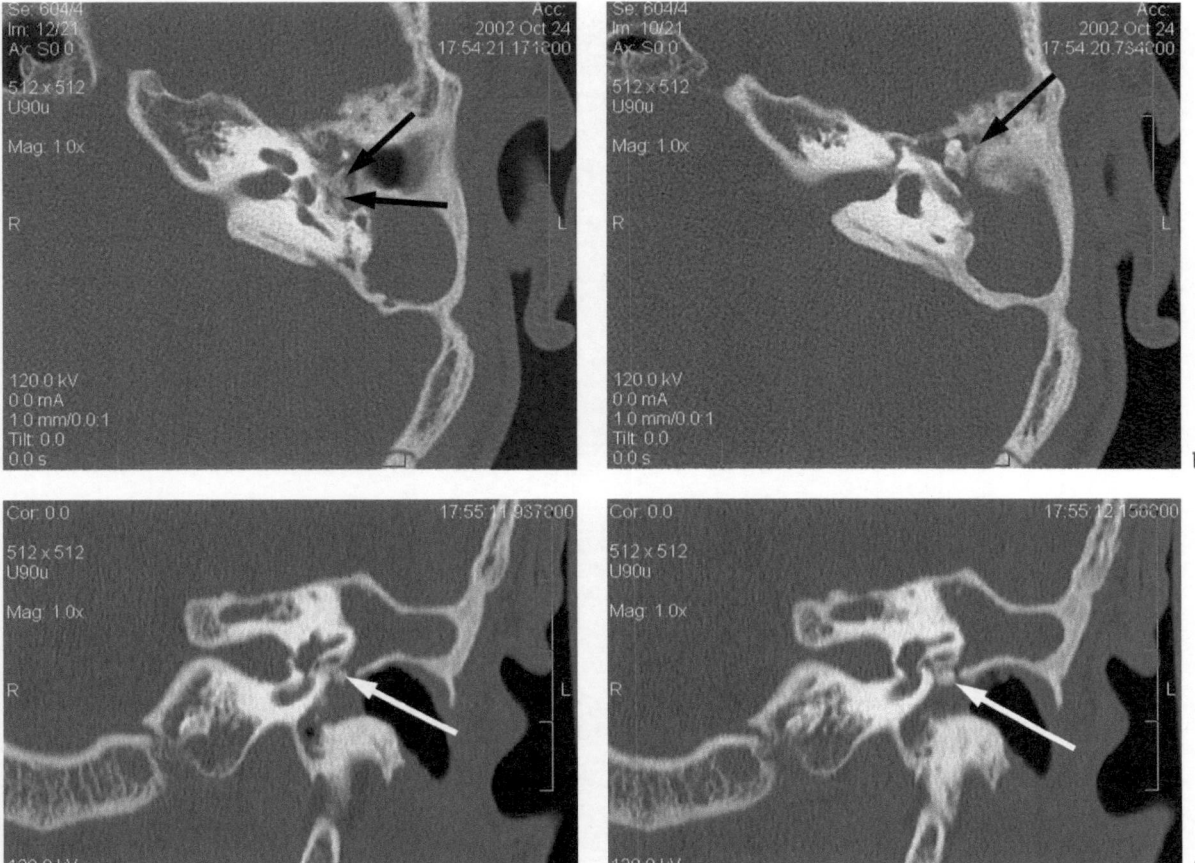

Fig. 3.7. a On the axial CT image new bone formation is seen lateral to the incus body, fixating the chain to the lateral tympanic cavity wall (*arrow*). **b** Ossific debris is also present in large portions of the mesotympanum and extending to the oval window (*arrows*). **c, d** This new bone formation (*arrow*) is also well seen on the coronal images

tensa cholesteatoma (also referred to as secondary acquired cholesteatoma, or sinus cholesteatoma). Both types of cholesteatoma differ from each other on many bases (Table 3.1).

Acquired cholesteatoma is seen on CT as a soft tissue mass with a homogeneous density of approximately 50 HU. Cholesteatoma consequently has no different appearance than that of granulation tissue or opacification of whatever origin (simple effusion, fibrous tissue formation, etc.). This means that the radiologist will often only be able to provide a detailed description of the extent and localization of the disease, and will take risks in trying to predict the histologic nature of what is seen. This is especially true in cases of beginning cholesteatoma formation. Once the cholesteatoma has become larger, and, besides the middle ear opacification, the erosion of the ossicles and other bony structures becomes clear, the diagnosis of cholesteatoma can be made with more confidence, since this combined finding indicates the presence of a cholesteatoma in 90% of cases (Figs. 3.8, 3.9; HARNSBERGER 1995).

Table 1. Comparison of two types of cholesteatoma

Characteristic	Pars flaccida cholesteatoma	Pars tensa cholesteatoma
Site of origin	Prussak's space	Posterosuperior retraction
Extension pattern	Posterolateral attic	Facial recess and sinus tympani
Extension to mastoid antrum	Lateral to incus	Medial to incus
Ossicular displacement	Medially	Laterally

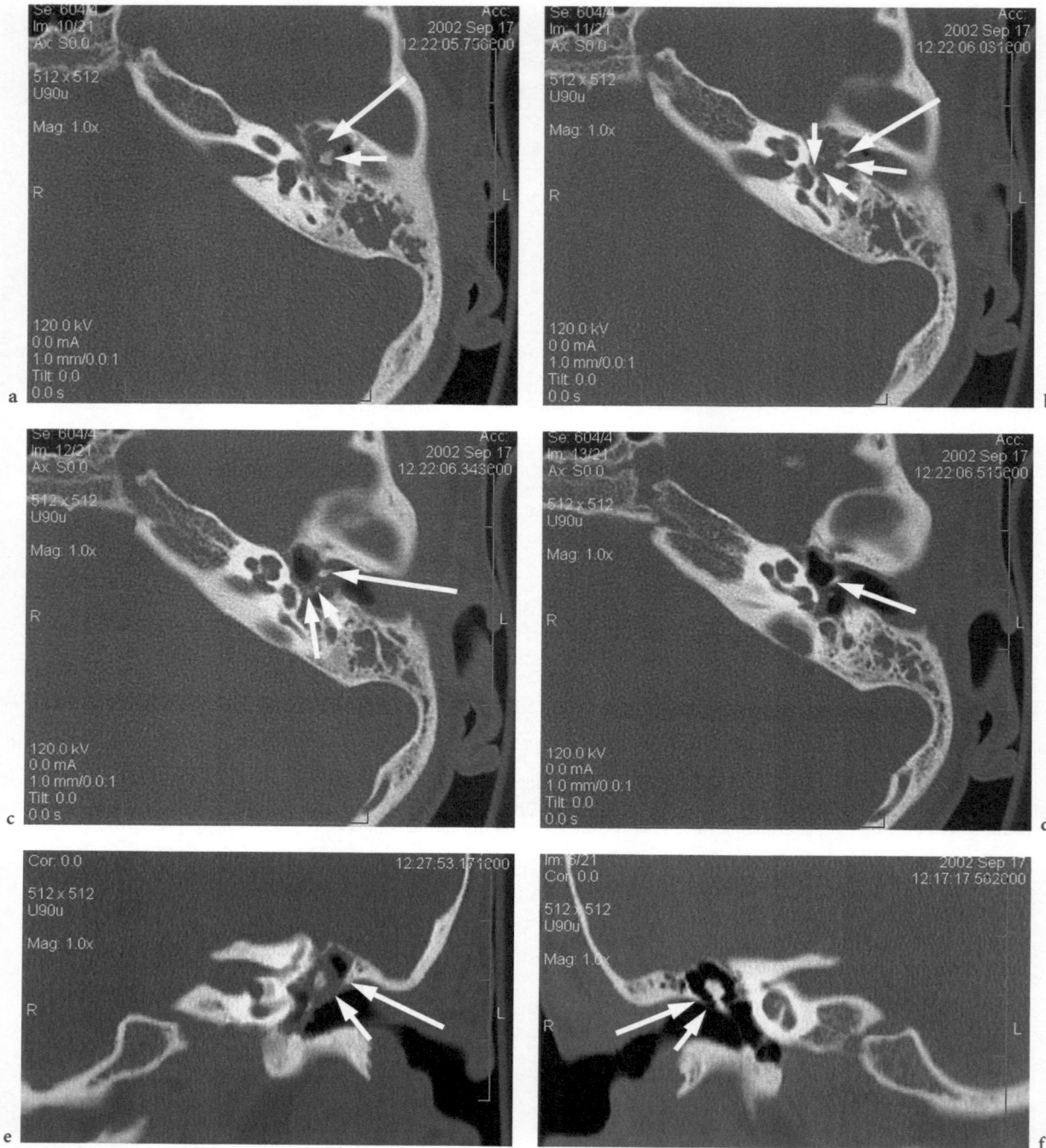

Fig. 3.8a–d. In this patient with cholesteatoma four consecutive axial CT images are shown from the left temporal bone. **a** On the most cranial axial image complete erosion of the head of the malleus is seen (*large arrow*), as well as an intact incus body and short process (*small arrow*). **b** On the image below the malleus neck is seen (*large arrow*), the incus long process (*middle arrow*), and both stapes crura (*two small arrows*). **c** More caudally the incudostapedial joint is seen composed of the incus lenticular process (*small arrow*), on one hand, and the capitulum stapedis (*middle arrow*), on the other hand. The transition between the malleus neck and handle (*large arrow*) is also visible. **d** An intact malleus handle (*arrow*). In this same patient the coronal images on the normal right side demonstrate the sharply delineated scutum (*large arrow*). Prussak's space (*small arrow*), the triangular space between the tympanic membrane, the malleus neck, and the lateral malleolar ligament, is normal and well aerated. In the left ear with cholesteatoma a soft tissue mass fills Prussak's space (*small arrow*), and the scutum (*large arrow*) is blunted

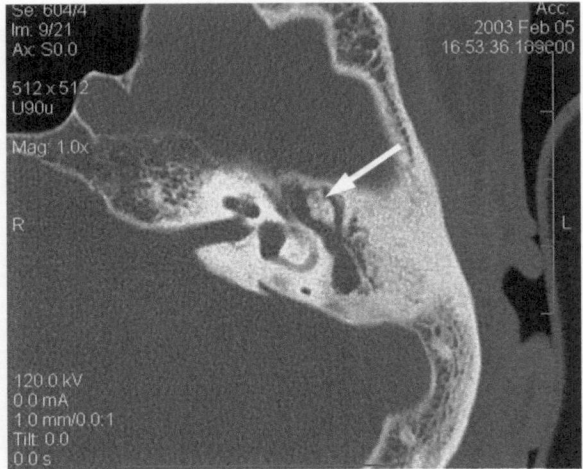

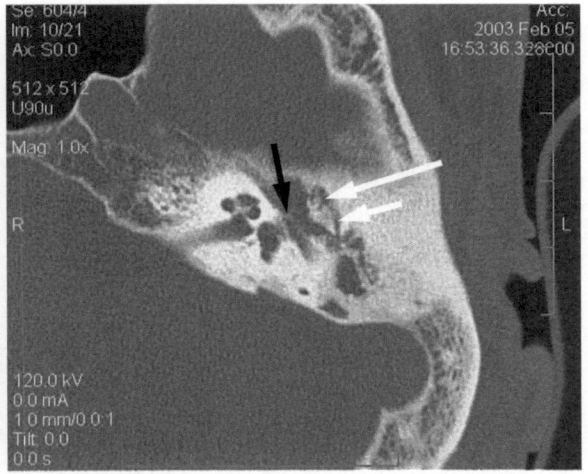

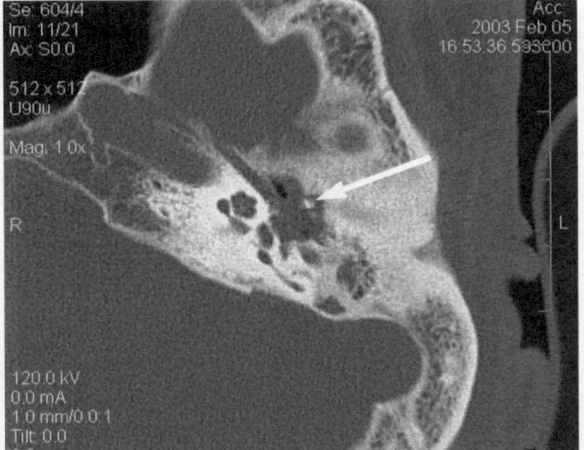

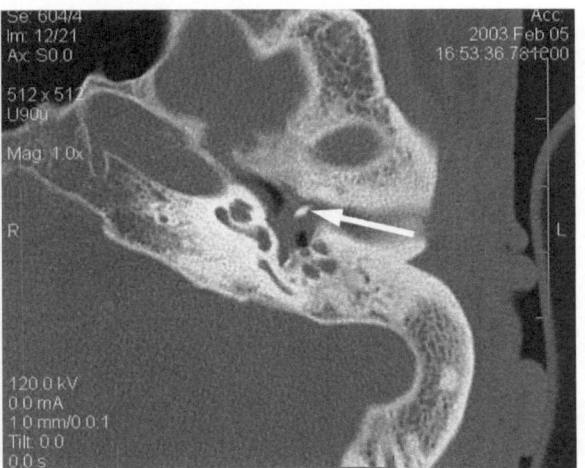

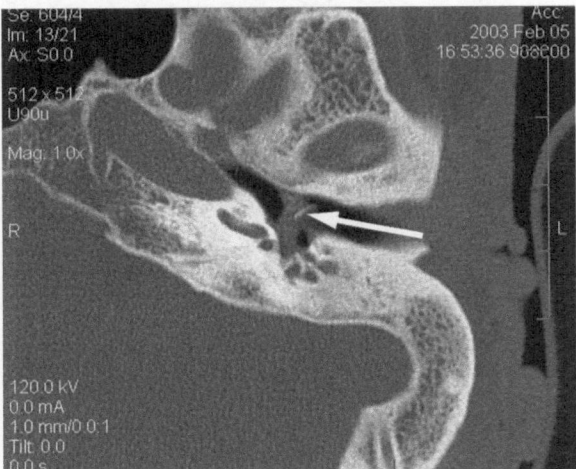

Fig. 3.9a–e. In this patient with sinus cholesteatoma five consecutive axial CT images are shown from the left temporal bone. Middle ear cavity opacification is seen on the basis of a combined presence of effusion and cholesteatoma. **a** An intact incudomalleal articulation (*arrow*) is seen. **b** The normal malleus head (*large white arrow*) and incus body (*small white arrow*), but no stapes crura are seen. The osseous ridge seen anterior to the oval window region is the cochleariform process (*black arrow*). **c** The middle image performed at oval window level confirms that the stapes is completely eroded. The incus long process is also eroded. The malleus neck is normally present (*arrow*). **d** On the image below oval window level no incudostapedial joint is seen, which indicates that the incus lenticular process and the capitulum stapedis are eroded. The malleus (*arrow*) is preserved. **e** The normal malleus handle (*arrow*)

3.3.2
Complications

Almost all complications of cholesteatoma are related to its erosive effect on the ossicles and other bony structures lining the tympanic cavity. An important role is reserved for the radiologist in the detailed description of such erosions. Pars flaccida cholesteatoma most frequently involves the incus long process, whereas pars tensa cholesteatoma primarily involves the incus long process and stapes superstructure. Fistula formation into the membranous labyrinth is another rare but well-known complication occurring in the presence of cholesteatoma. Labyrinthine fistula occurs with an incidence of 0.3 per 100,000 (KVESTAD et al. 2001). Presenting symptoms are subjective hearing loss (90%), otorrhea (65%), and dizziness (50%; KVESTAD et al. 2001; MOLLER et al. 2001). The most common fistula is the one to the lateral semicircular canal (SWARTZ 1984; SODA-MERHY et al. 2000; ROMA-

NET et al. 2001). On the basis of symptoms, signs, and CT imaging studies the diagnosis of fistula to the lateral semicircular canal can be preoperatively made in over 90% of cases (FUSE et al. 1996; SODA-MERHY et al. 2000). The exact invasion of the membranous labyrinth can be studied with MRI (SMADJA et al. 1999). The disease is to be considered as a very serious complication and can lead to important postoperative hearing loss, and even deafness (ROMANET et al. 2001). Labyrinthine fistula can also occur at the round and oval windows (SWARTZ 1984), and has even been described to involve the basal turn of the cochlea without combined disease occurring to the lateral semicircular canal (CHAO et al. 1996). In an important number of patients with labyrinthine fistula to the lateral semicircular canal the facial nerve canal is eroded (ROMANET et al. 2001).

Indeed, other important points that have to be studied in detail are eventual erosions of the facial nerve canal and of the tegmen tympani (Fig. 3.10).

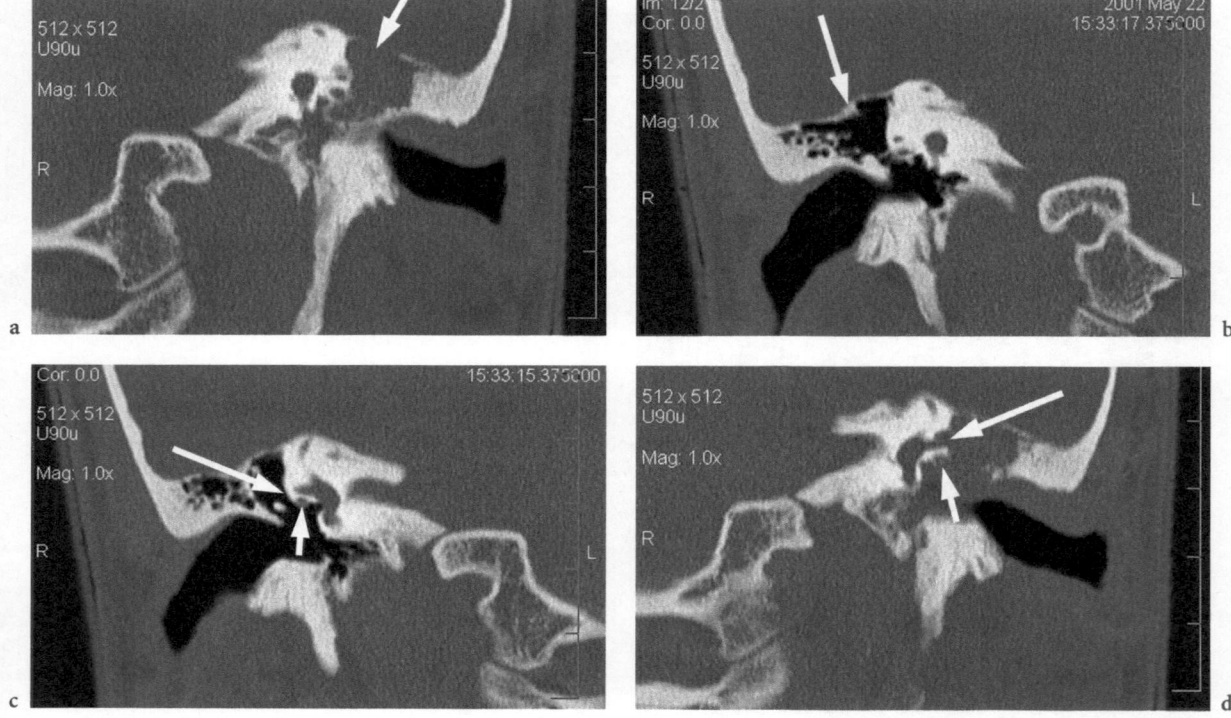

Fig. 3.10. In this patient with an aggressive cholesteatoma the coronal CT images show erosion of the tegmen tympani **b** on the ▷ left side (*arrow*), whereas the tegmen is intact in **a** the contralateral right ear (*arrow*). **c** More coronal images show intact bony structures covering the lateral semicircular canal (*large arrow*) and the second segment of the facial canal (*small arrow*) in the healthy right temporal bone. **d** In the left opacified middle ear the bony structure lateral to the lateral semicircular canal is no more present (*large arrow*) and dehiscence of the second segment of the facial canal (*small arrow*) is shown. This bony erosion (*arrow*) is also appreciated on **f, h** the axial images, whereas the lateral semicircular canal shows a normal bony cover (*arrow*) on **e, g** the corresponding images and performed on the normal right side. Also note important erosions of the incus, of which only a small portion is intact, articulating with an intact malleus head

Intracranial complications of cholesteatoma are very rare, and are the same as those seen in acute otomastoiditis without the presence of cholesteatoma: sigmoid sinus thrombosis, meningitis, and abscess formation in the cerebral temporal lobe. They are discussed in Chap. 6.

In the radiologic report on suspected cholesteatoma cases it is important that the radiologist mention whether the sinus tympani is aerated or not. The sinus tympani is difficult to visualize otoscopically and even surgically. Providing this information is especially important in cases of pars tensa cholesteatoma.

3.3.3
CT or MRI?

High-resolution computed tomography (HRCT) with bone window settings is considered the method of choice for examination of the middle ear structures. It provides excellent contrast between osseous structures, air, and soft tissues, together with a high spatial resolution. In most cases, HRCT can differentiate between inflammatory changes, cholesteatoma, and tumor. The high spatial resolution of the technique allows for demonstration of subtle osseous details and provides good identification of erosions of the ossicles, of the delineation of the tegmen and bony labyrinth, and enables reliable evaluation of the tympanic segment of the facial nerve; therefore, HRCT remains the primary examination tool for the evaluation of a suspected cholesteatoma and, more importantly, its extension.

However, magnetic resonance imaging (MRI) may provide additional information and lead to a more accurate diagnosis. Apart from an excellent soft tissue contrast, MRI offers the possibility of using various pulse sequences, including diffusion-weighted images, and the administration of intravenous contrast material. In some cases, HRCT remains unclear in the diagnosis of and description of the extension of a choles-

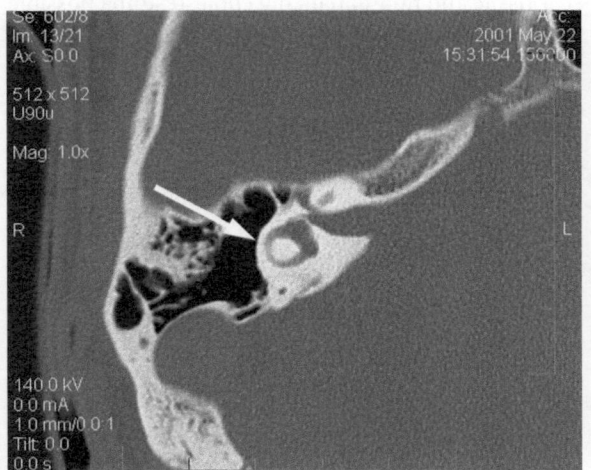
e

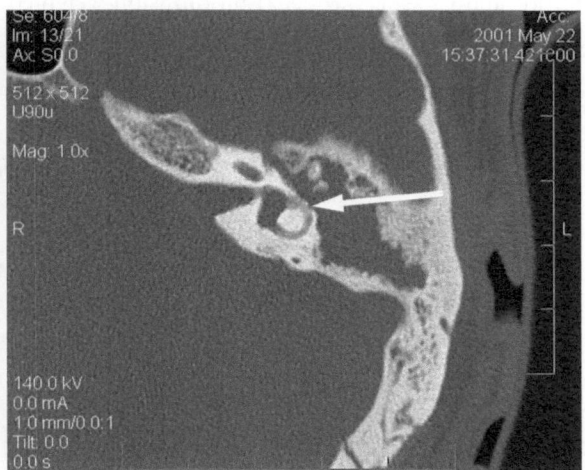
f

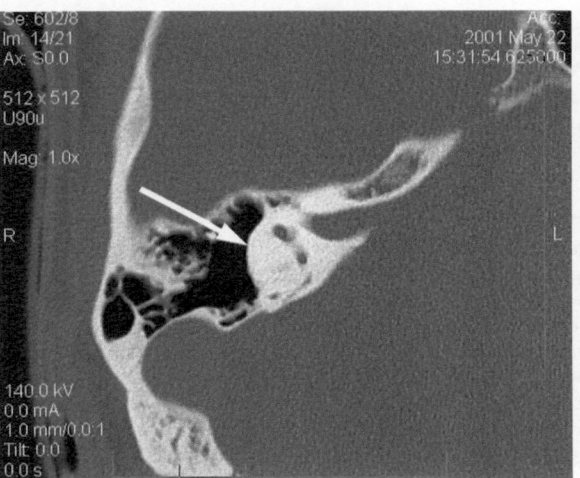
g

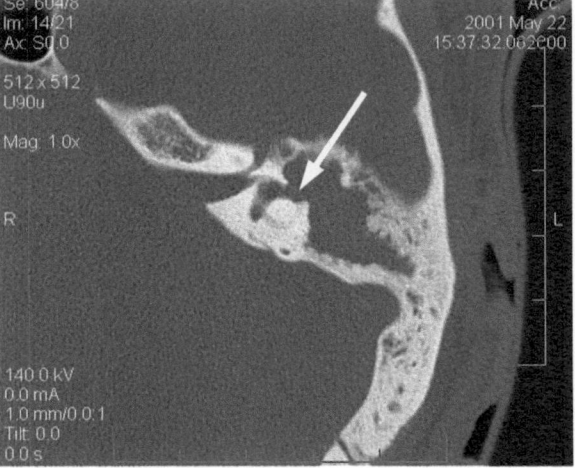
h

teatoma. According to recent technological evolutions, the importance of MRI will become more prominent in the future. Early reports demonstrated that granulation tissue can be differentiated from cholesteatomatous tissue because the former enhances after intravenous administration of gadolinium (MARTIN et al. 1990). Primary or congenital cholesteatoma and secondary cholesteatoma have a moderate hyperintense signal (compared with brain tissue) on T2-weighted images, with an isointense signal on T1-weighted images (ISHII et al. 1991; ROBERT et al. 1995), but they show no or only moderate peripheral enhancement after intravenous injection of gadolinium (Fig. 3.11; ROBERT et al. 1995); however, several reports have shown that the above-mentioned standard MRI sequences are no valid alternative to a second-look surgical intervention in the case of treated cholesteatoma (VAN DEN ABEELE et al. 1999; KIMITSUKI et al. 2001). Recently, initial reports have appeared discussing the appearance of primary cholesteatoma (FITZEK et al. 2002) and recurrent cholesteatoma (MAHESHWARI and MUKHERJI 2002; MARK and CASSELMAN 2002) on diffusion-weighted MRI images. Both cholesteatoma types appear to have a high signal on diffusion-weighted images (Fig. 3.11), and the reason for this remains unclear. It is thought to be a combination of a T2 shine-through effect, on one hand, and diffusion restriction, on the other

hand (MAHESHWARI and MUKHERJI 2002). Although cholesteatomas do not have a constantly high intensity on diffusion-weighted images, the combination of standard MRI sequences and diffusion-weighted MRI sequences appears to have the highest sensitivity and specificity in detecting and depicting middle ear cholesteatoma (Fig. 3.12). The major limitation for detecting cholesteatoma on standard MRI sequences and diffusion-weighted sequences is the size of a lesion (4 mm), and the association of chronic middle ear infection with cholesterol granuloma deposits (DE FOER et al. 2002). Other reports propose the use of delayed contrast-enhanced T1-weighted spin-echo MR images. It is stated that scar tissue and granulation tissue both show homogeneous enhancement on delayed T1-weighted imaging – contrary to the lack of enhancement on early contrast-enhanced T1-weighted images – and that this phenomenon makes the differential diagnosis of cholesteatoma difficult in the early phase. Delayed contrast-enhanced T1-weighted images make differentiation between the enhancing scar tissue and non-enhancing cholesteatoma possible (VEILLON et al. 2002; WILLIAMS et al. 2003). Further investigation regarding the role of MRI – as well with diffusion-weighted images as with delayed contrast-enhanced T1-weighted spin-echo images – seems to be necessary.

Fig. 3.11a–e. The typical MR characteristics are shown in a patient with a large middle ear cholesteatoma, with fistulization toward the lateral semicircular canal. **a** On the coronal T2-weighted MR image through the left middle ear a large nodular hyperintensity (*arrows*) is seen. Note the close relationship between the lesion and the lateral semicircular canal, suggesting the presence of a fistula to the canal (*arrowhead*). **b** The coronal T1-weighted MR image shows the same large nodular structure with an isointense signal (*arrows*). **c** On the coronal diffusion-weighted MR image the mass is hyperintense (*arrows*), suggestive of a large cholesteatoma. **d** The coronal contrast-enhanced T1-weighted MR image shows the large central non-enhancing cholesteatoma (*arrows*), with peripheral rim enhancement. **e** On the axial contrast-enhanced T1-weigthed MR image the same combined finding of a non-enhancing mass lesion (*arrows*) with peripheral rim enhancement is seen, and the enhancing extension is visualized into the lateral semicircular canal (*arrowhead*): cholesteatoma with fistulization into the membranous labyrinth

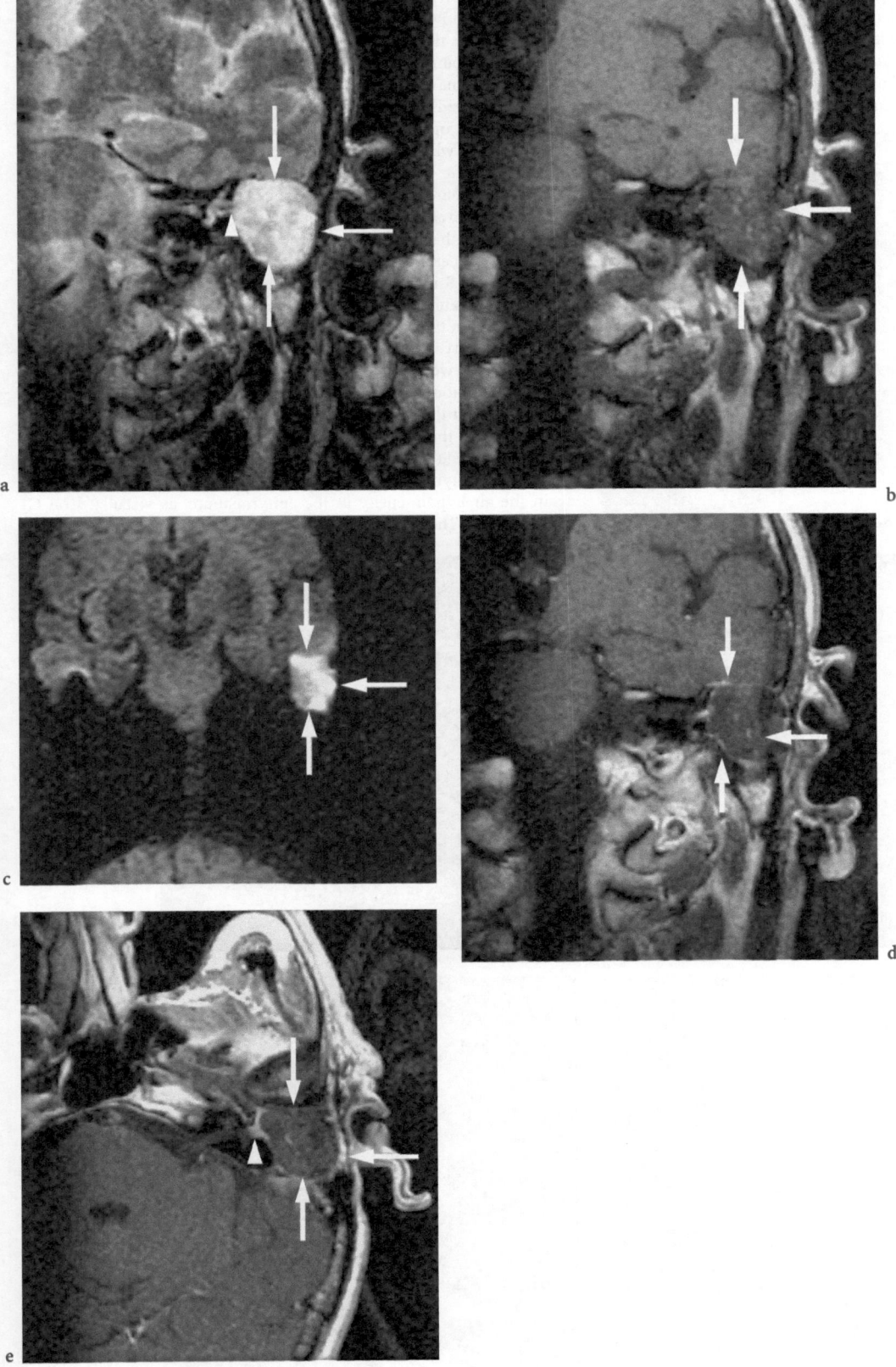

Fig. 3.12a–k. A series of CT and MR images is shown from a patient with cholesteatoma limited to the aditus ad antrum and antrum mastoideum, and with chronic inflammatory changes in the middle ear cavity and surrounding mastoid area. **a** The axial CT image at the level of the lateral semicircular canal shows diffuse soft tissue opacities in the middle ear cavity (*large arrows*), with subtotal opacification of the aditus ad antrum and antrum mastoideum (*small arrows*). Note presence of a central air lucency in the aditus ad antrum and antrum mastoideum. Possible cholesteatoma diagnosis can be suggested, but definitive differential diagnosis between cholesteatoma and inflammatory/granulation tissue is difficult. **b** On the coronal CT image through the middle

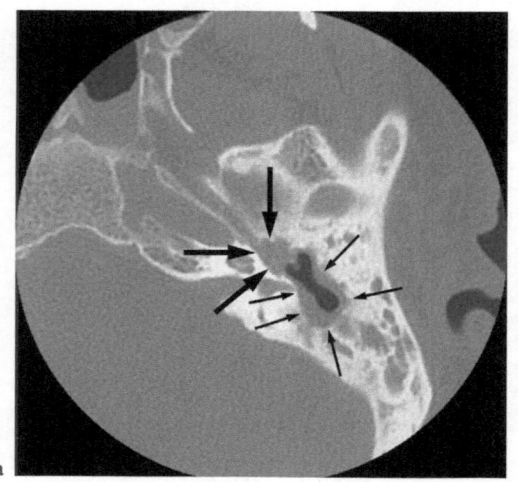

ear cavity total opacification of the hypo- and mesotympanum is seen (*large arrows*), whereas marginal opacification with central air lucency is present in the epitympanum and aditus ad antrum (*small arrows*). Only a small part of the malleus can is seen. Diagnosis of probable partial "auto"-evacuated cholesteatoma can be made. **c** The coronal CT image through the mastoid area at the level of the posterior semicircular canal shows a central soft tissue opacification (*arrows*). **d** The coronal T2-weighted MR image through the middle ear cavity (same level as **b**) shows a moderate hyperintense signal in the hypo- and mesotympanum (*arrows*), and in the epitympanum and aditus ad antrum. Note the same air hypointensity in the epitympanum as visualized on CT (*arrowhead*). **e** The coronal T2-weighted MR image through the mastoid area (same level as **c**) shows a moderate central hyperintensity (*arrows*). Note the higher (fluid) signal in the lower mastoid cells. **f** The coronal T1-weighted MR image through the middle ear cavity (same level as **b** and **d**) shows an isointense signal (in comparison with normal brain tissue) in the hypo-, meso-, and epitympanum and in the aditus ad antrum (*arrows*). Note again the air hypointensity in the epitympanum, as visualized on CT (*arrowhead*). **g** The coronal T1-weighted MR image centered on the left ... ▷

a

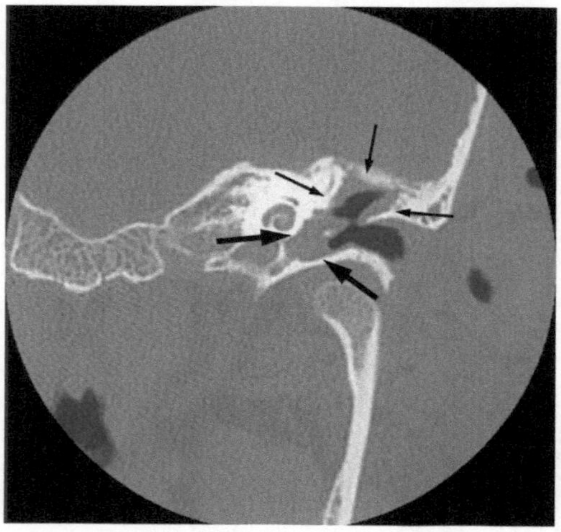

b 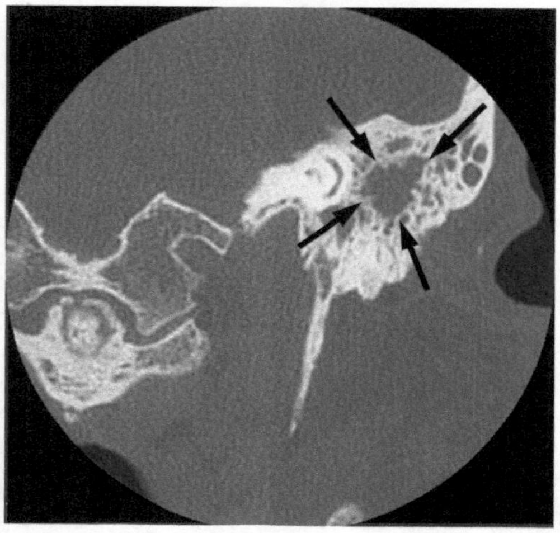   c

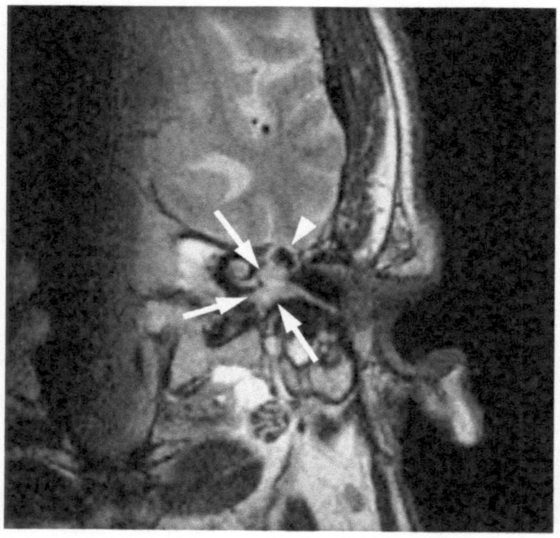

d 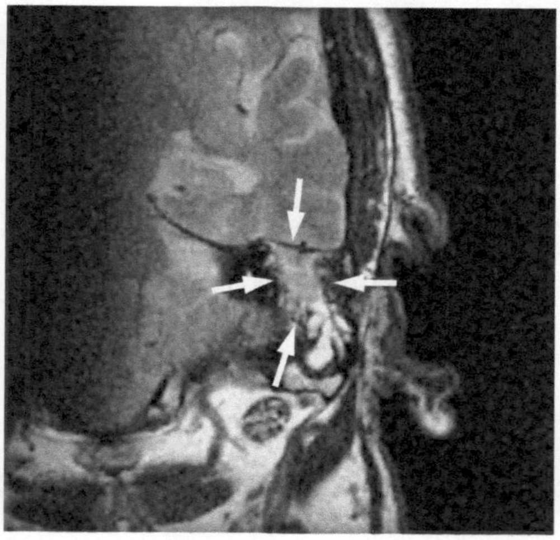   e

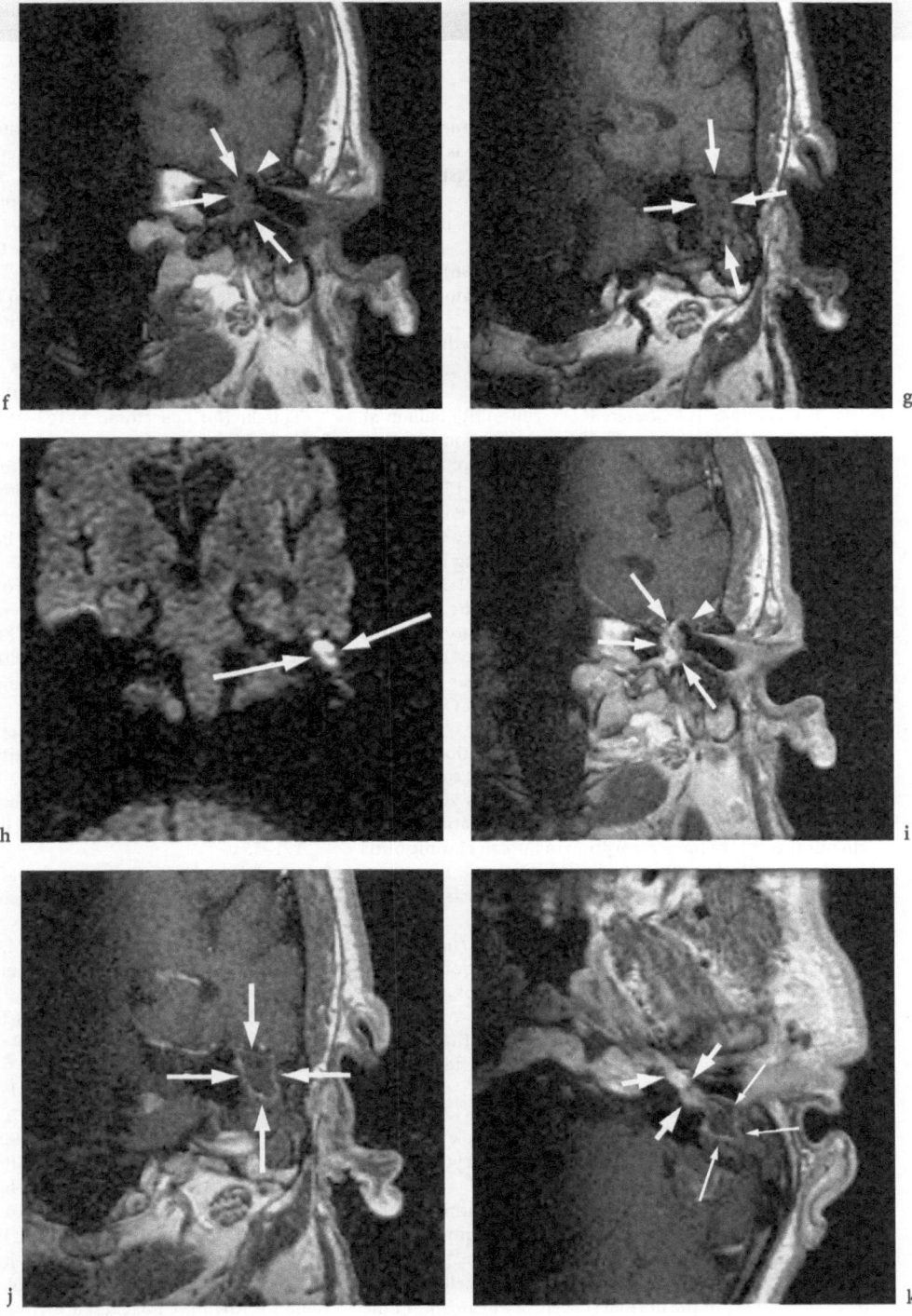

... ear through the mastoid area (same level as **c** and **e**) shows a central isointensity (*arrows*). **h** The coronal diffusion-weighted MR image (B1000) through the mastoid area (same level as **c, e,** and **g**) shows an obvious hyperintensity in the left mastoid area (*arrows*). No hyperintensity was present at the level of the middle ear cavity (not shown). **i** The coronal contrast-enhanced T1-weighted MR image through the middle ear cavity (same level as **b, d,** and **f**) shows diffuse enhancement of the pre-contrast isointensity in the hypo-, meso-, and epitympanum (*arrows*), suggesting the presence of inflammation/granulation tissue. Note again the central air hypointensity in the aditus ad antrum (*arrowhead*). **j** On the coronal contrast-enhanced T1-weighted MR image through the mastoid area (same level as **c, e, g,** and **h**) peripheral enhancement (*arrows*) is noted around a central non-enhancing structure, which represents the non-enhancing cholesteatoma. **k** The axial contrast-enhanced T1-weighted MR image (same level as **a**) again shows diffuse enhancement, suggesting the presence of middle ear granulation/inflammatory tissue (*large arrows*), whereas the aditus ad antrum and mastoid antrum are filled with non-enhancing hypointense tissue with a peripheral rim enhancement (*small arrows*), compatible with a cholesteatoma. Findings were surgically confirmed

References

Abramson M, Sugita T, Huang CC (1988) The natural history of cholesteatoma. In: Alberti PW, Ruben RJ (eds) Otologic medicine and surgery, vol I. Churchill Livingstone, New York, pp 803–811

Blevins NH, Carter BL (1998) Routine preoperative imaging in chronic ear surgery. Am J Otol 19:527–538

Chao YH, Yun SH, Shin JO, Yoon JY, Lee DM (1996) Cochlear fistula in chronic otitis media with cholesteatoma. Am J Otol 17:15–18

Chole RA (1988) Osteoclasts in chronic otitis media, cholesteatoma and otosclerosis. Ann Otol Rhinol Laryngol 97: 661–666

De Foer B, Casselman JW, Govaere F, Vercruysse JP, Pouillon M, Somers T (2002) The role of MRI and diffusion-weighted images in the diagnosis of middle ear cholesteatoma (paper). European Society of Head and Neck Radiology 15th Annual Meeting Refresher Course, Estoril. Acta Radiol Port 14:89

Falcioni M, Taibah A, De Donato G, Piccirillo E, Caruso A, Russo A, Sanna M (2002) Preoperative imaging in chronic otitis surgery. Acta Otorhinolaryngol Ital 22:19–27

Fitzek C, Mewes T, Fitzek S, Mentzel H-J, Hunsche S, Stoeter P (2002) Diffusion-weighted MRI of cholesteatomas of the petrous bone. J Magn Reson Imaging 15:636–641

Fuse T, Aoyagi M, Koike Y, Sugai Y (1992) Diagnosis of ossicular chain in the middle ear by high resolution CT. Nippon Jibbinkoka Gakkai Kaiho 95:247–252

Fuse T, Tada Y, Aoyagi M, Sugai Y (1996) CT detection of facial canal dehiscence and semicircular canal fistula: comparison with surgical findings. J Comput Assist Tomogr 20:221–224

Gantz BJ, Maynard J (1982) Ultrastructural evaluation of biochemical events of bone resorption in human chronic otitis media. Am J Otol 3:279–283

Garber LZ, Dort JC (1994) Cholesteatoma: diagnosis and staging by CT scan. J Otolaryngol 23:121–124

Harnsberger HR (1995) The temporal bone: external, middle and inner ear segments. In: Gay SM (ed) Handbook of head and neck imaging, 2nd edn. Mosby Year-Book, St. Louis, pp 426–458

Ishii K, Takahashi S, Kobayashi T, Matsumoto K, Tshibashi T (1991) MR imaging of middle ear cholesteatomas. J Comput Assist Tomogr 15:934–937

Kimitsuki T, Suda Y, Kawano H, Tono T, Komune S (2001) Correlation between MRI findings and second-look operation in cholesteatoma surgery. ORL J Otorhinolaryngol Relat Spec 63:291–293

Kvestad E, Kvaerner KJ, Mair IW (2001) Labyrinthine fistula detection: the predictive value of vestibular symptoms and computerized tomography. Acta Otolaryngol 121:622–626

Lemmerling MM, Stambuk HE, Mancuso AA, Antonelli PJ, Kubilis PS (1997a) CT of the normal suspensory ligaments of the ossicles in the middle ear. Am J Neuroradiol 18:471–477

Lemmerling MM, Stambuk HE, Mancuso AA, Antonelli PJ, Kubilis PS (1997b) Normal and opacified middle ears: CT appearance of the stapes and incudostapedial joint. Radiology 203:251–260

Maheshwari S, Mukherji SK (2002) Diffusion-weighted imaging for differentiating recurrent cholesteatoma from granulation tissue after mastoidectomy: case report. Am J Neuroradiol 23:847–849

Mark AS, Casselman JW (2002) Anatomy and disease of the temporal bone. In: Atlas SW (ed) Magnetic resonance imaging of the brain and spine, 3rd edn. Lippincot, Williams and Wilkins, Philadelphia, pp 1363–1432

Martin N, Stereckers O, Nahum H (1990) Chronic inflammatory disease of the middle ear cavities: Gd-DTPA-enhanced MR imaging. Radiology 176:399–405

Mishiro Y, Sakagami M, Takahashi Y, Kitahara T, Kajikawa H, Kubo T (2001) Tympanoplasty with and without mastoidectomy for noncholesteatomatous chronic otitis media. Eur Arch Otorhinolaryngol 258:13–15

Moller P, Molvaer OI, Lind O (2001) Perilymphatic fistula. Tidsskr Nor Laegeforen 20:162–165

Robert Y, Carcasset S, Rocourt N, Hennequin C, Dubrulle F, Lemaitre L (1995) Congenital cholesteatoma of the temporal bone: MR findings and comparison with CT. Am J Neuroradiol 16:755–761

Rocher P, Carlier R, Attal P, Doyon D, Bobin S (1995) Contribution and role of the scanner in the preoperative evaluation of chronic otitis. Radiosurgical correlation apropos of 85 cases. Ann Otolaryngol Chir Cervicofac 112:317–323

Romanet P, Duvillard C, Delouane M, Vigne P, De Raigniac E, Darantiere S, Brogniard P (2001) Labyrinthine fistulae and cholesteatoma. Ann Otolaryngol Chir Cervicofac 118: 181–186

Ruhl CM, Pensak ML (1999) Role of aerating mastoidectomy in noncholesteatomatous chronic otitis media. Laryngoscope 109:1924–1927

Schuknecht HF (1993) Infections. In: Bussy RK (ed) Pathology of the ear. 2nd edn. Lea and Febiger, Philadelphia, pp 191–253

Smadja P, Deguine O, Fraysse B, Bonafe A (1999) Preoperative evaluation of translabyrinthine cholesteatoma by MRI. J Radiol 80:933–937

Soda-Merhy A, Betancourt-Suarez MA (2000) Surgical treatment of labyrinthine fistula caused by cholesteatoma. Otolaryngol Head Neck Surg 122:739–742

Swartz JD (1984) Cholesteatomas of the middle ear: diagnosis, etiology and complications. Radiol Clin North Am 22: 15–35

Swartz JD, Wolfson RJ, Marlowe FI, Popky GL (1985) Postinflammatory ossicular fixation: CT analysis with surgical correlation. Radiology 154:697–700

Swartz JD, Laucks RL, Berger AS, Ardito JM, Wolfson RJ, Popky GL (1986) Computed tomography of the disarticulated incus. Laryngoscope 96:1207–1210

Van den Abeele D, Coen E, Parizel PM, Van De Heyning P (1999) Can MRI replace a second look operation in cholesteatoma surgery. Acta Otolaryngol (Stockh) 119:555–561

Veillon F, Riehm S, Enachescu B, Abu-Eid M, Naeve D, Greget M (2002) Diffusion versus delayed post gadolinium FATSAT T1-weighted imaging of cholesteatoms of the petrous bone (paper). European Society of Head and Neck Radiology 15th Annual Meeting Refresher Course, Estoril. Acta Radiol Port 14:89

Williams MT, Ayache D, Alberti C, Heran F, Lafitte F, Elmaleh-Bergs M, Piekarski JD (2003) Detection of postoperative residual cholesteatoma with delayed contrast-enhanced MR imaging: initial findings. Eur Radiol 13:169–174

The Clinician's View

I. Dhooge

Radiological documentation in cases of chronic ear disease serves two functions: firstly the evaluation of the extent and nature of the pathological change; and secondly the demonstration of underlying anatomical variation important when surgery is considered. In non-cholesteatomatous disease we want to know the extent and severity of disease, the presence of bone erosion suggesting development of mastoiditis, and the possible development of intratemporal and extratemporal (intracranial) complications.

Most cholesteatoma cases are eventually be treated surgically and the requirements for radiology have to be considered with this in mind. Preoperative imaging can influence the surgical approach. Elements of importance in the anatomy of the temporal bone is the extent of mastoid pneumatization, the position of the sigmoid sinus and the tegmen covering the middle fossa dura, the bony covering, and position of the bulbus jugulare. In a large and well-pneumatized mastoid, the surgeon will be more inclined to perform an intact canal wall approach. Considering the extent of the cholesteatoma, especially the possible involvement of a profound sinus tympani (tympanic recess), makes preservation of an intact canal wall difficult. Possible complications, such as fistulization of the lateral semicircular canal, denuded facial nerve, involvement of the inner ear, or intracranial extension, can be demonstrated and are helpful in guiding the surgeon and counseling the patient preoperatively. Also in patients with previous mastoid surgery radiological assessment is warranted.

Although useful information on the extent of cholesteatomata can be obtained, there is still some debate as to whether CT radiology is an absolute prerequisite in every patient.

4 Temporal Bone Trauma

S. S. KOLLIAS

4.1
Introduction

Temporal bone trauma, with or without associated fracture, is not uncommon in the context of severe trauma and frequently occurs in the context of closed head injury. It is estimated that approximately 5% of patients with closed head injury and 40% of patients with basilar skull fracture demonstrate a fracture of the temporal bone which is bilateral in 10–30% of cases (DAHIYA et al. 1999; GEAN 1994). More than 80% of patients are males and the most common mechanisms of injury are motor vehicle accidents, followed by falls and assaults. Despite the considerable attention that temporal bone fractures have received in the literature, their exact incidence is uncertain because they are frequently missed in the initial head CT.

S. S. KOLLIAS, MD
Institute of Neuroradiology, University Hospital of Zurich, Frauenklinikstrasse 10, 8091 Zurich, Switzerland

It is reported that approximately 30–60% of fractures are overlooked with routine 4- to 5-mm-thick sections even when imaged at bone windows (DAHIYA et al. 1999; HOLLAND and BRANT-ZAWADSKI 1984). Clinically, it may also be overlooked because symptomatology related to fracture is obscured by much more serious neurologic craniocerebral manifestations which dominate the attention of both the clinician and the neuroradiologist. The well-known "Battle's sign," ecchymosis over the mastoid process, is present in approximately 10% of cases and may provide a clinical clue to a temporal bone fracture (SWARTZ 1997). Bleeding from the external auditory canal occurs in 25–75% of cases (GEAN 1994).

4.2
Imaging Considerations

Optimal identification of a fracture in the setting of temporal bone trauma requires high-resolution CT (HRCT) with thin sections (<1.5 mm) in axial and coronal plane. For diagnosis, axial HRCT can demonstrate the fracture and identify ossicular derangements in almost every case, whereas coronal images provide more precise topographic analysis of the course of the fracture and subtle ossicular defects (HOLLAND and BRANT-ZAWADSKI 1984; SCHUBIGER et al. 1986; JOHNSON et al. 1984). If direct coronal imaging is not possible (e.g., associated injury of the cervical spine), overlapping thin-section axial images or a spiral acquisition should be reformatted in the coronal or other oblique planes. Magnetic resonance imaging is highly complementary particularly for the detection and precise demonstration of the consequences of the trauma. The fracture line and ossicular derangements are underestimated, unless outlined by cerebrospinal fluid (CSF) or blood within the fracture line (ZIMMERMANN et al. 1987); however, because of its greater ability to delineate cranial nerve injury, parenchymal abnormalities, and extracerebral collections, MRI plays an increasingly important role in the evaluation of these patients. Dural enhancement adjacent to the site of injury on high-resolution postcontrast MR images indicates microfractures of the temporal bone or microtears of the dura even in the absence of a fracture on CT (Sartoretti-Schefer et al. 1997). Traumatic injury involving the carotid canal or the sigmoid sinus should be further investigated with magnetic resonance angiography (MRA) to exclude carotid complications (i.e., dissection, carotid cavernous fistula) or dural sinus occlusive disease.

4.3
Temporal Bone Anatomy in the Context of Trauma

Evaluation of pathology in temporal bone trauma requires familiarization with normality. The temporal bone is composed of four segments: the squamosal and tympanic segments of membranous bone origin, and the petromastoid and styloid segments of cartilaginous origin. The segment most commonly involved in trauma is the petromastoid which is grossly triangular with its main axis oriented approximately 45° to the sagittal plane. The temporal bone is separated from the adjacent bones by extrinsic sutures, it contains intrinsic fissures separating its four segments, and it is pierced by several neurovascular foramina that can mimic a temporal bone fracture on neuroimaging studies; these include the temporoparietal, petrooccipital, sphenopetrosal, and occipitomastoid sutures, the tympanomastoid, tympanosquamous, petrosquamosal, and petrotympanic fissures, the vestibular and cochlear aqueducts, the petromastoid (subarcuate) and singular canals, and the mastoid and inferior tympanic canaliculi (Fig. 4.1). Knowledge of the location and radiographic appearance of these structures is essential to avoid confusion with a fracture (Swartz 1997).

4.4
Classification of Temporal Bone Fractures

Fractures most commonly involve the petromastoid (cartilaginous) segment of the temporal bone and have been traditionally categorized, according to their orientation relative to the main axis of the petrous pyramid, into two major types: longitudinal and transverse (Harvey and Jones 1980; Wright 1974; Gean 1994; Swartz 1997). An anterior and a

posterior longitudinal subtype, and a medial and a lateral transverse subtype, have been described in these two major fracture-line orientations. Complex fractures exhibit both transverse and longitudinal components and occur in 10% of cases. Atypical fractures are the only fractures that partially involve the petrous bone, such as fractures of the temporomandibular joint or purely mastoidal fractures. Styloid process fracture is another variant of temporal bone injury usually associated with upper neck pain, temporal headaches, and temporomandibular joint complaints (Wong et al. 1995).

4.4.1
Longitudinal Fractures

Longitudinal fractures are by definition parallel to the long axis of the temporal bone, caused by blows to the temporoparietal region of the skull and representing the most common type with estimates ranging from 70 to 90% (Hough and Stuart 1968). The fracture line usually originates in the squamosal portion of the temporal bone, extends medially through the middle ear, and terminates in the vicinity of the petrous apex sparing the labyrinth (Fig. 4.2a, b; Gean 1994). The middle ear is commonly involved resulting in conductive hearing loss in 50% of cases. The labyrinthine structures are rarely involved as the fracture line extends along the path of least resistance toward the petrous apex, sparing the otic capsule (57 S). Occasionally, a longitudinal fracture can extend across the midline to the contralateral side (Gean 1994), may involve the carotid canal resulting in dissection or pseudoaneurysm (Swartz 1997), or may involve the glenoid fossa, particularly with the more anterior variant of transverse fracture (Fig. 4.2c, d; Bonafe et al. 1995).

4.4.2
Transverse Fractures

Transverse fractures are by definition perpendicular to the long axis of the temporal bone, caused by blows to the occipital or frontal area, and account for 10–30% of all temporal bone fractures (Cannon and Jahrsdoerfer 1983; Fritz et al. 1989; Goodwin 1983; Hasso and Ledington 1988; Wright 1974). The fracture line commonly originates in the vicinity of the jugular fossa and crosses the petrous portion of the temporal bone to its anterior surface in the middle cranial fossa passing either through the fundus of the internal auditory canal medial to the arcuate eminence (medial variety), or through the bony labyrinth lateral to the arcuate eminence (lateral variety; Fig. 4.3a, b; SWARTZ 1997). The middle ear usually remains intact. Sensorineural hearing loss is present in approximately 50% of cases and is often complete and permanent either due to involvement of the labyrinthine structures or due to transection of the cochlear nerve (Fig. 4.3c, d; GENTRY 1991; SCHUBIGER et al. 1986). Transverse fractures may also involve the carotid canal (Fig. 4.3e) with vascular complications similar to the transverse fractures, and may associate with other cranial nerve deficits due to their extension in the jugular foramen (Fig. 4.3f; GEAN 1994).

4.4.3
Otic Capsule Sparing Versus Otic Capsule Violating Fractures

The classification of fractures by using the transverse-longitudinal scheme is forcing a complex fracture line into a limited geometric category and it was based on simulated impact studies on cadaver skulls (GURDJIAN and LISSNER 1946), which is not representative for the present temporal bone trauma, resulting most frequently from motor vehicle crashes. In recent years, experience with HRCT has shown that in most cases fracture lines do not fall into strict transverse or longitudinal categorization. For this reason, some investigators have proposed alternative classification schemes including oblique, mixed, complex, and atypical fracture line orientations, or a classification based on which part of the temporal bone was involved, i.e., the mastoid, external auditory canal, inner ear, etc. (HOLLAND and BRAND-ZAWADSKI 1984; SCHUBIGER et al. 1986; HASSO and LEDINGTON 1988; ZIMMERMANN et al. 1987; KHAN et al. 1985; CANNON and JAHRSDOERFER 1983; BRODIE and TOMPSON 1997; GHORAYEB and YEAKLEY 1992; YANAGIHARA et al. 1997). A more recent study, assessing the practicality and utility of the traditional classification scheme in a large number of patients, found that in a large number of patients the classic characterization of transverse versus longitudinal fracture was not possible and therefore clinical correlation to complications related to this categorization was not possible (DAHIYA et al. 1999). They also reported that use of a classification system that emphasizes violation or lack of violation of the otic capsule offers the advantage of radiographic utility and correlation to clinical severity. Compared with otic-capsule-sparing fractures, patients with

otic-capsule-violating fractures were approximately two times more likely to develop facial paralysis, four times more likely to develop CSF leak, and seven times more likely to experience profound hearing loss, as well as more likely to sustain intracranial complications including epidural hematoma and subarachnoid hemorrhage (Fig. 4.4; DAHIYA et al. 1999).

4.5
Consequences of Temporal Bone Fractures

Temporal bone fractures can be associated with complications that can significantly decrease the patient's quality of life. These complications include hearing loss, facial nerve injury, vertigo, CSF fistulas, labyrinthine hydrops, and vascular complications.

Uncomplicated temporal bone fractures need no surgical therapy. The conductive hearing loss caused by hematotympanum will eventually disappear with resorption of the hematoma or with healing of the ruptured tympanic membrane. Complete hearing loss caused by transection of the cochlear nerve or severe labyrinthine trauma due to a transverse fracture of the inner ear will be permanent and cannot be treated. Other complications, such as disruption of the ossicular chain, damage to the facial nerve canal, or otorhinoliquorrhea, are accessible to surgical therapy and detailed imaging is critical for appropriate management. Potential vascular complications, such as internal carotid artery dissection or pseudoaneurysm, laceration, or occlusion of the jugular vein–sigmoid–transverse sinus, or development of posttraumatic fistulas, may also represent medical emergencies and should not escape the attention of the neuroradiologist (SWARTZ 1995, 1997; GENTRY 1991; GEAN 1994; SCHUBIGER et al. 1986; KOLLIAS 2000).

4.5.1
Hearing Loss

It is a common consequence of temporal bone trauma and audiometry may reveal a conductive, sensorineural, or mixed deficit.

4.5.1.1
Conductive Hearing Loss

Conductive hearing loss is usually of immediate onset and can be caused by hematotympanum result-

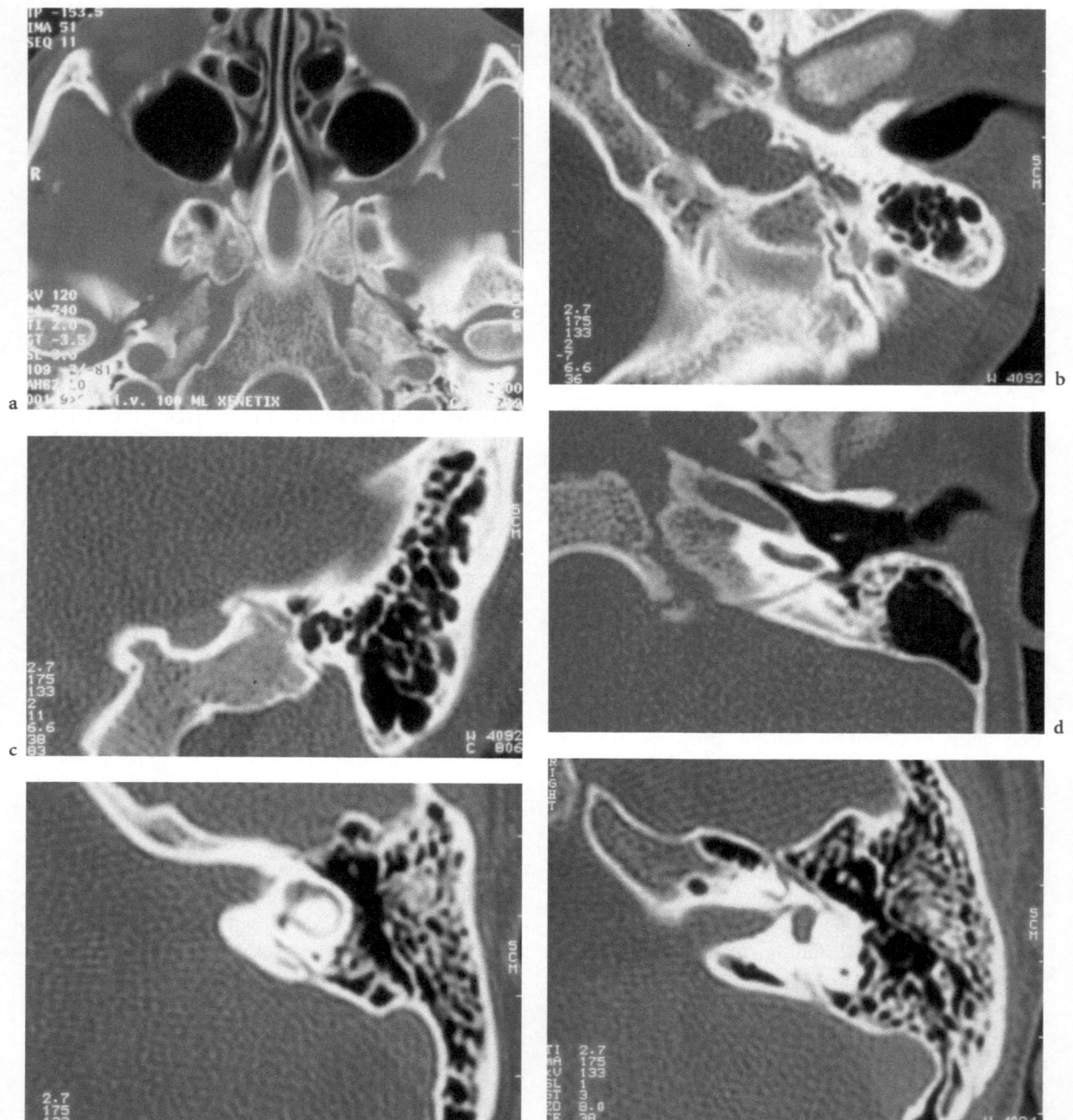

Fig. 4.1a–k. Normal anatomical structures that should not be confused with skull base fractures. The petrooccipital fissure (**a**) is seen coursing obliquely between the petrous apex and the clivus from the foramen lacerum anterior to the jugular foramen (pars nervosa) posterior. The sphenopetrosal suture borders the anterior surface of the petrous apex extending obliquely behind the foramen ovale and in front of the carotid canal. The occipitomastoid suture is consistently seen on axial (**b**) and coronal (**c**) images as an irregularly shaped linear lucency between the mastoid process of the petrous bone and the occipital bone. The cochlear canal (**d**) is a cerebrospinal fluid (CSF)-filled bony channel oriented mediolateral in the posterior surface of the petrous pyramid extending from the posterior fossa to basal cochlear turn (in the vicinity of the round window). The vestibular aqueduct (**e**) is another intrinsic ▷▷

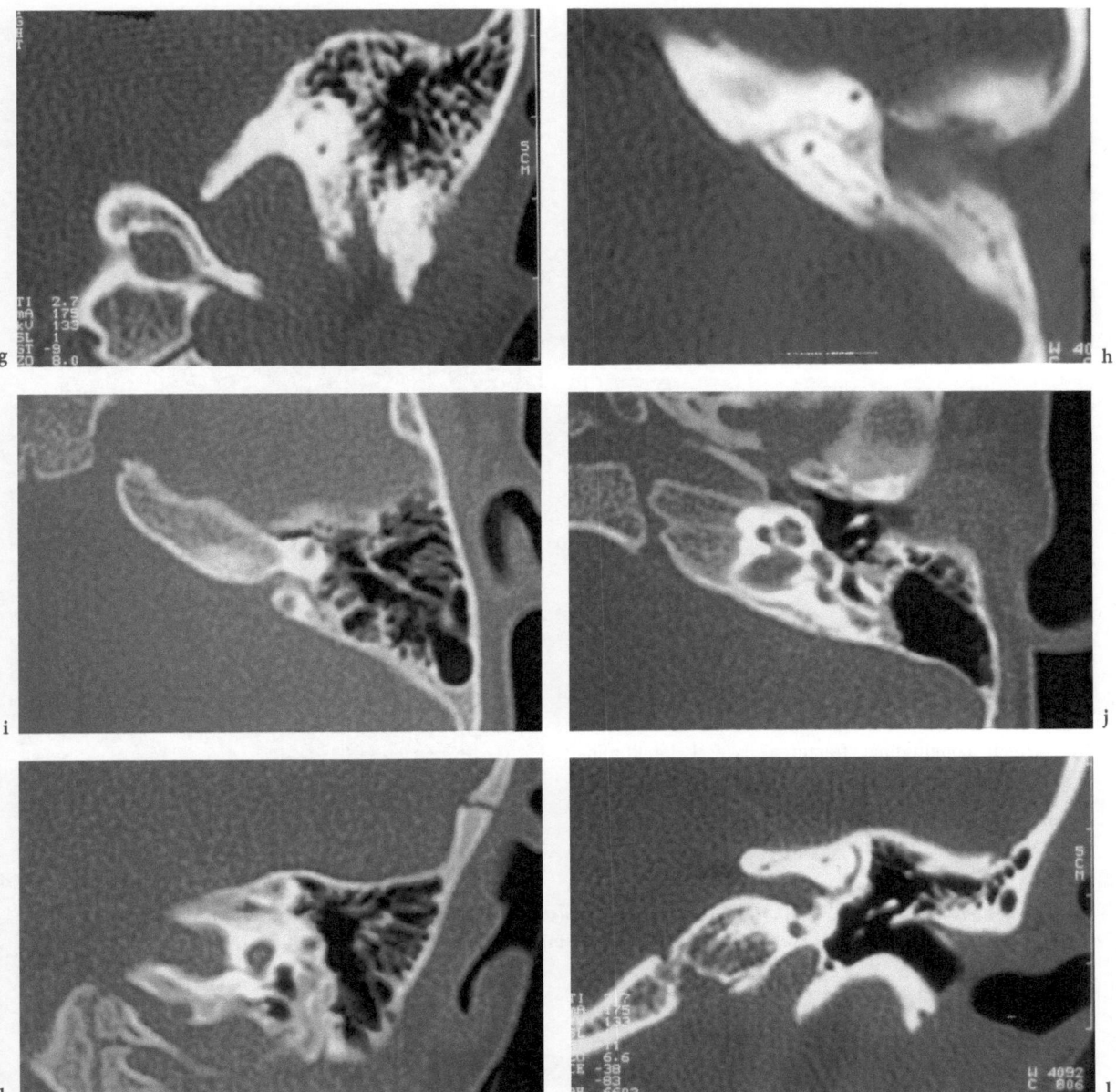

channel in the petrous pyramid, containing the endolymphatic duct and partially the endolymphatic sac, and it is distinct by the lateromedial orientation and the course parallel to the posterior semicircular canal. The fallopian canal with its vestibular, tympanic (f), and mastoidal (g) segments provides a bony conduit for the corresponding intratemporal segments of the facial nerve. Note also in this coronal image (g) the mastoid canaliculus, a mediolaterally oriented channel between the jugular foramen and the mastoid segment of the fallopian canal that transmits the nerve of Arnold, a branch of the vagus allowing communication between the vagus and the facial nerve. The petromastoid canal (h) is a dura-lined channel crossing as an anterior convex curvilinear structure below the superior semicircular canal. It is a remnant of the voluminous subarcuate fossa (i) seen more prominently in infants and young children. The singular canal can be identified in axial (j) and coronal (k) images parallel and posteroinferior to the internal auditory canal (IAC) and contains the posterior ampullary nerve (a branch of the inferior vestibular nerve) for the posterior semicircular canal. The inferior tympanic canaliculus is seen on coronal images, almost perpendicularly oriented between the jugular foramen and the hypotympanum which transmits the nerve of Jacobson, the inferior tympanic branch of the XI (glossopharyngeal) nerve

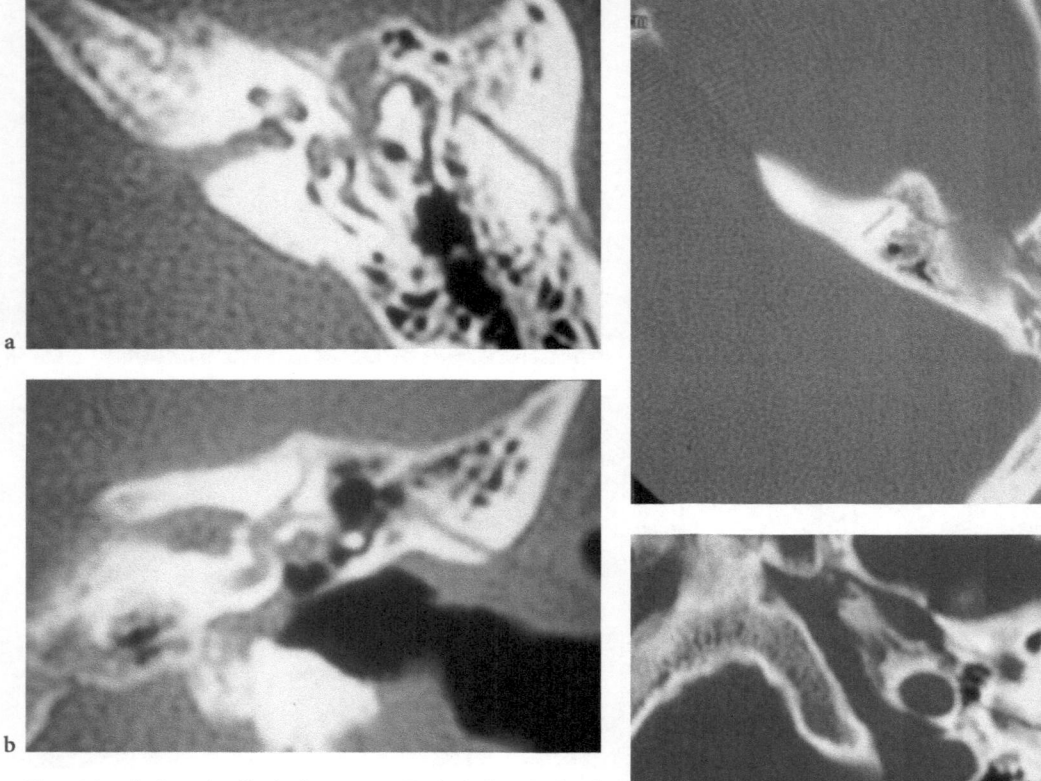

Fig. 4.2a–d. Longitudinal fractures. Typical longitudinal fracture in axial (**a**) and coronal (**b**) projection. The fracture line passes through the epitympanic space extending to the vicinity of the petrous apex in the region of the geniculate ganglion. Debris are present in the tympanic cavity, whereas the labyrinthine structures are spared. Anterior subtype of longitudinal fracture (**c**) extending from the anterior portion of the squamous temporal bone and terminating in the petrous apex with sparing of the otic capsule. A longitudinal fracture may involve the carotid canal (**d**) and thus be associated with injury of the petrous segment of the IAC

ing in disturbance of the conductive mechanism, or damage of the tympanic membrane with or without a fracture of the tympanic ring (Fig. 4.5; SCHUBIGER et al. 1986; SWARTZ 1997; BELLUCI 1983; CANNON and JAHRSDOERFER 1983; GOODHILL 1971). In these cases it is very likely that CT can establish a specific diagnosis. A persistent conductive hearing deficit after membrane healing or repair and resorption of the middle ear debris raises the clinical suspicion of ossicular derangement which may occur with or without temporal bone fracture (SCHUBIGER et al. 1986; SWARTZ et al. 1985; SWARTZ 1997; HASSO and LEDINGTON 1988; HOUGH and STUART 1968). Occasionally, conductive hearing loss can be caused by a displaced fracture of the anterior aspect of the external auditory canal wall and consequent stenosis (Fig. 4.6; GEAN 1994).

Detailed knowledge of the normal bony and ligamentous anatomy of the middle ear, and HRCT images in the coronal and axial planes, are crucial for evaluating the integrity of the ossicular chain and the diagnosis of a potential disruption (Fig. 4.7). The ice-cream-cone configuration of the incudomalleal articulation at the level of the attic is produced by the short process and body of the incus (the cone) which is located within the fossa incudis, and the head of the malleus (the ice cream). A faint semicircular lucency represents their articulation and is best evaluated on axial CT images. The incudostapedial articulation and the stapes superstructure are also best seen on axial sections due to the horizontal orientation of the anterior and posterior crura (SWARTZ 1989, 1997). Coronal images are best suited for the evaluation of the long process of the incus and the manubrium

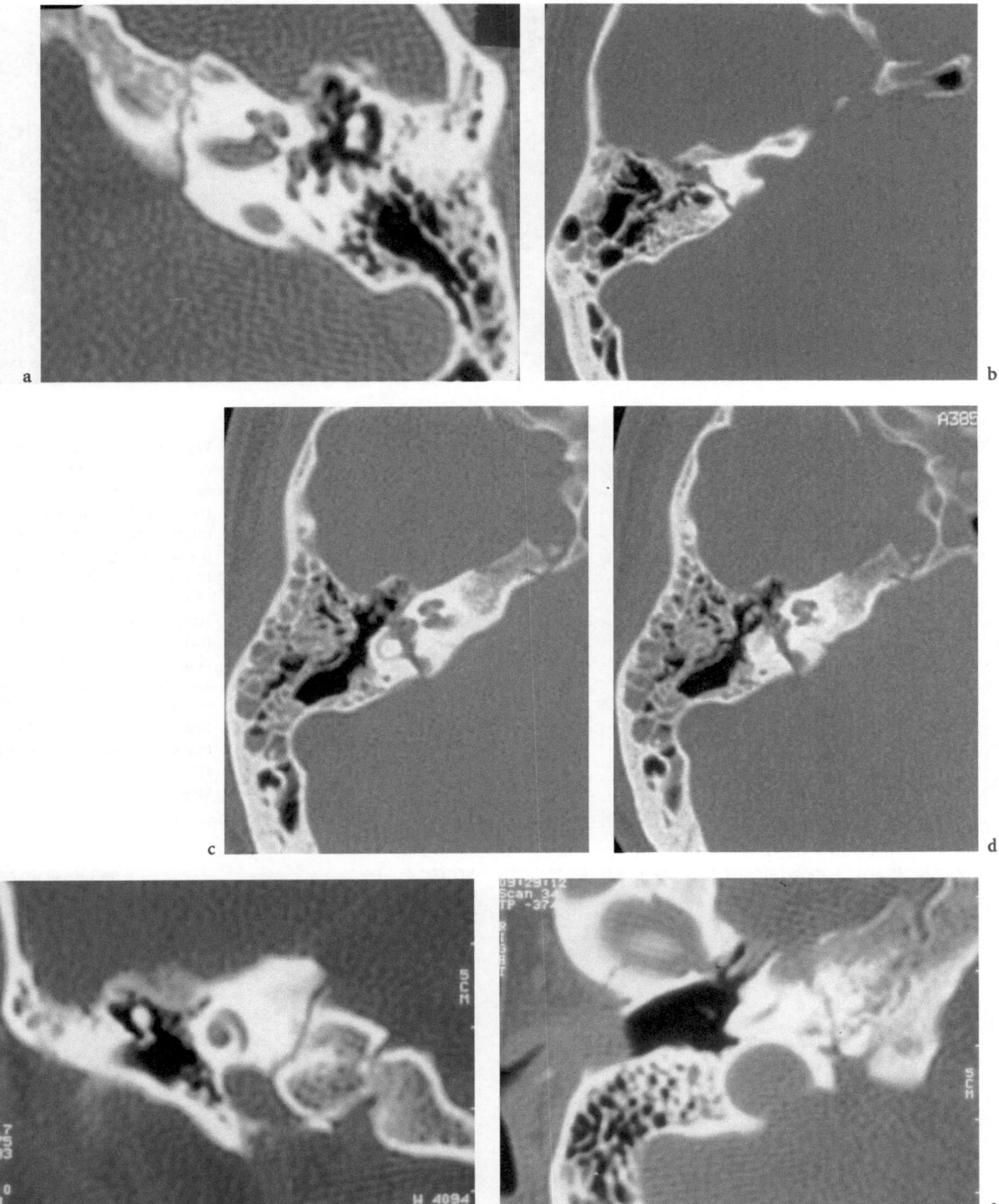

Fig. 4.3a–f. Transverse fractures. Axial section at the level of the IAC shows a medial subtype transverse fracture (**a**) coursing from the posterior surface of the petrous bone through the porus of the IAC to the anterior surface in the middle cranial fossa. In another patient, a lateral subtype transverse fracture (**b**) courses trough the superior semicircular canal just lateral to the arcuate eminence (note also the perpendicular midline fracture of the clivus). The labyrinthine structures in the transverse fractures are commonly involved, whereas the middle ear usually remains intact (**c, d**). The fracture line may also involve the carotid canal resulting in injury of the artery (**e**) and commonly it extends to the jugular foramen causing additional cranial nerve deficits (**f**)

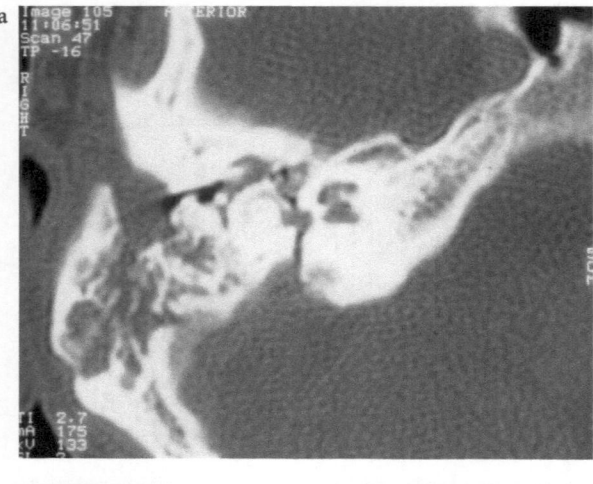

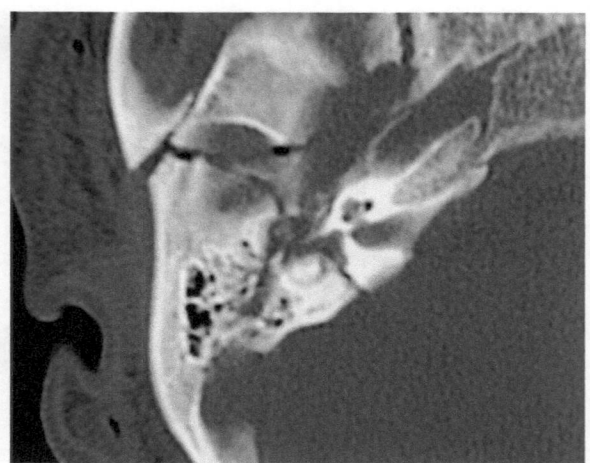

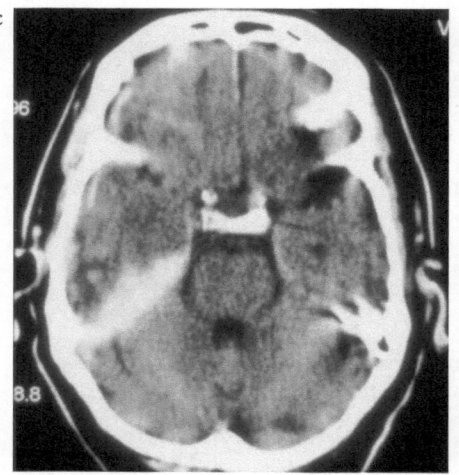

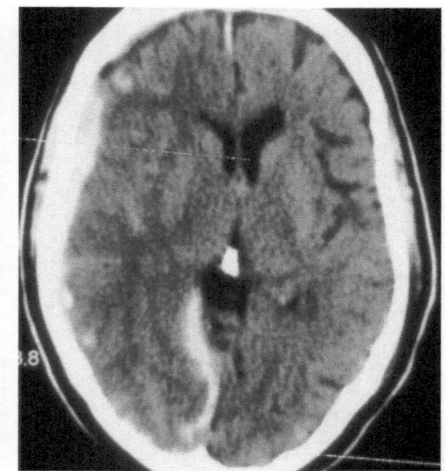

Fig. 4.4a–d. Mixed fractures. Axial sections from two cases of temporal bone trauma exhibiting both longitudinal and transverse fracture components (**a, b**). In these cases the violation of the otic capsule represents the most important feature correlating to the clinical severity. Presence of associated intracranial complications, such as epidural hematomas and parenchymal contusions, is also more common with otic capsule violating fractures (**c, d**)

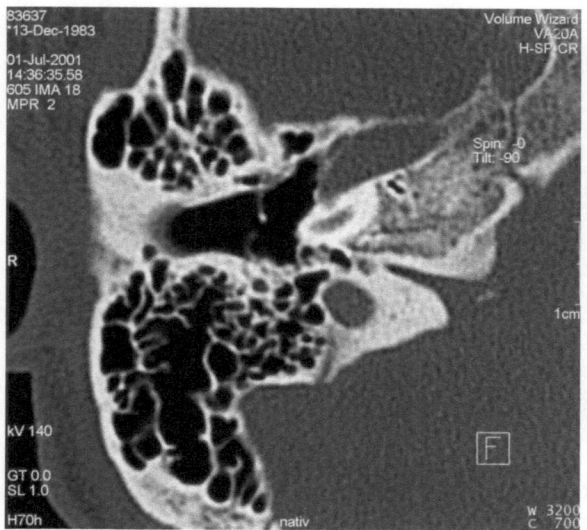

Fig. 4.5. Axial high-resolution CT scan demonstrating posttraumatic disruption of the tympanic membrane

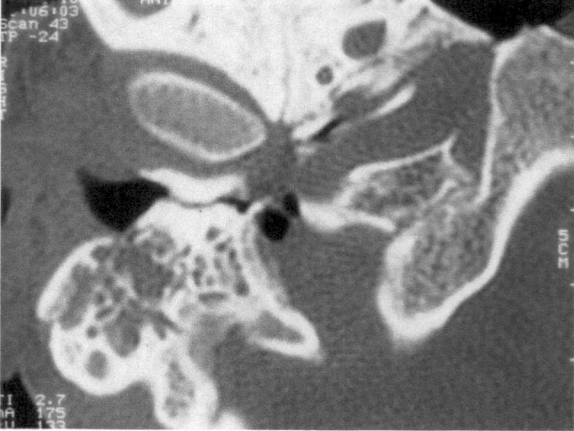

Fig. 4.6. Complex temporal bone trauma associated with fracture of the glenoid fossa and posterior displacement of the anterior wall of the external auditory canal and consequent obliteration

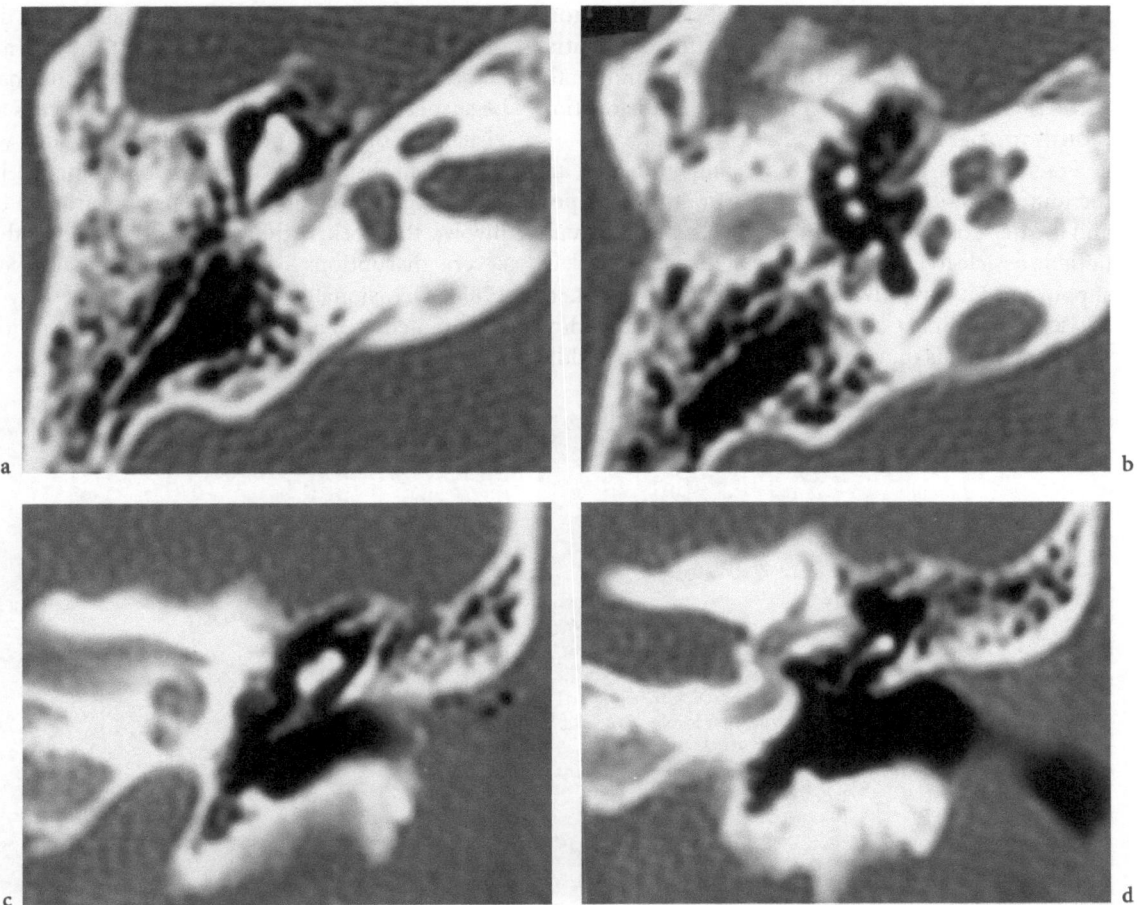

Fig. 4.7a–d. Normal ossicular anatomy. Axial images better demonstrate the integrity of the incudostapedial articulation (**a**) and the stapes superstructure(**b**), whereas coronal images are best suited for the evaluation of the long (**c**) and lenticular (**d**) processes of the incus

of the malleus which course superoinferior almost parallel to each other, and for the lenticular process of the incus which is a continuation of the long process forming a 90° angle before it articulates with the capitulum of the stapes (SWARTZ 1997).

The malleus is the least likely to be injured because it receives broad support from the attachment of the manubrium to the tympanic membrane and is further stabilized by the anterior, posterior, superior, and lateral malleolar ligaments, as well as by the tensor tympani tendon. The stapes is firmly anchored to the oval window by its annular ligament and is stabilized posteriorly by the stapedius tendon. In contrast, the incus is suspended between the malleus and the stapes, and its only firm support is the posterior incudal ligament thus being the most vulnerable ossicle to injury even following minor trauma (SWARTZ 1983, 1997; VIGNAUD 1974; SCHUCKNECHT 1974). The ossicular chain can be disrupted at multiple sites by a variety of derangements. Fractures are less frequent than luxations. Subluxation of the incudostapedial joint is considered the most common posttraumatic ossicular derangement followed by complete incus dislocation from both its incudomalleolar and incudostapedial articulations (SWARTZ 1997; HOUGH 1970; BELLUCCI 1983; MARQUET and OFFECIERS 1980; SWARTZ et al. 1986; WRIGHT 1974). Disruption of the incudomalleal articulation results in an easy-to-diagnose alteration of the normal ice-cream-cone appearance of the malleolar head and the incus within the attic of the middle ear (GEAN 1994; SWARTZ 1989, 1997). The eccentric location of the head of the malleus and of the body of the incus in the epitympanic recess is an important indirect sign of luxation or fracture. Widening of this joint space may indicate a partial subluxation of the incudomalleal articulation and comparison with the opposite side is always useful in diagnosing subtle disruptions (Fig. 4.8a).

Dislocation of the incudostapedial joint is more difficult to diagnose because of insufficient spatial resolution and often can be diagnosed only indirectly with HRCT by evidence of a major incus dislocation (SCHUBIGER et al. 1986).

Fracture sites, in order of decreasing frequency, are the long process of the incus, the crura of the stapes, and the neck of the malleus. The incus is the most vulnerable ossicle to fracture because of its relative lack of support and it is relatively easy to diagnose (Fig. 4.8b; SWARTZ 1995; BELLUCCI 1983). The dislocated and/or fragmented incus may be identified within the middle ear cavity, the external auditory canal, or may disintegrate and not be visible. Fractures of the crura of the stapes are difficult to demonstrate at CT and may only be suspected if the anterior and posterior crus are not visualized on overlapping axial images and when a significant dislocation of the incudostapedial joint is present. Fractures of the malleus are rare and usually involve the neck region being associated with other severe disruptions of the ossicular chain (SWARTZ 1983). Occasionally, the ossicular chain may be so fragmented that it defies a specific description and categorization of the injury (Fig. 4.8c, d).

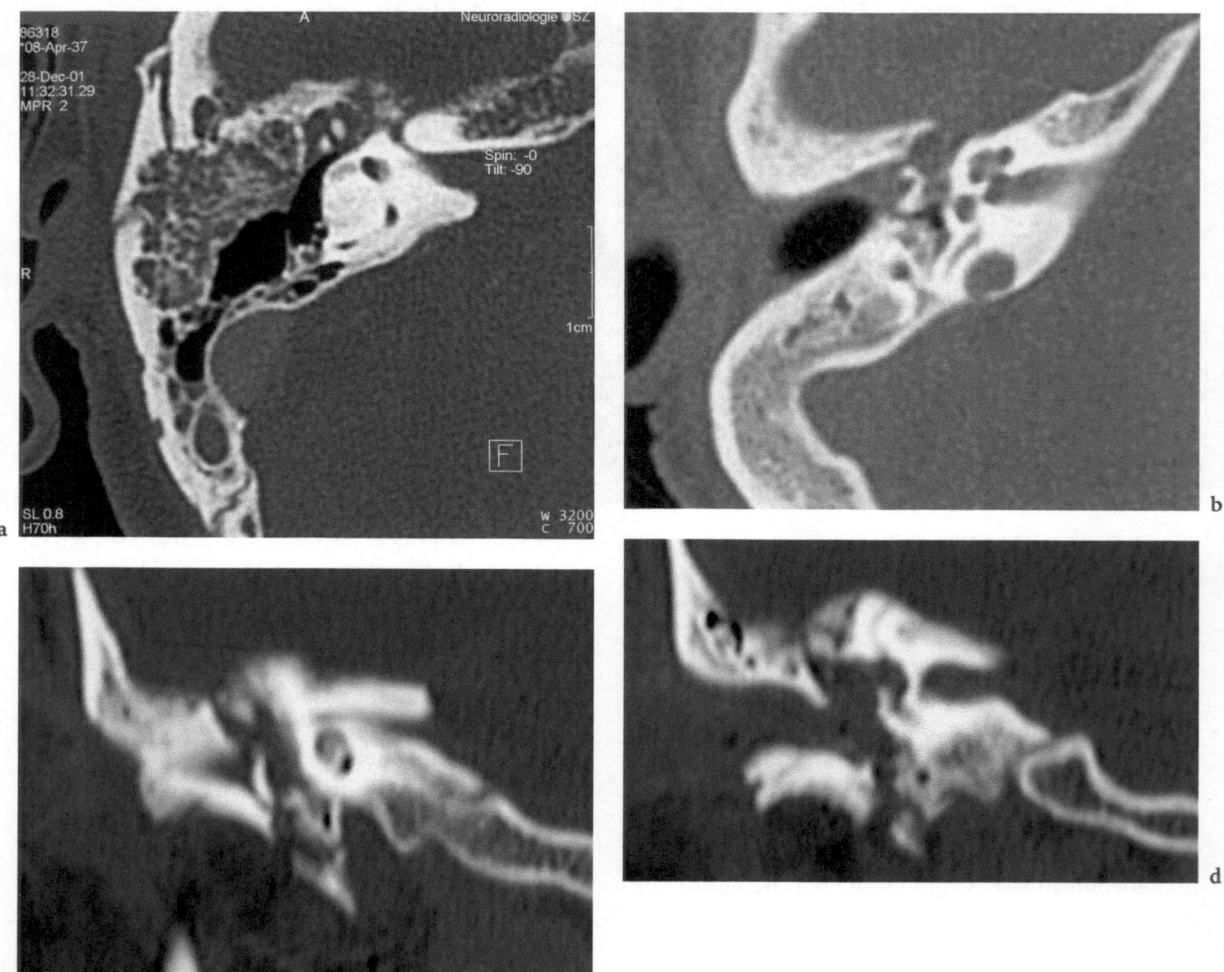

Fig. 4.8. Posttraumatic disruptions of the ossicular chain (**a**) subluxation of the incudomalleal articulation is indicated in this axial image showing a pathologic widening of this articulation in the epitympanic space; (**b**) axial image in a patient with longitudinal temporal bone fracture passing through the lateral tympanic cavity with hematotympanum throughout the attic and antrum. The incus is fractured, malrotated, and displaced in the lateral tympanic cavity, and the incus cannot be identified. **c, d** Coronal images of a patient with lateral-type transverse fracture, passing through the tympanic cavity, demonstrate severe fragmentation of the ossicular chain that defies exact categorization. The malleus is probably fragmented at the neck region (**c**), the incus is displaced inferior and probably ruptured as well, and the stapes cannot be identified. Opacification of the middle ear cavity from the hematotympanum (**d**)

4.5.1.2
Posttraumatic Sensorineural Hearing Loss

Posttraumatic Sensorineural Hearing Loss (SNHL) is less common than conductive hearing loss but has a worse prognosis. It may result from a direct injury to cochlear nerve in the cerebellopontine angle cistern, at the root entry zone or within the internal auditory canal, or from a fracture through the bony labyrinth (Fig. 4.9). The SNHL may also result from a traumatic contusion involving the auditory pathway at the level of the cochlear nuclei within the posterolateral aspect of the upper medulla, at the level of the lateral lemniscus in the brain stem, or rarely from contusions involving the inferior colliculi. Unilateral lesions of the auditory pathway rarely result in complete hearing loss, because most of the pathway is made up of crossed fibers (GEAN 1994; SWARTZ 1997; JANE et al. 1991; KHAN et al. 1985). Magnetic resonance imaging has an important role in these patients. Precontrast T1-weighted images of the temporal bone are essential for the diagnosis of intralabyrinthine hemorrhage by demonstrating the hyperintense signal of methemoglobin in the labyrinth even in the absence of a demonstrable fracture (SWARTZ 1997; WEISSMAN et al. 1992). Contrast-enhanced images should also be obtained to exclude development of posttraumatic labyrinthitis (Fig. 4.10). T1- and T2-weighted images of the intraaxial auditory pathway are also necessary for the exclusion of intraparenchymal contusion (SWARTZ 1995); however, even after thorough imaging, posttraumatic SNHL may be not associated with a demonstrable pathology in which case patients are often given the diagnosis of labyrinthine concussion, implying SNHL of variable severity and persistence resulting from a severe concussive force (SWARTZ 1995, 1997; LINDEMAN 1979; CANNON and JAHRSDOERFER 1983; GOODWIN 1983).

Hearing loss may also be associated with a posttraumatic perilymphatic fistula (see later).

4.5.2
Facial Nerve Injury

The facial nerve is the most commonly injured cranial nerve and a fracture of the temporal bone must be assumed in patients with posttraumatic facial nerve palsy even when a fracture can not be identified radiologically. Posttraumatic facial nerve palsy is the most common cause for facial nerve paralysis after Bell's palsy. It is associated with approximately 50% of transverse temporal bone fractures and 10–20%

of longitudinal fractures (HARKER and MCCABE 1974; FISCH 1974, 1980; MCCABE 1972; MCCOVERN 1968). Intraoperative investigations established different etiologies for facial nerve damage including nerve transection, impingement by an adjacent bony fragment or a hematoma, and compression by an intraneural hematoma or edema (Fig. 4.11; FISCH 1974, 1980; MURAKAMI et al. 1990). Trauma may also be iatrogenic secondary to otologic, parotid, or cerebellopontine angle surgery (SWARTZ 1997). The nerve may be injured anywhere along its course from the root exit zone within the inferolateral aspect of the pons, along the fallopian canal, and finally to its intraparotid segment, and therefore its entire course should be studied in axial, coronal, and eventually sagittal sections. Clinically, the location of injury to the proximal, middle, or distal portion of the nerve can be determined by the presence of associated symptoms, such as lacrimation, taste, and stapedius function, related to various facial nerve branches. Most commonly longitudinal fractures are associated with lesions in the region of the geniculate ganglion, the greater superficial petrosal nerve, and the proximal tympanic portion of the nerve, whereas transverse fractures more often involve the labyrinthine segment of the nerve (lateral subtype of transverse fracture) or the intracanalicular portion (medial subtype; FISCH 1974; SWARTZ 1997). The labyrinthine segment is the narrowest portion of the fallopian canal and intraneural edema in this region (i.e., due to traction and stretching of the greater superficial petrosal nerve) leads to compression of the nerve within the narrow bony conduit with secondary ischemia and eventually nerve degeneration via a pathogenic mechanism similar to that described in inflammatory palsy clearly making this segment of the nerve the most vulnerable to injury (Fig. 4.12; FISCH 1974, 1980; ANDERSON et al. 1991).

Posttraumatic partial or complete facial paralysis can have either immediate onset (within 24 h) often caused by nerve transection or compression by a bony fragment or delayed onset (>24 h after the trauma) caused by edema, swelling, and hematoma with or without associated fracture (FISCH 1974, 1980; POTTER 1964). Patients with immediate complete paralysis have only 50% chance of spontaneous recovery, whereas patients with delayed-onset facial paralysis have a high incidence of nearly total spontaneous recovery. In the latter case, an early (within the first 72 h from the onset of the symptoms) decompression is advocated by several investigators to prevent wallerian degeneration of the nerve (MCKENNAN and CHOLE 1992; MAY 1986; COKER et al. 1989).

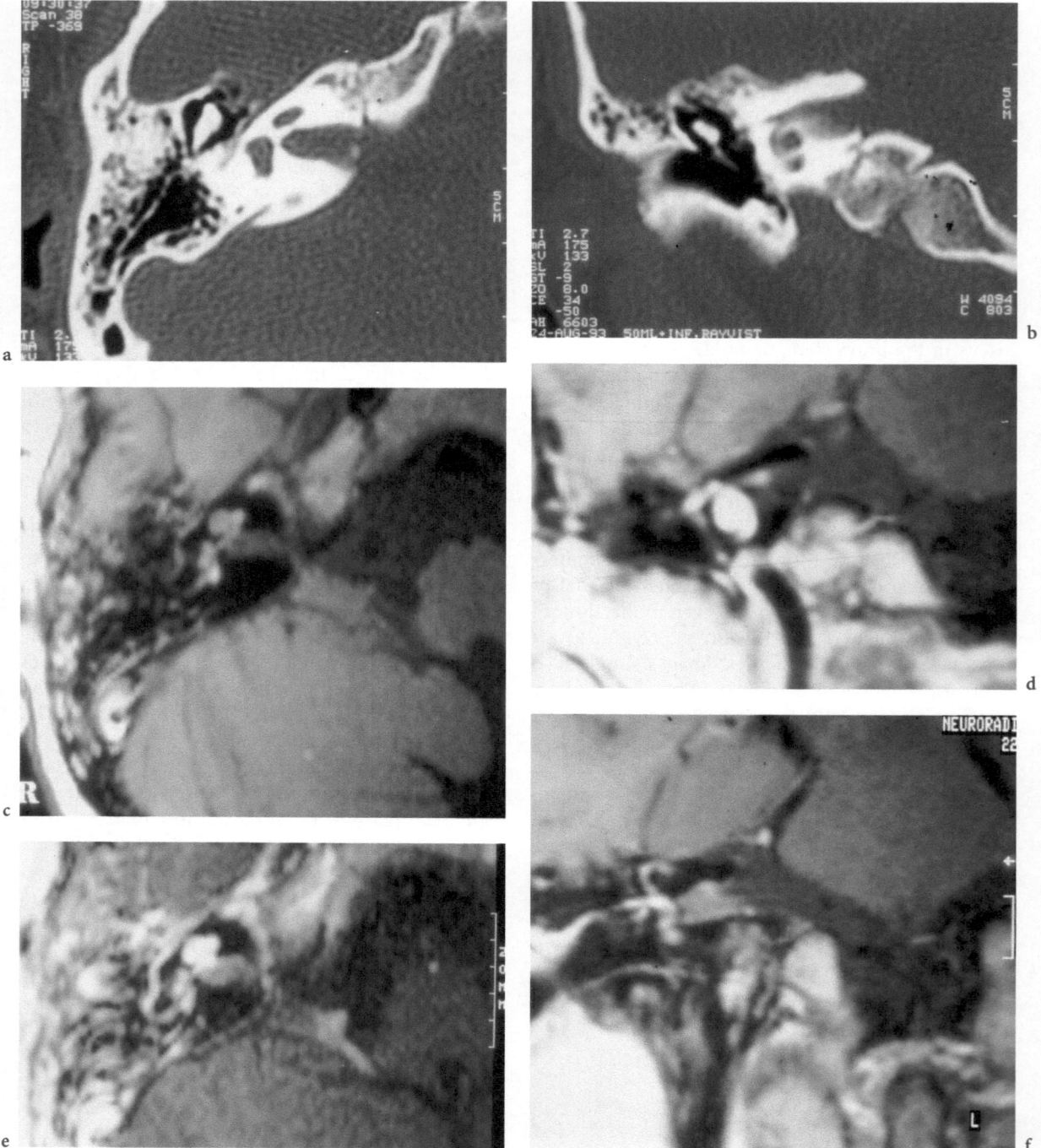

Fig. 4.9a–f. Sensorineural hearing loss associated with labyrinthine hemorrhage. Axial (**a**) and coronal (**b**) CT images in a patient with a medial subtype transverse fracture. The fracture line passes through the porus of the IAC and a small bony fragment is identified at the level of the porus. Axial (**c**) and coronal (**d**) MRI without contrast shows hyperintense signal of methemoglobin indicating posttraumatic labyrinthine hemorrhage within the cochlea and the labyrinth. Axial (**e**) and coronal (**f**) MR follow-up images show diffuse enhancement of the cochlea and the vestibule indicating development of posttraumatic labyrinthitis

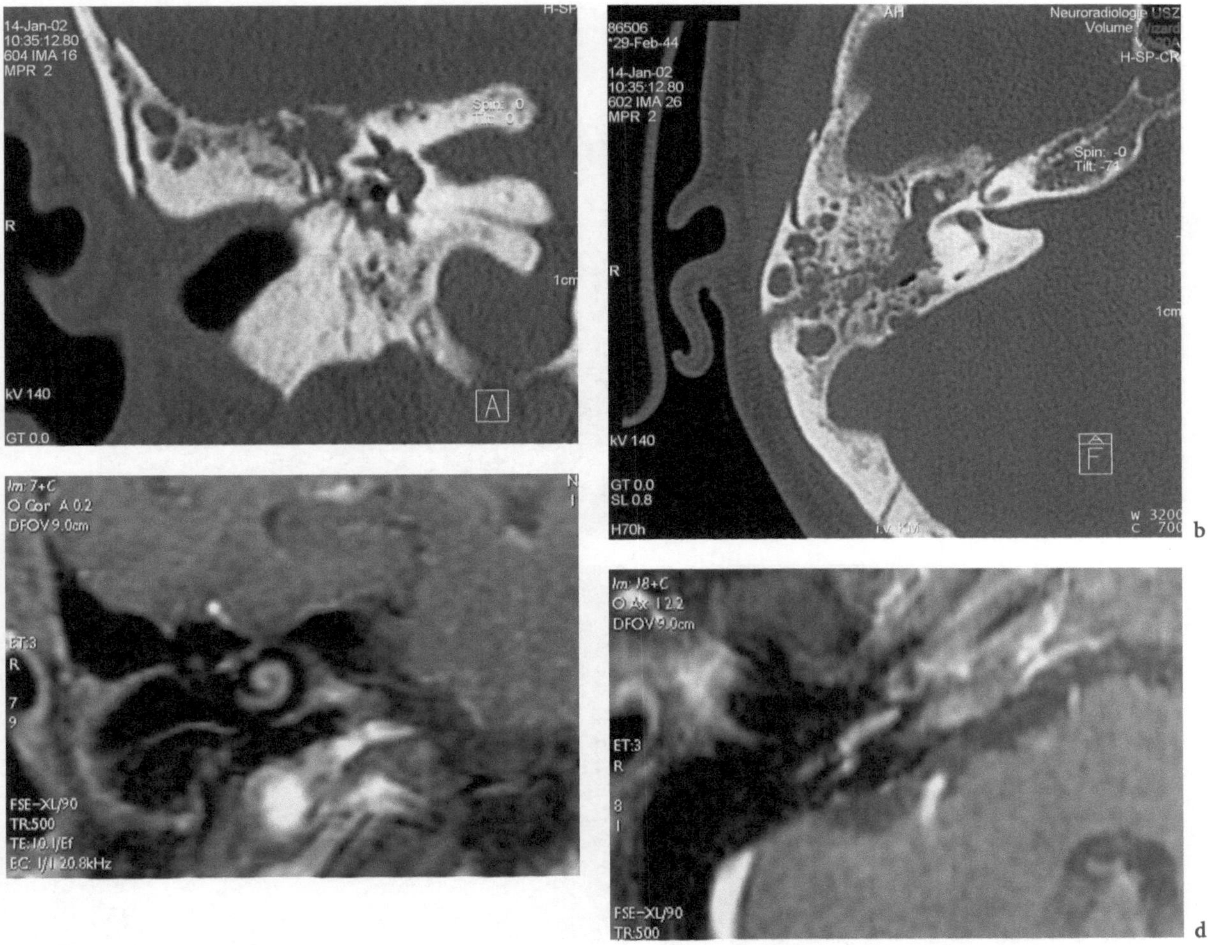

Fig. 4.10a–d. Sensorineural hearing loss associated with posttraumatic labyrinthitis. Coronal (a) and axial (b) CT images in a patient with a complex fracture of the temporal bone. One of the fracture lines involves the labyrinthine structures. Postcontrast T1-weighted axial (c) and coronal (d) MR images demonstrate intense enhancement of the cochlea indicating the development of posttraumatic labyrinthitis

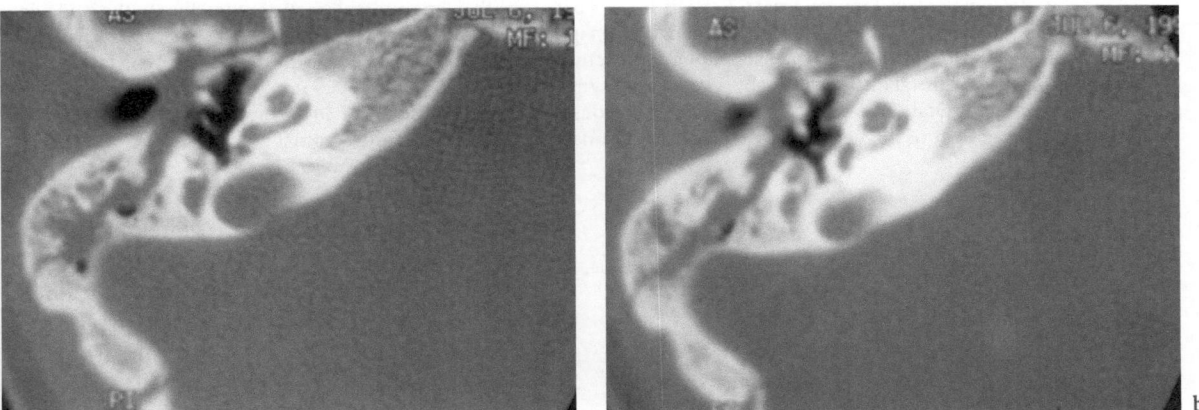

Fig. 4.11. Posttraumatic facial nerve palsy. Axial CT images in a patient with a longitudinal fracture extending to the anterior surface of the temporal bone. A bony fragment impinges the nerve in the region of the geniculate ganglion. Note also the associated multiple fractures and the disruption of the ossicles in the middle ear

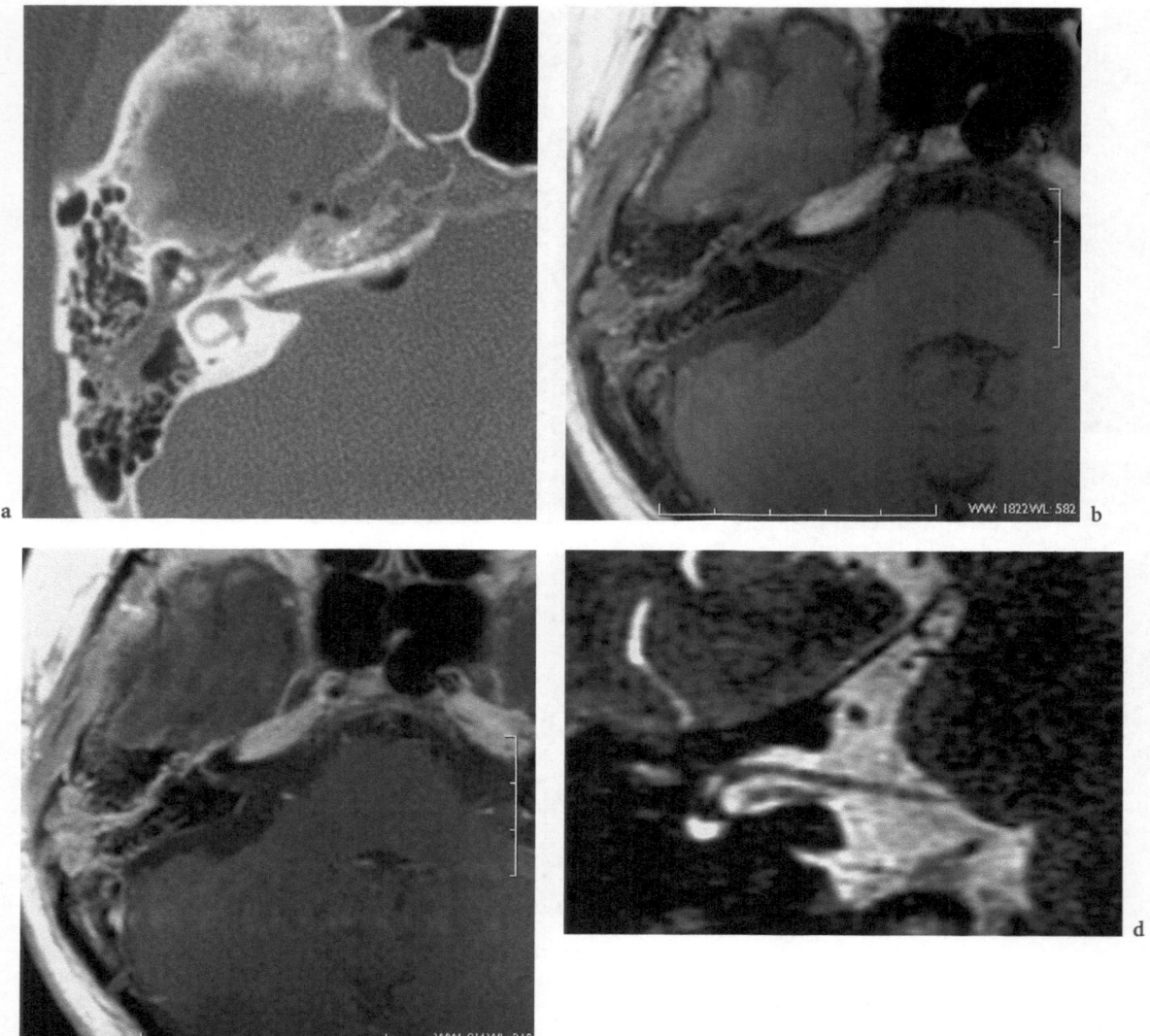

Fig. 4.12a–d. Posttraumatic facial injury. Axial CT image (**a**) in a patient with a longitudinal fracture extending to the geniculate ganglion and the tympanic portion of the fallopian canal. T1-weighted axial MR image without contrast (**b**) shows the obliteration of the mastoid and the fluid signal intensity along the fracture line. After contrast administration (**c**), there is intense contrast enhancement in the distal intrameatal, labyrinthine, and tympanic segments of the facial nerve, as well as in the geniculate ganglion. Three-dimensional, T2-weighted, fast-spin-echo reconstruction along the nerve (**d**) shows a focal thickening in the distal intrameatal segment of the nerve corresponding to the anatomical location of the contrast enhancement

Imaging in the patients with posttraumatic facial nerve injury represents a particular challenge. High-resolution CT may correctly depict the fracture line and occasionally an adjacent hematoma or a bony fragment compressing the nerve; however, the facial nerve itself is not visible and a potential injury can be delineated only indirectly (SARTORETTI-SCHEFER et al. 1997). High-resolution, contrast-enhanced MRI nearly always detects abnormal enhancement in the distal intrameatal segment and often in the laby-rinthine segment, the geniculate ganglion, and the proximal tympanic segment indicating damage to the nerve itself despite the fact that this enhancement does not correlate with the percentage of nerve-fiber degeneration as determined by electroneurography (SARTORETTI-SCHEFER et al. 1997). The abnormal contrast enhancement can last for up to 2 years after the trauma and is explained by a long-lasting damage to the blood/peripheral nerve barrier related to degeneration and regeneration of the myelinated nerve fibers (SARTORETTI-SCHEFER et al. 1997). Additional endoneural and perineural fibrosis of variable extent and scarring surrounding the regenerated axons, as identified in histologic studies, lead to thickening and intense enhancement of the affected nerve segments (Fig. 4.12; SARTORETTI-SCHEFER et al. 1997; FELIX et al. 1991). High-resolution T1-weighted MR images without contrast may show a hematoma in the region of the geniculate ganglion or a hematotympanum compressing the nerve at the mid-tympanic segment beneath the lateral semicircular canal. Transection of the nerve within the internal auditory canal is presently difficult to detect by conventional MRI. Newer three-dimensional, T2-weighted MR acquisitions by providing a cisternogram-like contrast may yield useful information on the integrity of this minute structure in the future.

4.5.3
Vertigo

Vertigo is generally defined as hallucination of linear or angular movement and is associated clinically with nausea, vomiting, and spontaneous nystagmus (GEAN 1994). It typically follows damage to the vestibular apparatus (utricle, semicircular ducts), or the vestibular nuclei in the inferolateral pons and upper medulla. It may be related to a temporal bone fracture (most commonly of transverse type) transecting the vestibule, the vestibular nerves, or the vestibular aqueduct (Fig. 4.13), but may also be related to a shearing injury at the root entry zone of the nerve or a contusion involving the vestibular nuclei in the brain stem in the absence of a fracture (SWARTZ 1997; FITZGERALD 1996; CANNON and JAHRSDOERFER 1983; GRAY and BARTON 1981; RIZVI and GIBBON 1979). Both CT of the temporal bone and MRI of the brain stem are necessary in the assessment of these patients, although its exact cause may often defy any imaging evaluation. In these cases, vertigo may be the result of perilymphatic fistula, labyrinthine concussion, or cupololithiasis (KHAN et al. 1985; ALTHAUS 1982; SCHUKNECHT 1969). The latter entity occurs when the otoliths (calcium carbonate deposits on the membranous labyrinth) detach (i.e., as a consequence of a blow) and move freely within the endolymph. Until they adhere or absorb they stimulate the sensory epithelium with various head motions causing benign positional vertigo. Although vertigo is a common complaint after temporal bone trauma, it is usually self-limited and requires only symptomatic treatment generally resolving after

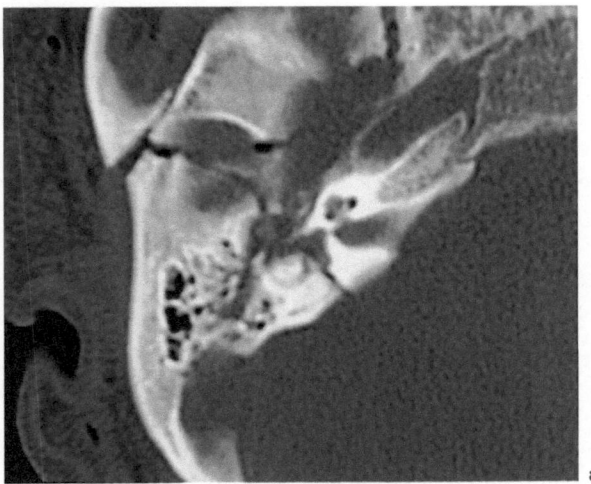

a

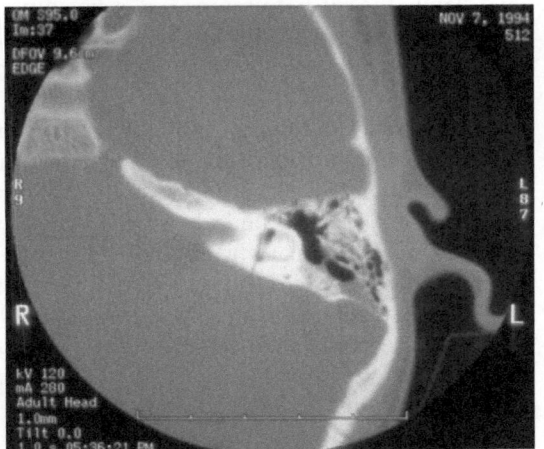

b

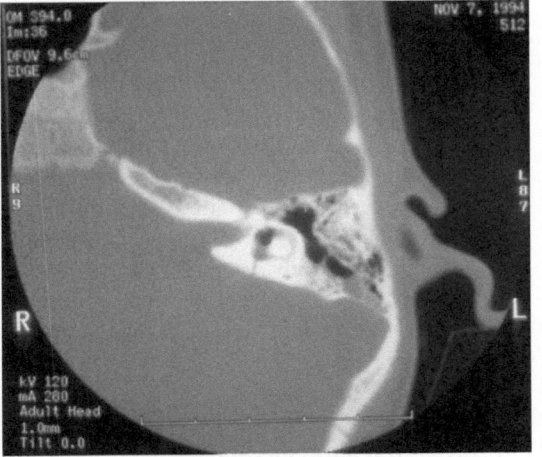

c

Fig. 4.13. Axial image (**a**) in a patient with a complex fracture of the temporal bone. The transverse fracture line courses through the vestibule disrupting the vestibular apparatus. Axial images (**b, c**) in a child with a transverse fracture coursing through the labyrinth, lateral semicircular canal, and through the proximal tympanic segment of the facial nerve. Note the presence of air within labyrinthine cavity (pneumolabyrinth)

several months (Cannon and Jahrsdoerfer 1983; Schubiger et al. 1986). If it persists and is quite incapacitating, patients may require ablation of the labyrinth or transection of the vestibular nerve (Fitzgerald 1996).

4.5.4
Perilymphatic Fistula/Endolymphatic Hydrops

It consists of an aberrant leakage of perilymph from the inner ear to the middle ear cavity through the oval or round window. It can be associated with a labyrinthine fracture leading to rupture of these inner ear seals, but more often is the consequence of a more common etiology such as sneezing, coughing, openhand slap to the ear, barotrauma (i.e., scuba diving or rapid ascent/descent within an airplane), or may be iatrogenic (Gean 1994; Fee 1968; Healy et al. 1974; Fitzgerald 1996). The loss of perilymph from the labyrinth into the middle ear cavity will result in endolymphatic hydrops (dilatation of the membranous labyrinth accompanied by degeneration of the sensory epithelium) with similar clinical manifestations to that produced in posttraumatic hydrops after disruption of the endolymphatic sac/duct (i.e., a transverse fracture through the vestibular aqueduct; Shea et al. 1995). The patients present with fluctuating SNHL associated with vertigo (occurring especially when a Valsalva maneuver transmits pressure through the fistula to the inner ear) and they are usually treated as an otologic emergency sometimes necessitating surgical exploration of the oval and round windows (Gean 1994; Althaus 1982; Fitzgerald 1996; Gussen 1981). Radiographically, the direct identification of the fistula is difficult or even impossible. In the absence of a fracture, indirect findings indicating an open communication between the labyrinth and the middle ear cavity are the presence of pneumolabyrinth (Fig. 4.13) and unexplained effusion within the middle ear and mastoid which are easily detected by HRCT (Mafee et al. 1984; Lipkin et al. 1985; Nurre et al. 1988; Weissman and Curtin 1992).

4.5.5
Cerebrospinal Fluid Fistulas

Cerebrospinal Fluid fistulas are an immediate or delayed complication of temporal bone trauma resulting from a disruption of the bone and the overlying dura most commonly in the region of the tegmen tympani (Neeley et al. 1982). This leads to a direct communication between the subarachnoid space in the middle cranial fossa and the middle ear with egress of CSF in the middle ear cavity. If the tympanic membrane is also ruptured, the CSF leakage manifests as otoliquorrhea. When the tympanic membrane is intact, the CSF drains from the middle ear via the eustachian tube to the nasopharynx and nasal cavity resulting in rhinoliquorrhea (Schubiger et al. 1986). Longitudinal fractures that extend into the tegmen tympani are the most common cause of otorhinoliquorrhea (Schubiger et al. 1986). The CSF fistula between the posterior cranial fossa and the mastoid (particularly if extensively pneumatized) may also result in otorhinoliquorrhea, but it is more rare (Swartz 1997). The dura overlying the skull base is easily torn during trauma and nearly 50% of fractures of the tegmen tympani are associated with otorhinoliquorrhea (Tamakawa and Hanafee 1980; Manelfe et al. 1982).

A persistent CSF leak can serve as a pathway for central nervous system infection and facilitate the development of meningitis, probably the most devastating sequelae of posttraumatic CSF fistula. When a bony defect of sufficient size is associated with intact dura, delayed complications include development of meningocele or meningoencephalocele with herniation of dura and/or brain into the middle ear cavity (Martin et al. 1989). High-resolution bone algorithm CT images are necessary for precise characterization of the fracture. The diagnosis is best established in the coronal projection, which demonstrates the fracture and the associated depression of the tegmen tympani (Fig. 4.14; Schubiger et al. 1986). If the patient is unable to undergo the positioning for direct coronal images, high-quality reformations in the coronal and sagittal planes can be obtained from contiguous axial sections that may help significantly in the delineation of the fistula. The demonstration of a depressed fracture in the tegmen tympani with clinically unequivocal otoliquorrhea is sufficient for planning the operative approach (Schubiger et al. 1986); however, in most cases the bony defect is small or it is transiently sealed off by mucosal swelling, herniated cerebral tissue, or bone prolapse allowing only minimal and intermittent escape of CSF into the middle ear making the neuroradiologic diagnosis of a CSF fistula difficult (Gean 1994). The presence of pneumocephalus may also imply a CSF fistula and sometimes may indicate the site of the bony/dural defect (Rothfus et al. 1987). Computed tomographic cisternography with water-soluble contrast material injected via lumbar puncture intrathecally and subsequently manipulated into the basal cisterns, followed by HRCT, may directly delineate the site of the fistula and the accumulation of the contrast

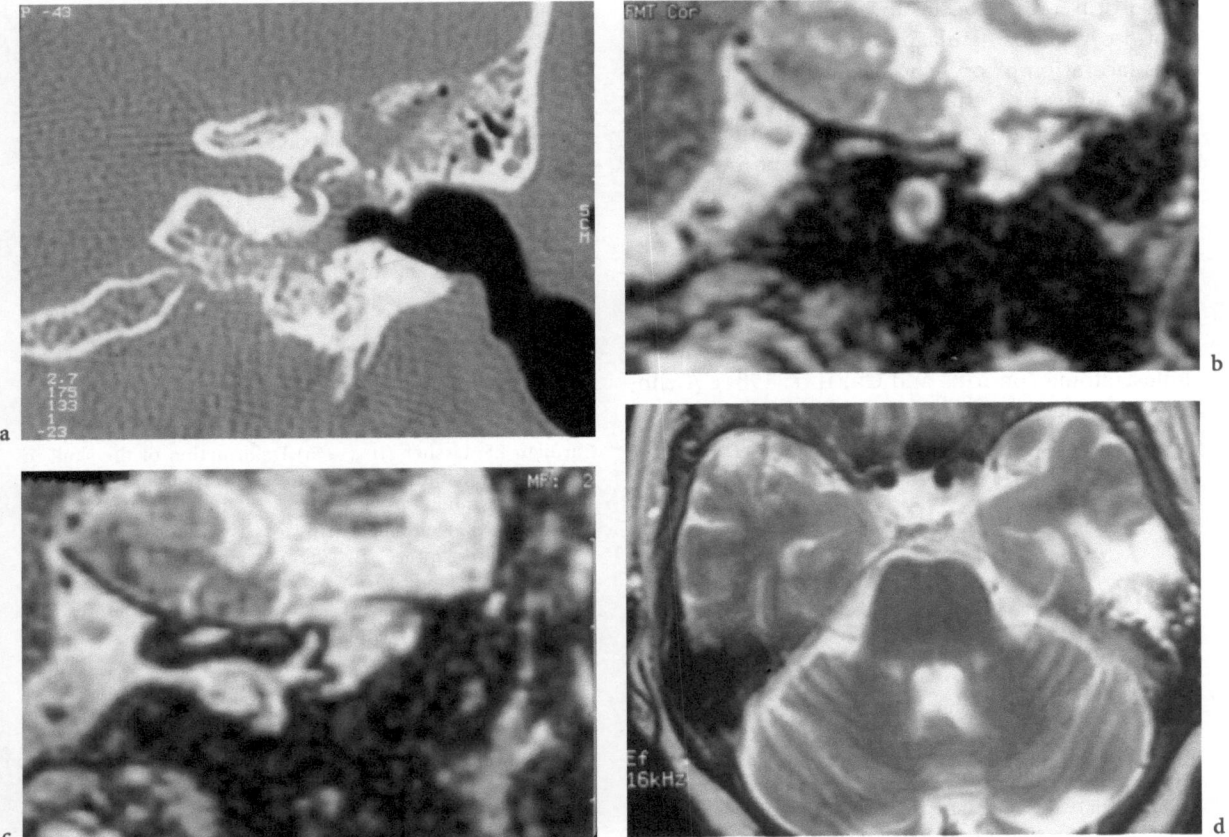

Fig. 4.14a–c. Patient with transverse fracture associated with cerebrospinal fluid fistula. Coronal CT image (**a**) demonstrates the fracture associated with a defect in the tegmen tympani and associated obliteration of the middle ear cavity. Coronal, heavily T2-weighted MR images (**b, c**) demonstrate the defect in the tegmen tympani and the communication of the subarachnoid space on the middle cranial fossa with the tympanic cavity. Axial T2-weighted image demonstrates the associated parenchymal damage of the basal temporal lobe

material in the middle ear cavity (SCHUBIGER et al. 1986). It is always useful to perform the imaging study during periods of actual leakage rather than during the quiescent period, and to place the patient in a position that would facilitate detection of the leakage (GEAN 1994). Magnetic resonance imaging plays an increasingly important role in the evaluation of these patients. High-resolution, heavily T2-weighted MR sequences provide non-invasively cisternogram-like images and may directly demonstrate the aberrant communication, because the overlying dural/bony defect can be directly visualized (Fig. 4.14). Magnetic resonance imaging is also more accurate than CT for delineation of associated meningocele or meningoencephalocele and detecting potential parenchymal damage to the basal temporal lobe (Fig. 4.14). In most cases, a CSF fistula will close spontaneously within 1 week due to cerebral adhesions or local inflammation (GEAN 1994). In rare instances, CSF leak can be delayed for several

months or even years after trauma. A potential explanation for that is that fractures of the enchondral layer of the labyrinthine capsule heal via fibrous union rather than callus formation, thus increasing the potential for fistula (LUNDY et al. 1996). If the leak persists longer than 2 weeks, or if it is of delayed onset, or if the patient experiences repeated episodes of meningitis, surgical exploration and repair of the fistula is indicated in which case the exact location of the fistula should be neuroradiologically determined prior to the intervention (MANELFE et al. 1982; NAGERIS et al. 1995).

4.5.6
Other Complications

It is emphasized that the observer should be careful to not overlook potential vascular complications associated with temporal bone fracture such as internal carotid artery occlusion or pseudoaneurysm, carotid cavernous fistula, and jugular vein–sigmoid sinus laceration or occlusion (GENTRY 1991). These complications are especially common when these vessels are in the path of the fracture line and the onset of clinical manifestations may be immediate or delayed.

During traumatic perforation of the tympanic membrane, squamous epithelial debris may be embedded in the mesotympanum and invade the tympanic membrane or the fracture line predisposing the patient for the development of an acquired cholesteatoma (BROOKS and GRAHAM 1984). A cholesteatoma developing in this clinical context may be quite aggressive and dangerous because these individuals often have well-developed mastoids.

References

Althaus SR (1982) Perilymph fistulae. Laryngoscope 91: 538–562

Anderson J, Awas IA, Hahn JF (1991) Delayed facial nerve palsy after temporal lobectomy for epilepsy: report of four cases and discussion of possible mechanisms. Neurosurgery 28:453–456

Bellucci RJ (1983) Traumatic injuries of the middle ear. Otolaryngol Clin North Am 16:633–650

Bonafe A, Laval C, Arrue P, Manelfe C (1995) Temporal bone fractures. Riv Neuroradiol 8:847–854

Brodie HA, Thomson TC (1997) Management of complications of 820 temporal bone fractures Am J Otol 19:188–197

Brooks BG, Graham MD (1984) Post-traumatic cholesteatoma of the external auditory canal. Laryngoscope 94:667–670

Cannon CR, Jahrsdoerfer RA (1983) Temporal bone fractures: review of 90 cases. Arch Otolaryngol 109:285–288

Coker NJ, Kendall KA, Jenkins HA, Alford BR (1989) Traumatic intratemporal facial nerve injury: management rationale for preservation of function. Otolaryngol Head Neck Surg 97:26–29

Dahiya R, Keller JD, Litofsky NS et al. (1999) Temporal bone fractures: otic capsule sparing versus otic capsule violating. Clinical and radiographic considerations. J Trauma 47:1079–1085

Fee GA (1968) Traumatic perilymph fistulae. Arch Otolaryngol 88:47

Felix H, Eby TL, Fisch U (1991) New aspects of facial nerve pathology in temporal bone fractures. Acta Otolaryngol (Stockh) 111:332–336

Fisch U (1974) Facial paralysis in fractures of the petrous bone. Laryngoscope 84:2141–2154

Fisch U (1980) Management of intratemporal facial nerve injuries. J Laryngol Otol 94:129–134

Fitzgerald DC (1995) Persistent dizziness following head trauma and perilymphatic fistula. Arch Phys Med Rehabil 76:1017–1020

Fitzgerald DC (1996) Head trauma: hearing loss and dizziness. J Trauma 40:488–496

Fritz R, Rieden K, Lenarz T, Haels J (1989) Radiological evaluation of temporal bone disease: high resolution CT versus conventional X-ray diagnosis. Br J Radiol 62:107–113

Gean AD (1994) Scalp and skull injury. In: Gean AD (ed) Imaging of head trauma. Raven Press, New York, pp 51–73, 542, 556

Gentry LR (1991) Temporal bone trauma: current perspectives for diagnostic evaluation. Neuroimaging Clin North Am 1:319–340

Ghorayeb BY, Yeakley JW (1992) Temporal bone fractures: longitudinal or oblique? The case for oblique temporal bone fractures Laryngoscope 102:129–233

Goodhill V (1971) Sudden deafness and round window rupture. Laryngoscope 81:1462–1467

Goodwin WJ (1983) Temporal bone fractures. Radiol Clin North Am 16:651–659

Gray RF, Barton RP (1981) Round window rupture. J Laryngol Otol 95:165–177

Gurdjian ES, Lissner HR (1946) Deformation of the skull in head injury studied by the "stresscoat" technique, quantitative determinations. Surg Gynecol Obstet 83:219–233

Gussen R (1981) Sudden hearing loss associated with cochlear membrane rupture. Two human temporal bone reports. Arch Otolaryngol 107:598–600

Harker LA, McCabe BF (1974) Temporal bone fractures and facial nerve injury. Otolaryngol Clin North Am 2:425–428

Harvey FH, Jones AM (1980) "Typical" basal skull fracture of both petrous bones: an unreliable indicator of head impact site. J Forensic Sci 25:280–286

Hasso AN, Ledington JA (1988) Traumatic injuries of the temporal bone. Otolaryngol Clin North Am 21:295–316

Healy GB, Strong MS, Campagna D (1974) Ataxia, vertigo and hearing loss: a result of rupture of the inner ear window. Arch Otolaryngol 100:130–135

Holland BA, Brant-Zawadski M (1984) High resolution CT of temporal bone trauma. AJNR 5:291–295

Hough JVD (1970) Fractures of the temporal bone and associated middle and inner ear trauma. Proc R Soc Med 63:245–256

Hough JVD, Stuart WD (1968) Middle ear injuries and skull trauma. Laryngoscope 78:899–937

Jane NN, Laureno R, Mark AS et al. (1991) Deafness after bilateral midbrain contusion: a correlation of magnetic resonance imaging with auditory brainstem evoked responses. Neurosurgery 29:106–1101

Johnson DW, Hasso AN, Stewart CE, Thompson JR, Hinshow DR (1984) Temporal bone trauma: high resolution computed tomographic evaluation. Radiology 151:411–415

Khan AA, Marion M, Hinojosa R (1985) Temporal bone fractures: a histopathologic study. Otolaryngol Head Neck Surg 93:177–186

Kollias SS (2000) Traumatisms of the skull base and their consequences. Riv Neuroradiol 13 (Suppl 1):209–212

Lindeman RC (1979) Temporal bone trauma and facial paralysis. Otolaryngol Clin North Am 12:403–413

Lipkin AF, Bryan RN, Jenkins HA (1985) Pneumolabyrinth after temporal bone fracture: documentation by high resolution CT. AJNR 6:294–297

Lundy LB, Graham MD, Kartush JM, LaRouere MJ (1996) Temporal bone encephalocele and cerebrospinal fluid leaks. Am J Otol 17:461–469

Mafee MF, Valvassori GE, Kumar A et al. (1984) Pneumolabyrinth: a new radiologic sign for fracture of the stapes foot plate. Am J Otol 5:374–375

Manelfe C, Cellelier P, Sobel D et al. (1982) Cerebrospinal fluid rhinorrhea: evaluation with metrizamide cisternography. AJR 138:471–476

Marquet J, Offeciers E (1980) Dislocation of the incus: a radiologic diagnosis? J Belg Radiol 63:225–233

Martin N, Sterkers O, Murat M, Hahum N (1989) Brain herniation into the middle ear cavity: MR imaging. Neuroradiology 31:184–186

May M (1986) Trauma to the facial nerve. In: May M (ed) The facial nerve. Thieme , New York, pp 421–440

McCabe BF (1972) Injuries to the facial nerve: symposium on trauma in otolaryngology. Laryngoscope 82:1891–1896

McCovern FH (1968) Facial nerve injuries in skull fractures. Arch Otolaryngol 88:102–108

McKennan KX, Chole RA (1992) Facial paralysis in temporal bone trauma. Am J Otol 13:167–172

Murakami M, Ohtani I, Aikawa T, Anzai T (1990) Temporal bone findings in two cases of head injury. J Laryngol Otol 104:986–989

Nageris B, Hanson MC, Lavelle WG, VanPelt FA (1995) Temporal bone fractures. Am J Emerg Med 13:211–214

Neeley JG, Neblett CR, Rose JE (1982) Diagnosis and treatment of spontaneous cerebrospinal fluid otorrhea. Laryngoscope 92:609–612

Nurre JW, Miller GW, Ball JB (1988) Pneumolabyrinth as a late sequela of temporal bone fracture. Am J Otol 9:489–493

Patay Z, Lourgans, Baleriaux D (1995) Early complications of petrous bone fractures. Riv Neuroradiol 8:855–866

Potter JM (1964) Facial palsy following head injury. J Laryngol Otol 78:654–657

Rizvi SS, Gibbon KP (1979) Effective transverse temporal bone fracture on the fluid compartment of the inner ear. Ann Otol Rhinol Laryngol 88:741–748

Rothfus WE, Deeb ZL, Daffner RH, Prostko ER (1987) Head-hanging CT: an alternative method for evaluating traumatic CSF rhinorrhea. AJNR 8:155–156

Sartoretti-Schefer S, Scherler M, Wichmann W, Valavanis A (1997) Contrast-enhanced MR of the facial nerve in patients with posttraumatic peripheral facial nerve palsy. Am J Neuroradiol 18:1115–1125

Schubiger O, Valavanis A, Stuckmann G, Antonucci F (1986) Temporal bone fractures and their complications: examination with high resolution CT. Neuroradiology 28:93–99

Schuber O, Valavanis A, Stuckmann G, Antonucci F (1986) Examination with high resolution CT. Neuroradiology 28: 93–99

Schuknecht HF (1969) Cupulolithiasis. Arch Otolaryngol 90: 765–778

Schucknecht HF (1974) Pathology of the ear. Harvard University Press, Cambridge, pp 291–318, 351–414

Shea JJ, Ge X, Orchik DJ (1995) Traumatic endolymphatic hydrops. Am J Otol 16:235–240

Swartz JD (1983) High resolution CT of the middle ear and mastoid. I. Normal anatomy including normal variations. Radiology 148:449–454

Swartz JD (1989) Current imaging approach to the temporal bone. Radiology 171:309–317

Swartz JD (1995) Temporal bone trauma. In: Som PM, Curtin HD (eds) Head and neck imaging, 3rd edn, vol 2. Mosby, St. Louis, pp 1425–1431

Swartz JD (1997) Trauma. In: Swartz JD, Harnsberger HR (eds) Imaging of the temporal bone, 3rd edn. Thieme, New York, pp 318–344

Swartz JD, Swartz NG, Korsvik H et al. (1985) CT evaluation of the middle ear and mastoid for post-traumatic hearing loss. Ann Otol Rhinol Laryngol 94:263–266

Swartz JD, Laucks RL, Berger AS et al. (1986) Computed tomography of the disarticulated incus. Laryngoscope 96: 1207–1210

Tamakawa Y, Hanafee WN (1980) Cerebrospinal fluid rhinorrhea: significance of an air-fluid level in the sphenoid sinus. Radiology 135:101–104

Vignaud J (1974) Traité de radiodiagnostic, tome 17–1: temporal, fosses nasales, cavités accessoires. Masson, Paris

Weissman JL, Curtin HD (1992) Pneumolabyrinth: a computed tomographic sign of temporal bone fracture. Am J Otolaryngol 13:113–114

Weissman JC, Curtin HD, Hirsch BE et al. (1992) High signal from the otic labyrinth on enhanced magnetic resonance imaging. AJNR 13:1183–1187

Wong E, Lee G, Mason DT (1995) Temporal headaches and associated symptoms related to the styloid process and its attachments. Ann Head Med Singapore 24:124–128

Wright JW (1974) Trauma of the ear. Radiol Clin North Am 12:527–532

Yanagihara N, Murakami S, Nishihara S (1997) Temporal bone fractures including facial nerve paralysis: a new classification and its clinical significance. Ear Nose Throat J 76: 79–86

Zimmermann RA, Bilaniuk LT, Hackney DB et al. (1987) Magnetic resonance imaging in temporal bone fracture. Neuroradiology 29:246–251

The Clinician's View

I. DHOOGE

Head injury is one of the most frequently suffered traumatic events. In approximately 20% of cases temporal bone injury is associated. Head trauma can be classified into three major categories: blunt trauma; penetrating trauma; and iatrogenic trauma.

Motor vehicle accidents are the chief cause of blunt head injury resulting in temporal bone fractures. Because patients have often associated head, spine, and body injuries which are more life-threatening, the diagnosis of temporal bone fractures is made with some delay; however, immediate bedside evaluation can give valuable information and direct the management. Immediate facial paralysis, due to temporal bone fracture, necessitates surgical exploration; late onset paralysis can be managed expectantly. Tuning-fork testing in a non-comatous patient can differentiate between sensorineural and conductive hearing loss which can be related to the type of fracture, transversal or longitudinal. The presence of cerebrospinal fluid otorrhea or rhinorrhea indicates a more severe trauma. Computed tomography can document and localize the fracture within the temporal bone. When a patient is comatous, the site and type of fracture can predict the sort of lesions to be expected. When surgical intervention is considered in a case of posttraumatic facial nerve damage, it is important to identify single or multiple areas of nerve damage. Similarly, the degree of mastoid pneumatization and other anatomical elements are important when planning nerve exploration. In severe blunt and penetrating trauma an assessment of the vascular structures of the temporal bone may be necessary. Occlusion of the jugular bulb and transverse sinus, impingement on or injury to the carotid artery, traumatic carotid aneurisms, and arteriovenous malformations are identified in this way.

5 Tumorous Lesions of the Temporal Bone

H. Imhof, C. Czerny, A. Dirisamer, E. Oschatz

CONTENTS

5.1
Introduction

Tumorous lesions of the temporal bone excluding tumors of the cerebellopontine angle (CPA) are relatively rare. The publications of these lesions are mostly in the form of case reports.

The lesions are classified as congenital (primary cholesteatomas) or as acquired tumorous lesions. The acquired lesions are divided into benign and malignant blastomas (Table 5.1). Furthermore, the tumorous lesions can be classified as primary or secondary malignant blastomas. The benign and malignant tumors can again be separated depending on their localization and origin. The localization may be either the external ear or external acoustic meatus (EAM), the middle ear, the inner ear, or other locations. The origin of these tumorous lesions may be either epithelial, osseous, vascular, or nervous, or it is unclear. Benign lesions of the external ear usually do not need any imaging, except if they are growing into the inner parts of the temporal bone.

Aggressive lesions usually need imaging for the pretherapeutic staging and follow-ups (therapy control; Wenig 1993; Valvassori et al. 1995).

5.2
Imaging

Up-to-date imaging of the temporal bone consists of spiral computed tomography (spiral CT) obtained at high-resolution bone-window-level settings (HRCT) and MRI with various pulse sequences and intravenously applied contrast-media-enhancing soft tissue structures of the temporal bone and neighboring structures (brain and meninges, vessels, nerves, joints, etc.). Digital subtraction angiography has its only place before embolization of glomus tympanicum tumors.

5.2.1
High-resolution computed tomography

High-resolution computed tomography of the temporal bone is usually performed in the axial (parallel to the orbito-meatal line) and eventually in the coronal plane (perpendicular to the hard palate). The slice thickness should be max. 1.0 mm with no gap. The scans are performed without intravenous application of contrast material and by the use of post-processing in a high-resolution bone-window-level setting. The field of view should be max. 20 cm, and the matrix 512×512. With single- and multi-detector spiral CT

H. Imhof, MD; C. Czerny, MD; A. Dirisamer, MD;
E. Oschatz, MD
Osteologie/Radiodiagnostik AKH Wien, Währinger Gürtel 18–20, 1090 Vienna, Austria

Table 5.1. Tumors of the temporal bone and their locations

Lesion	External ear + meatus acusticus externus	Middle ear	Inner ear	Other locations
Exostosis osteoma	++	+	0	+
Basal cell carcinoma	+++	0	0	0
Squamous cell carcinoma	++	+	0	0
Ceruminal gland adenocarcinoma	++	0	0	0
Middle ear adenoma/adenocarcinoma	0	+	0	0
Primary cholesteatoma	+	+	+	+
Glomus tympanicum tumor	0	++	0	0
Middle ear schwannoma (facial nerve, chorda tympani, Jacobson nerve)	0	+	0	0
Endolymphatic sac tumor	0	0	+	0
Inner ear schwannoma (cochlearis, nerve, vestibular nerve)	0	0	+	0
Rhabdomyosarcoma	0	0	0	++ (pediatric population)
Ewing, osteo-, chondro-, fibrosarcoma, lymphoma				+
Osteoblastoma, chondroblastoma, hemangioma				+
Metastasis				+

++ Uncommon, + common, +++ very common, 0 not present

scanners, the coronal sections can also be obtained by reconstructions from the axial slices thus reducing radiation dose and patient examination time.

The HRCT images provide an excellent bone contrast, which is important to evaluate the bony structures of the temporal bone and demonstrate calcifications. It also enables excellent 3D reconstructions (MAROLDI et al. 2001; CASSELMAN et al. 2001).

5.2.2
Magnetic resonance imaging

Magnetic resonance imaging of the temporal bone in cases of suspected tumorous lesions should be performed with a head coil which offers the possibility to examine both temporal bones simultaneously – which allows an easy comparison – and also gives the best information about a potential involvement of intracerebral structures.

The MRI examination should start with axial T2-weighted fast-spin-echo or fluid-attenuated inversion recovery sequences over the whole brain to exclude any other gross brain pathology. Then, a 3D T2-weighted fast-spin-echo sequence (potentially with fat saturation) in axial planes may be obtained. After these sequences, axial 3D T1-weighted gradient-echo (GRE) sequences before and after i.v. application of gadolinium compounds are performed. In cases with a proven tumor, additional coronal 3D T1-weighted GRE sequences are performed or reconstructed, particularly to visualize the tumor extension in all dimensions.

The slice thickness of the sequences should be 1 mm or less, the field of view approximately 20–25 cm, and the matrix 512×512. With MRI, visualization of soft tissue structures is excellent. Moreover, discrimination of cartilaginous and bony structures is easily done. Local bone marrow or brain edema can be a first sign of tissue invasion. Magnetic resonance angiography with i.v. contrast application allows delineation of normal and abnormal vessel structures and flow within the vessels (MAROLDI et al. 2001; SOM and CURTIN 1994; CASSELMAN et al. 2001; SABNIS et al. 2000).

5.3
Principles of Tumor Extension

Usually any tumor grows in the directions in which there is less resistance and sufficient vascularization. The resistance increases step by step from sutures, canals to soft tissue, cartilage, bone, and ending with the hardest structure around the otic capsule; therefore, in aggressive lesions the otic capsule will be the last involved structure, whereas tumor growth against the outer ear and into soft tissues will be found very often. Anteriorly, the borders are presented by the temporomandibular joint and the eustachian tube and carotid artery as well. Posteriorly, we find the mastoid and facial canal. Medially, the borders are represented by the middle ear or by the extreme hard bone of the inner ear (otic capsule). Superiorly, rain and relatively thin bony structures are found. Tumor ingrowth into the brain is one of the worst clinical scenarios and is the most feared. The growth into the inferior direction passes through relatively thin bone into the soft tissues of the neck. Finally, the specific anatomy of the external auditory canal must also be recognized: the external auditory canal has no subcutaneous tissue. Aggressive (malignant) lesions of the external auditory canal infiltrate very early the periosteum and the neighboring bone.

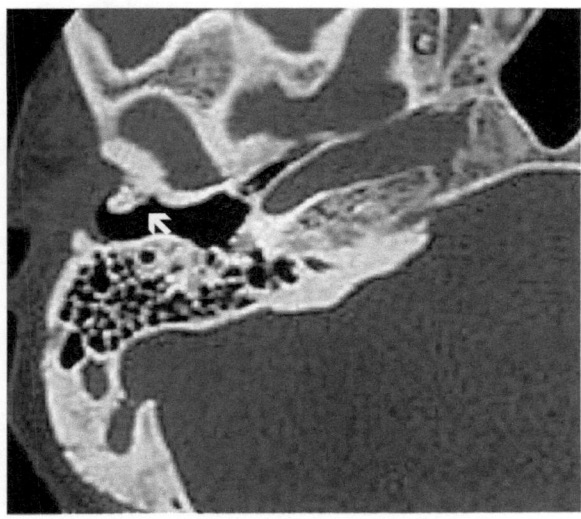

Fig. 5.1. Axial high-resolution computed tomographic (HRCT) image shows an exostosis within the external auditory canal (*arrow*). No bone marrow within the tumor

5.4
Pathology and Imaging

5.4.1
External Ear and External Auditory Canal

Imaging of the external ear may be of great clinical interest in any aggressive lesion. The most common neoplastic aggressive lesions of the external ear are the basal cell carcinoma, squamous cell carcinoma, and local metastasis. These neoplastic aggressive lesions must be differentiated from malignant otitis externa and aggressive ingrowth of adenoid-cystic carcinoma and melanoma metastasis. Furthermore, imaging of the external ear may also be of interest in cases of locally space-occupying lesions within the meatus externus. The most common lesions are exostosis and osteomas.

5.4.1.1
Exostoses and Osteoma

Exostoses are far more common than osteomas (Fig. 5.1). They are predominantly broad based and in the medial half of the bony outer canal near the tympanic annulus. The have no bone marrow and as a rule they are asymptomatic, but occasionally they become large enough to cause retention of epithelial debris and obstruction ending up in external otitis. A definite relationship between frequent swimming in cold water and the formation of meatal exostosis has long been recognized (VAN GILSE 1938). They develop between 20 and 50 years of age.

Osteoma, contrary to exostosis, have all layers of a normal bone including bone marrow (Fig. 5.2). They are usually situated near the tympano-mastoid or tympano-squamous suture. Similar to the exostosis, debris may accumulate, as they obliterate the lumen. This may result in the formation of an external cholesteatoma.

In both cases imaging is important to locate the disease within the external auditory canal and visualize the medial part of the external meatus.

Osteomas may also arise occasionally within the mastoid and from the medial aspect of the petrous pyramid near porus of the internal auditory canal (Figs. 5.3, 5.4).

5.4.1.2
Basal cell carcinoma

The basal cell carcinoma is a slow-growing, locally infiltrative malignant neoplasm of the skin and subcutaneous adnexal tissue. It is the most common cutaneous malignancy, affects particularly Caucasians, and affects males more than females. It is most commonly seen in the fifth to seventh decades of life (WENIG 1993; NAGER 1993).

The sun-exposed areas of head and neck are the most frequent sites of occurrence (nose, eyelids, nasolabial area, auricular area; Fig. 5.5). Basal cell carcinoma are asymptomatic in general. Complete surgical excision is the treatment of choice. The prognosis is excellent after complete excision. Local recurrences are not uncommon, and metastasis is

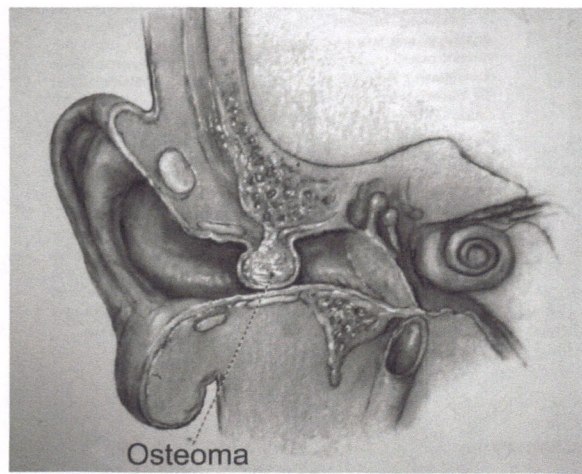

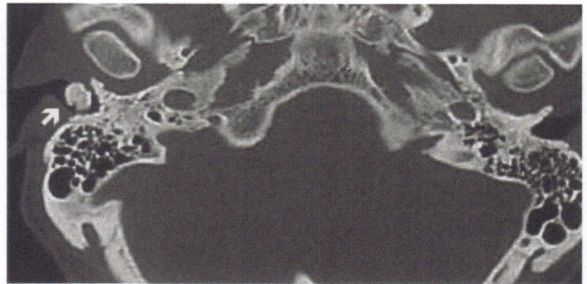

Fig. 5.2. a An osteoma within the external auditory canal. The bone marrow continues directly into the osteoma. **b** Axial HRCT image shows a narrowing of the external auditory canal by an osteoma of the external auditory canal. Note the bone marrow within the tumor (*arrow*)

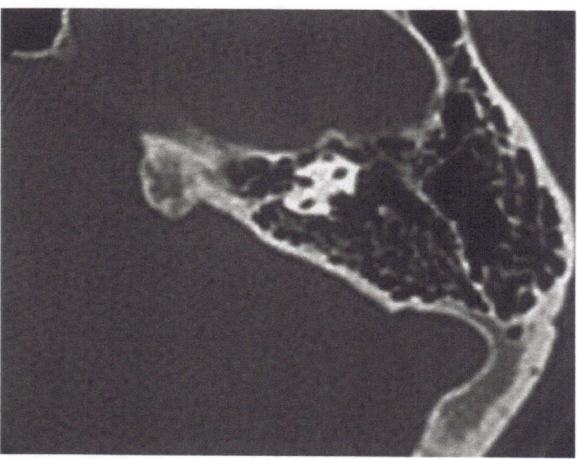

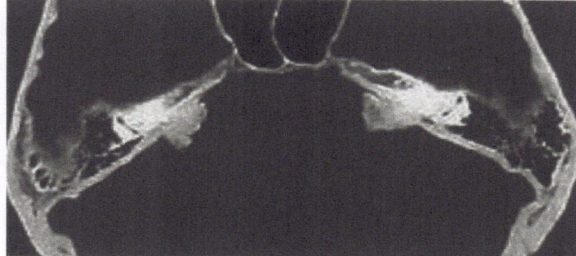

Fig. 5.4. Axial HRCT image with symmetrical osteomas near the porus acusticus internus

Fig. 5.3. Axial HRCT image presenting an osteoma at the medial border of the pyramid

rare except for neglected and long-standing tumor that attains large sizes and becomes deeply and extensively infiltrative. Basal cell carcinoma of the external auditory canal is uncommon but tends to have extensive subcutaneous involvement, which may not be clinically appreciated.

Indications for imaging of the soft tissue (MRI with contrast application) and the neighboring bone (CT) exist only in cases of unclear involvement of the neighboring tissues or posttherapeutic follow-up.

5.4.1.3
Squamous cell carcinoma

Squamous cell carcinoma is a malignant epithelial tumor arising from the surface of the epithelium. It accounts for approximately 25% of all squamous cell carcinomas of the head and neck. While the squamous cell carcinoma of the external ear affects more often males than females, the opposite is true in squamous cell carcinomas of the external ear (Figs. 5.6, 5.7). As with basal cell carcinoma, it is a tumor of the older

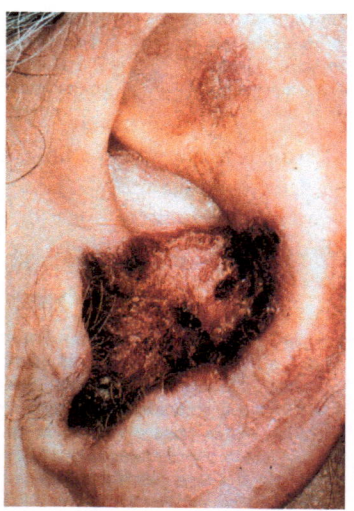

Fig. 5.5. Photo of the external ear: typical basal cell carcinoma with signs of chronic dermatitis

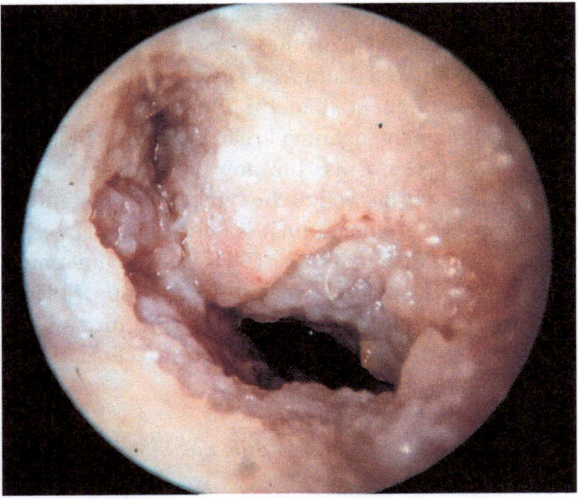

Fig. 5.6. Photo of the external auditory meatus (otoscopy): irregular, knob-like lesion representing a squamous cell carcinoma

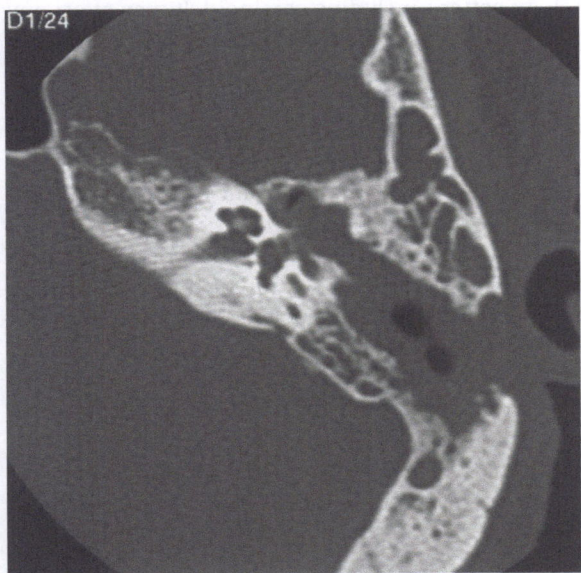

Fig. 5.7. Axial HRCT image with a huge soft tissue mass with extensive bony destruction and soft tissue masses within the middle ear. There is beginning erosion of the otic capsule

generation (max. between 50 and 70 years). Clinically, it may be misdiagnosed as chronic otitis media with pain, otorrhea, and hearing deficits.

The treatment of choice is complete surgical excision. This often requires a radical procedure such as mastoidectomy or temporal resection. Depending on the extent of the disease, additional radiotherapy may be indicated. The 5-year survival rate is only 25%. Regional

lymph node metastasis is seen infrequently and death is in most cases due to intracranial extension.

Imaging is indicated in unclear cases for local lymph node staging of the tumor and posttherapeutic follow-up (WENIG 1993; NAGER 1993).

5.4.1.4
Ceruminal Gland Adenocarcinoma

Ceruminal gland adenocarcinoma is a malignant neoplasm of cerumen-secreting modified apocrine glands, located in the external auditory canal. It affects more males than females with an age peak between 50 and 60 years. Clinically characteristic is a cerumen discharge with pain and hearing loss. Complete surgical excision is the treatment of choice, which may be supplemented with radiotherapy.

Similar to the basal cell carcinoma and squamous cell carcinoma, imaging is indicated to define the extent of the disease and in the posttherapeutic follow-up (WENIG 1993; NAGER 1993; BENJAMIN et al. 1995).

5.4.2
Middle Ear

Signs and symptoms of middle ear tumors are nonspecific. They include conductive (or mixed) hearing loss, (pulsatile) tinnitus, vertigo, and less commonly earache or discharge. By otoscopy a mass in seen which may be reddish or bluish in cases of vascular tumors. Pulsation of the mass is rarely appreciated.

5.4.2.1
Glomus Tympanicum Tumor

The glomus tympanicum tumor arises from the extra adrenal, neural crest-derived paraganglia, specifically located in the middle ear or temporal bone. It is the most common tumor of the middle ear and affects more females than males, most commonly seen in the fifth to seventh decades of life. It is associated with the tympanic branch of the glossopharyngeal nerve (Jacobson's nerve), which represents 80% of all glomus tumors, within the temporal bone (the other 20% concern Arnold's nerve in the external auditory meatus). The tumor may be locally destructive. It is mostly located at the level of the mucosa overlying the promontory. Typical clinical symptoms are conductive hearing loss, tinnitus, and pain. The drum is typically blue (Fig. 5.8). With CT a small soft tissue mass is shown, often with evidence of extensive destruction

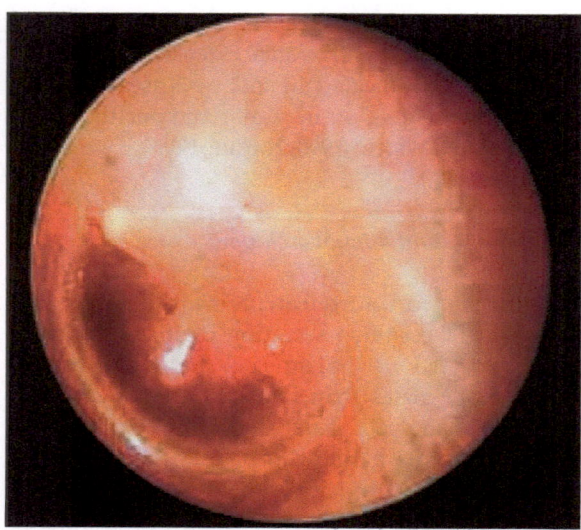

Fig. 5.8. Otoscopy photo of the ear drum: there is a small red mass on the medial surface of the tympanic membrane with some bluish color

The local recurrence rate reaches 50%. Malignant transformation is rare. In these cases metastasizing to cervical lymph nodes, lungs, and liver may be observed. Much more frequent than the glomus tympanicum tumor is the paraganglioma arising within the jugular foramen. Because of its common propensity to grow through the inferior wall of the tympanic cavity and to invade the mesotympanum, it is referred to as glomus jugulo-tympanicum tumor (Fig. 5.10). Differential diagnosis between the two entities is impossible at otoscopy. Imaging is therefore mandatory for surgical planning (NOUJAIM et al. 2000; MANOLIDIS et al. 1999).

5.4.2.2
Middle Ear Adenoma and Middle Ear Adenocarcinoma

Middle ear adenoma is a rare neoplasm arising from the middle ear mucosa. Its complete name is middle ear adenomatous tumor of non-papillary mixed histology pattern including carcinoid. It may affect any portion of the middle ear – preferentially the middle part, however – including the Eustachian tube, mastoid air spaces, ossicles, and chorda tympani nerve. Clinically, the patients complain about unilateral conductive hearing loss, tinnitus, and dizziness. There is no known relationship to chronic otitis media. It is a slow-growing tumor (Fig. 5.11).

Magnetic resonance imaging shows a well-circumscribed soft tissue mass within the middle ear, which shows almost no enhancement after i.v. application of contrast medium. There are no signs of destruction or invasion. With CT the soft tissue mass is also well outlined. No bony destructions or calcifications are demonstrated (Fig. 5.12).

In very rare instances a malignant middle ear adenocarcinoma may be found. This rare neoplasm should

of adjacent structures (Fig. 5.9). With MRI the soft tissue tumor is hyperintense on T2-weighted images and excellently outlined. It enhances extensively after i.v. application of contrast medium (Fig. 5.9), also demonstrating local bony invasion. The typical soft and pepper pattern due to the serpentine and punctuate flow voids of vessels known from glomus jugulare tumors is not appreciated in small paragangliomas. There also may be invasion of the epitympanic recess, eustachian tube, or mastoid, whereas ossicular destruction is rare. Treatment of choice is complete surgical excision. In cases of inoperability radiotherapy is useful resulting in a decrease or ablation of vascularity and promotes fibrosis. Preoperative embolization has been advocated as useful to decrease vascularity, too.

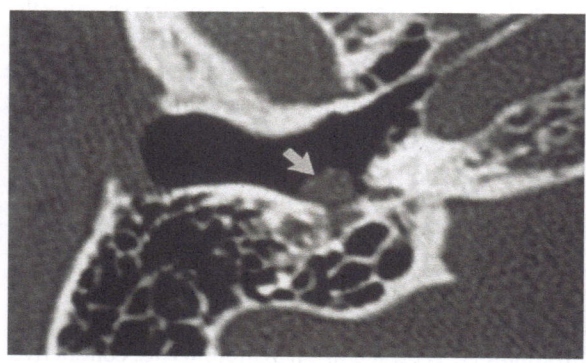
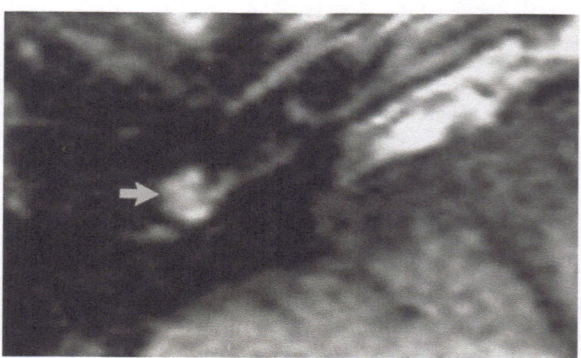

a

b

Fig. 5.9. a Coronal HRCT image shows a soft tissue mass (*arrow*) in the hypotympanum adjacent to the promontory representing a glomus tympanicum tumor. **b** Axial contrast-enhanced T1-weighted MRI shows a hyperintense mass (*arrow*) in the hypotympanum adjacent to the promontory compatible with a glomus tympanicum tumor

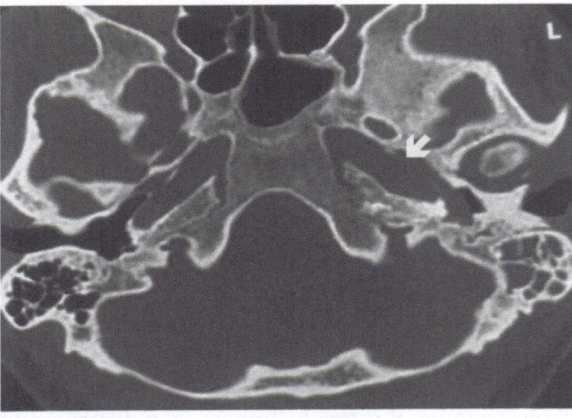

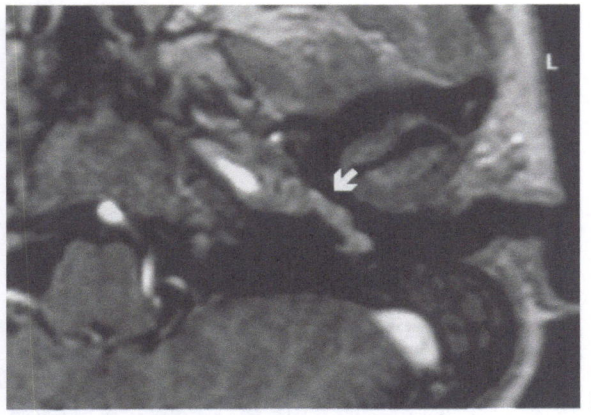

Fig. 5.10. a Axial HRCT image: mass within the left hypotympanum (*arrow*). **b** Axial T1-weighted MRI with contrast: enhancing mass in the left hypotympanum representing a glomus jugulo-tympanicum tumor

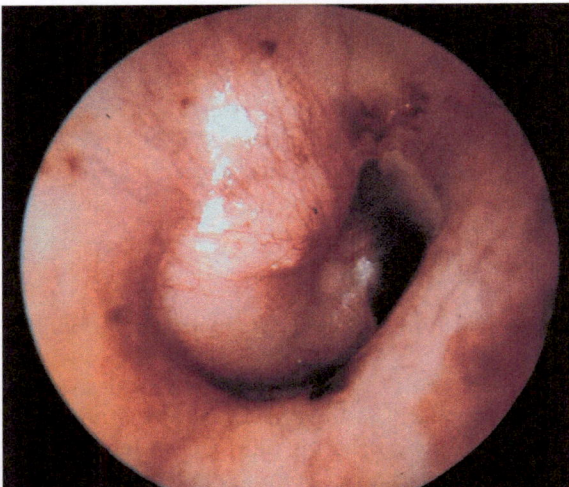

Fig. 5.11. Otoscopy photo: white mass filling parts of the middle ear. Histology: adenoma of middle ear

be differentiated from metastasis of adenocarcinomas of other sites. With MRI and CT the tumor may show aggressiveness against the surrounding tissue. In cases of brain invasion prognosis is worse even in this slow-growing tumor which does not metastasize (Fig. 5.13; WENIG 1993; DADAS et al. 2001).

5.4.2.3
Squamous Cell Carcinoma of the Middle Ear

Squamous cell carcinoma of the middle ear is an epithelial neoplasm of epidermoid cells arising from the middle ear mucosa. It is most commonly seen in the sixth and seventh decades of life. The patients have a long history of chronic otitis media. In up to 25% of patients concomitant cholesteatomas are seen. The treatment is radical surgery with radiotherapy. The prognosis is poor. The 5-year survival rate is 39%.

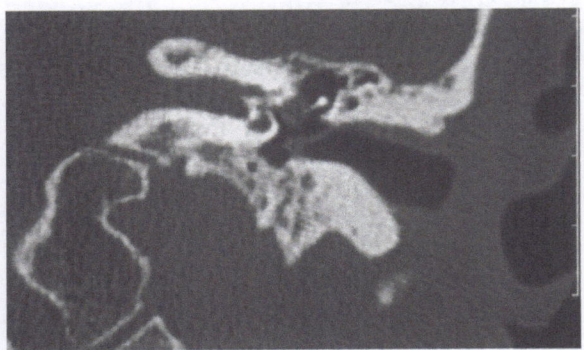

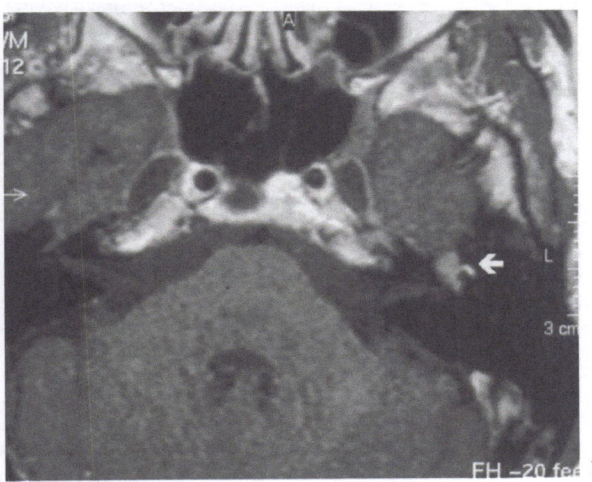

Fig. 5.12. a Coronal HRCT image visualizing a 5-mm soft tissue mass near the stapes and round window. **b** Axial T1-weighted MRI with contrast shows enhancement of the soft tissue mass. Histology proved an adenoma (carcinoid; *arrow*)

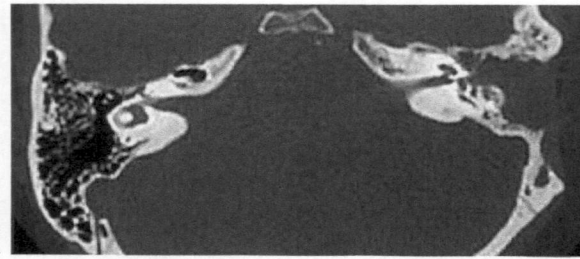

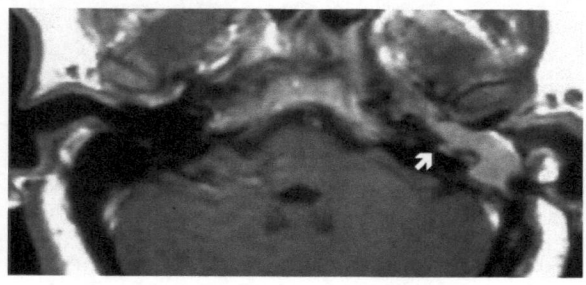

Fig. 5.13. a Axial HRCT image: huge soft tissue mass in the left tympanum with extensive bony destruction. **b** Axial T1-weighted MRI with contrast: the soft tissue is well delineated. There is not much enhancement. *Arrow* points to soft tissue mass within the tympanum. Histology revealed an adenocarcinoma of the middle ear

Imaging is necessary to evaluate the tumor extension and therapy control. Lymph node metastases are found in 25% of cases.

5.4.2.4
Middle Ear Schwannoma

Middle ear schwannomas are benign neoplasms arising from the facial nerve (Fig. 5.14), chorda tympani, or Jacobson's nerve – or may originate from the VIII

to XI cranial nerves extending into the tympanic cavity, bulging through the round window or eroding the jugular foramen (KERTESZ et al. 2001).

In 59% of cases it is found in the mastoid segment, and in 20% in the intracanalicular and labyrinthine segment (LILIEQUIST et al. 1972). Facial nerve schwannoma are the most common primary neural neoplasm within the middle ear. Usually, the clinical presentation consists of conductive hearing loss and facial nerve dysfunction. Taste abnormalities are described in lesions involving the chorda tympani.

The CT appearance is non-specific and does not allow differential diagnosis from paraganglioma or cholesteatoma. But this technique may demonstrate ossicular erosion and the involvement of the lateral semicircular canal. Magnetic resonance imaging characterizes the lesion better. Intravenous contrast-medium application causes relevant enhancement, although not as intensely as in paraganglioma. The pattern of growth along the course of the facial nerve (Jacobson's nerve or chorda tympani) further raises the probability of a schwannoma (Fig. 5.14).

Malignant transformation is exceedingly rare and, if present, neurofibromatosis should be suspected (JÄGER and REISER 2001).

5.4.2.5
Congenital (Primary) Cholesteatoma (Epidermoid)

Congenital cholesteatomas arise from sequestrations of epidermal cells at the time of closure of the medullary groove, between the third and fifth embryonic weeks. They are far less common than their acquired counterpart (only 2% of all cholesteatomas). Within the temporal bone, congenital cholesteatomas may arise in the petrous apex, the area of the geniculate

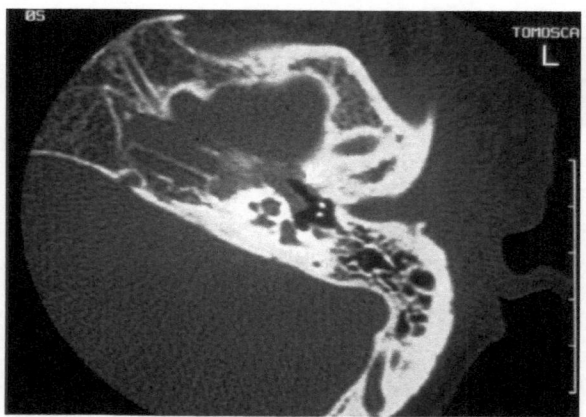

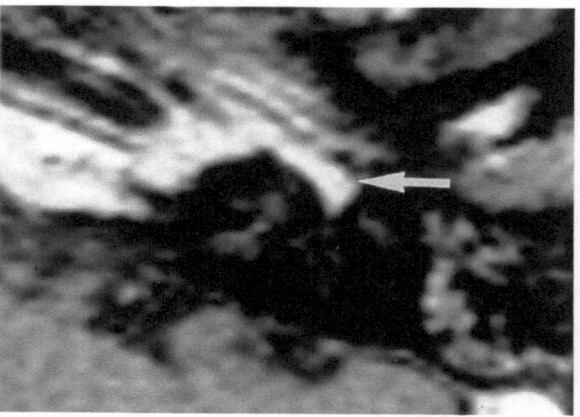

Fig. 5.14. a Axial HRCT image: elongated soft tissue mass along the facial nerve in the segment (*arrow*). **b** Axial T1-weighted MRI with contrast reveals an elongated hyperintense lesion compatible with facial nerve schwannoma (*arrow*)

ganglion, the middle ear, and mastoid process. Two typical sites within the middle ear are described: the anterior epitympanum, in the proximity of the eustachian tube opening; and the posterior mesotympanum, close to the incudostapedial joint. Progressive conductive hearing loss may be the patient's complaint. In almost all patients there is no history of chronic otitis media. The tympanic membrane is uninterrupted and the mastoid cells are clear. Facial nerve impairment results from anterior epitympanum lesions, undetectable at otoscopy. The age-incidence range is from birth to 80 years with gender equality, but 75% of the tumors are found in young children. The CT density is comparable to that of acquired cholesteatomas, but there are no signs of abnormal mastoid aeration. With MRI, on T2-weighted images hyperintensity exists, whereas on T1-weighted images low intensity is shown. There is no contrast enhancement (Fig. 5.15). Cholesteatomas impinge on and gradually may destroy the ossicular chain.

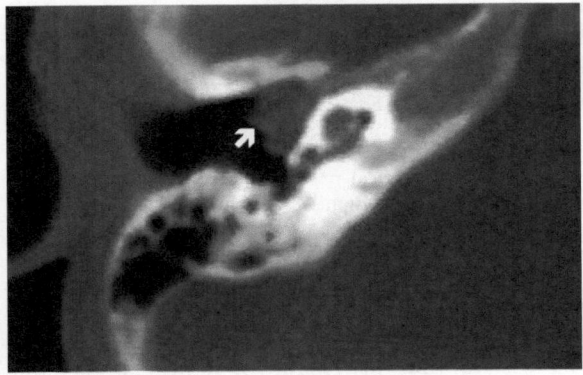

Fig. 5.15. Axial CT image (6-year-old child): soft tissue mass in the anterior portion of the mesotympanum (*arrow*). The mastoid cells are clear and intact

Within the petrous apex congenital cholesteatomas are typically large, expansible unilobulated, or multilobulated well-demarcated lesions that tend to elevate and thin the petrous ridge. It may extend in the middle or posterior cranial fossa and expand the bone around it into an egg-shell-thin, incomplete capsule. The margins always remain clearly defined, scalloped, and sclerotic. Erosions of the vestibular or cochlear or internal meatus acusticus are not uncommon. With CT a well-defined soft tissue mass is seen, which shows no contrast enhancement (Fig. 5.16).

5.4.3
Inner Ear

5.4.3.1
Schwannoma

Primary tumors of the inner ear are exceedingly rare. This statement is also right for the cochlear nerve or vestibular nerve schwannomas. They show the typical imaging findings already described in schwannomas of the facial nerve. Computed tomography may outline a local bony destruction of the cochlea or parts of the semicircular canal or vestibulum. Characteristic is the strong contrast enhancement on T1-weighted MR images (Figs. 5.17, 5.18). On T2-weighted images they are depicted as a round-shaped slightly hypointense mass.

5.4.3.2
Endolymphatic Sac Tumor

Endolymphatic sac tumor (ELST) is a very rare tumor (less than 100 cases worldwide have been described). Its full name is adenoma or adenocar-

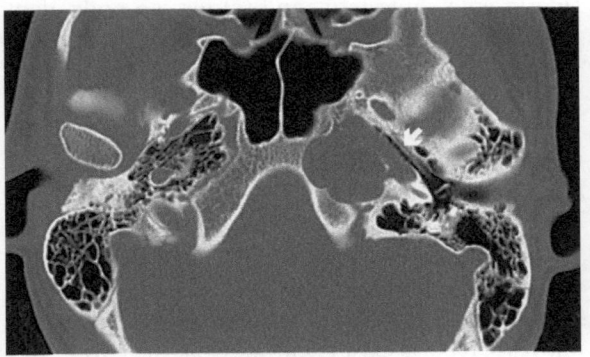
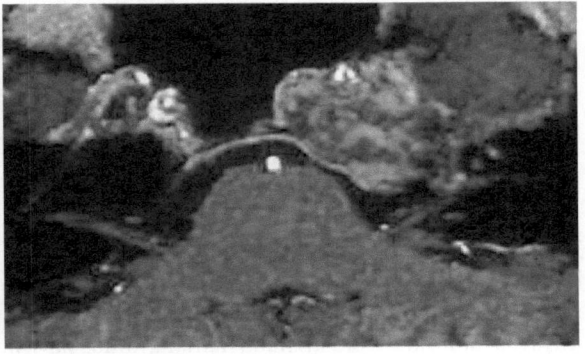

a b

Fig. 5.16. a Axial HRCT image shows a large soft tissue mass in the anterior part of the pyramid. The margins of the expansive tumor are well defined and the thin sclerotic margins are compatible with extreme slow growth (*arrow*). **b** Axial T1-weighted MRI with contrast: inhomogeneous tumor in the anterior part of the pyramid. No enhancement! Histology: primary cholesteatoma

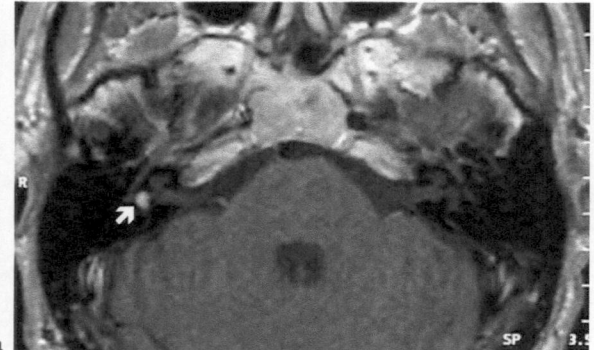

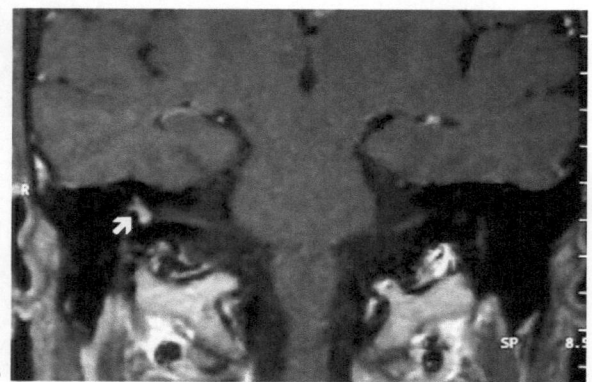

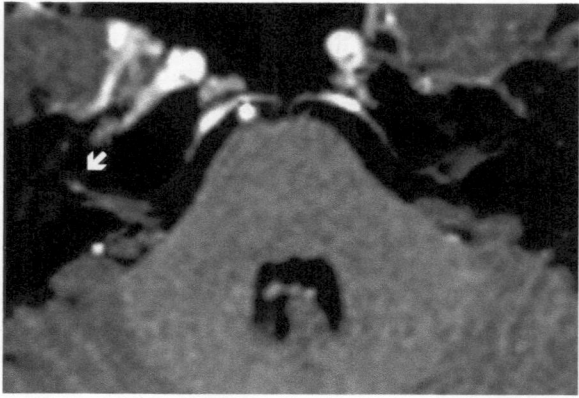

Fig. 5.18. Axial T1-weighted MRI with contrast: tiny enhancement within the cochlea representing a N. cochlearis schwannoma (*arrow*)

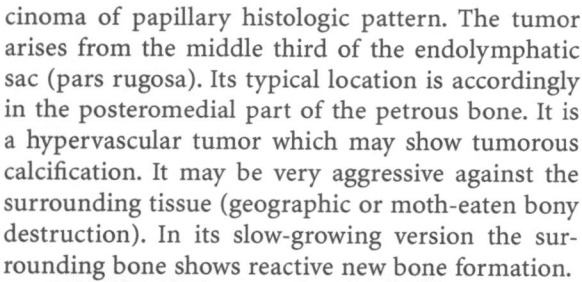

Fig. 5.17. **a** Axial T1-weighted MRI with contrast: strong enhancement within the vestibulum (*arrow*). **b** Coronal T1-weighted MRI with contrast: strong enhancement in the vestibulum representing a N. vestibularis schwannoma (*arrow*)

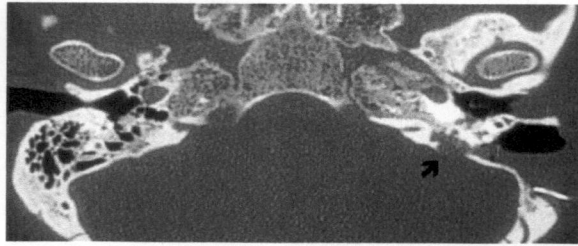

Fig. 5.19. Axial HRCT revealing an irregular defect (osteodestruction) in the typical position of the endolymphatic sac representing an endolymphatic sac tumor (ELST; *arrow*)

cinoma of papillary histologic pattern. The tumor arises from the middle third of the endolymphatic sac (pars rugosa). Its typical location is accordingly in the posteromedial part of the petrous bone. It is a hypervascular tumor which may show tumorous calcification. It may be very aggressive against the surrounding tissue (geographic or moth-eaten bony destruction). In its slow-growing version the surrounding bone shows reactive new bone formation.

With CT the above-mentioned tumoral calcification, new bone formation bone, and/or destruction (Fig. 5.19), and the enhancing soft tissue mass in the typical location, are well delineated. Magnetic resonance imaging allows outlining of the complete soft tissue tumor mass with enormous enhancement after i.v. contrast-medium application (Fig. 5.20). Such lesions must be differentiated from paragangliomas, hemangiomas, meningiomas, chondrosarcomas, and metastasis. Paragangliomas show with MRI a typical intravascular flow-void artifact, hemangiomas have a different typical location. Meningioma and chondrosarcoma cannot be ruled out because of their imaging features. Metastases are rare in this location.

The ELST is found in patients between the ages of 20 and 80 years. Females and males are equally involved. Clinically, the patients show unilateral hearing loss and tinnitus. Therapy is radical surgery, but there is a high recurrence rate. There is a well-known higher incidence in von Hippel-Lindau disease.

From some authors three different phases of an ELST are differentiated: (a) hemorrhage; (b) hemosiderin with cholesterol; and (c) foreign body giant cells and bone destruction (MUKHERJI et al. 1997).

5.4.4
Other Tumors (Not Originating from the External Ear, Middle Ear, or Inner Ear)

These tumors are in the vast majority of cases of mesenchymal origin and include benign and malignant lesions. Altogether they are exceedingly rare; for some, only case reports exist (TARHAN et al. 2000; ALLEYNE et al. 2000; RAMIREZ-CAMACHO et al. 1998).

Clinically important is the rhabdomyosarcoma, which is highly aggressive. Among the pediatric

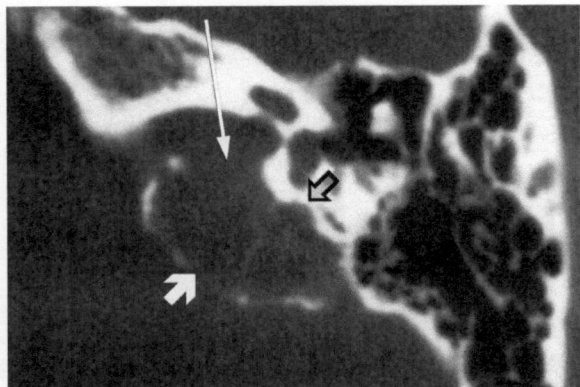

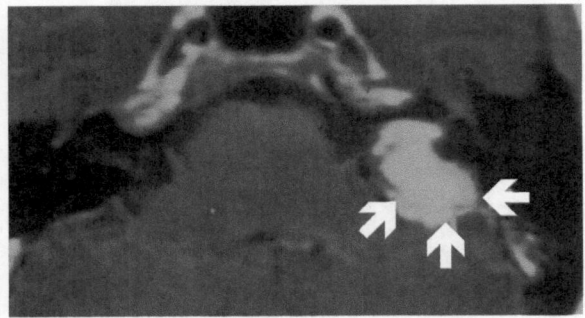

Fig. 5.20. a Axial CT: large retrolabyrinthine soft tissue mass (*long arrow*) with geographic marginal calcification (*white arrow*). Porus acusticus internus (*open black arrow*). **b** Axial T1-weighted MRI with contrast: strong enhancement of the tumor (*white arrow*). Histology: ELST tumor

population it accounts for the second most common head and neck malignancy. It is much more common in whites than in blacks or Asians. The average age at onset is 4.4 years. Most case reports support the middle ear origin in the muscle cells near the eustachian tube or the mastoid. Its aggressive pattern of growth leads to marked bone destruction with early involvement of the facial nerve and potential intracranial spread. Distant metastases are found in the lungs, bones, and liver (SWARTZ and HAMSBERGER 1998; SOM and CURTIN 1994). Regional lymph node involvement is found in 5–20% of cases. Treatment includes non-radical surgery as well as radio- and chemotherapy. The survival rate is directly related to the extent of disease at diagnosis (Table 5.2), which

Table 5.2. Clinical grouping: classification of rhabdomyosarcoma

Group I	Localized disease, complete resection
Group II	Microscopic residual disease after regional resection
Group III	Incomplete resection with gross residual disease
Group IV	Distant metastasis

makes imaging very important. The 5-year survival rate varies between 20 and 83%.

Computed tomography shows a soft tissue mass with extensive bony destruction, MRI a T1-weighted hypointense heterogeneous mass which enhances after contrast application. The mass is irregularly demarcated and poorly defined and may show hemorrhage. The presence of parameningeal involvement is important for staging; therefore, MRI with contrast application is the imaging modality of choice.

Non-Hodgkin's lymphoma may very rarely involve the temporal bone. The tumor is on CT and MRI a relative homogenous soft tissue mass that destroys all bony structures (Figs. 5.21, 5.22). There may be regressive changes with bleeding and cyst formation.

Other tumors reported are Ewing-, fibro-, osteo-, and chondrosarcomas. Benign lesions include osteoblastoma, giant cell tumor, chondroblastoma, and hemangiomas. Of these tumors, Ewing, chondro-, and osteosarcomas; osteoblastomas and chondroblastomas may show intratumoral calcification as well (Fig. 5.23; DOSHI et al. 2001). Cartilage tumor calcification may be differentiated by MRI because of its high hyperintensity on T2-weighted images.

Secondary tumors to the temporal bone are not as uncommon as would be expected. They may be found in patients with squamous cell carcinoma of the head and neck as well as with mammary gland, lung, kidney, and prostate carcinoma, and with melanomas as well. Due to the high vascularization of the apex of the petrous bone it is usually involved. The lesion may be either lytic or blastic, or mixed, depending on the structure of the primary tumor. The metastasis my invade the middle ear and/or mastoid (Figs. 5.24, 5.25).

Finally, the temporal bone may be invaded by neighboring aggressive lesions, most commonly from nasopharyngeal tumors which may grow in through foramina, fissures, along vessels, or nerves.

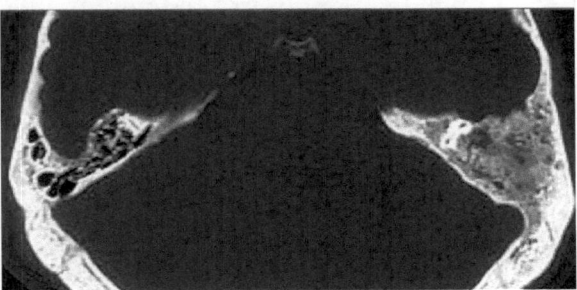

Fig. 5.21. Axial HRCT: left-sided irregular bony destruction within the petrous bone representing a lymphoma

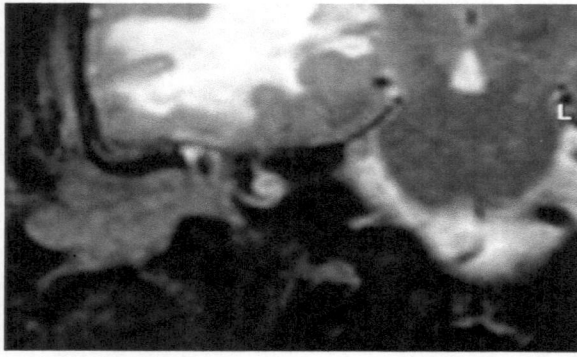
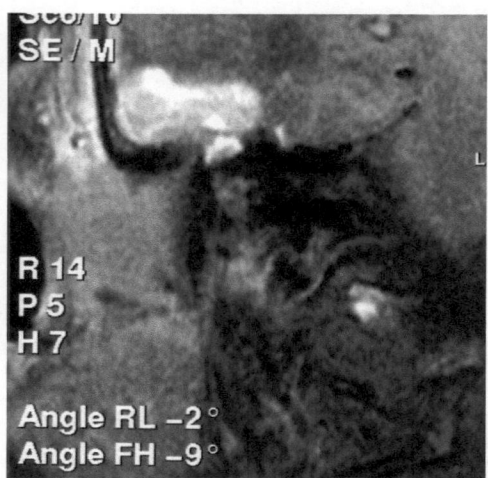

Fig. 5.22. a Coronal T2-weighted MRI showing a soft tissue mass within the middle ear. Brain edema. **b** Coronal T1-weighted MRI with contrast showing enhancement in the neighboring brain structures representing an infiltrative lymphoma

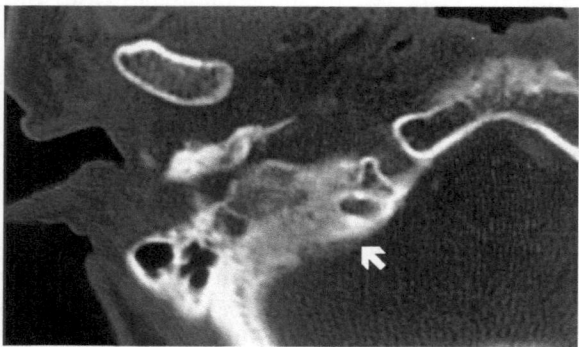

Fig. 5.23. Axial HRCT revealing a sclerosing formation within the petrous bone with irregular margins (*arrow*). Histology: osteosarcoma

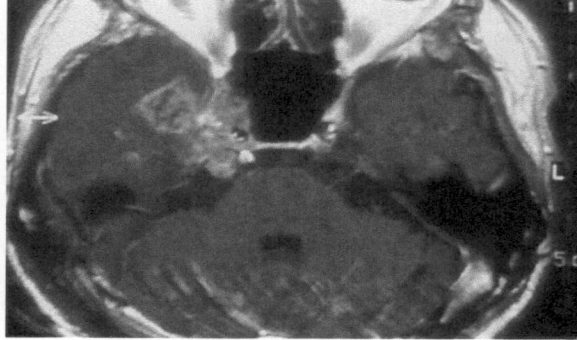

Fig. 5.24. Axial HRCT: irregular sclerotic tumor near the anterior part of the pyramid. Histology: metastases from squamous cell carcinoma of the tonsilla

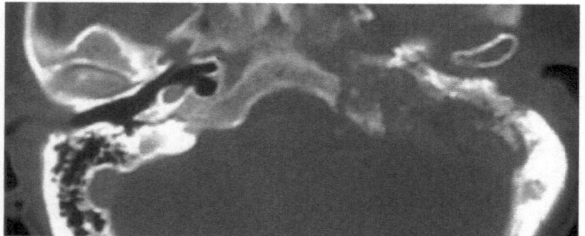

Fig. 5.25. Axial HRCT: osteolytic process with the petrous bone. Metastasis from mammary carcinoma

References

Alleyne CH, Theodore N, Spetzler RF, Coons SW (2000) Osteosarcoma of the temporal fossa with hemorrhagic presentation: case report. Neurosurgery 47:447–451

Benjamin B, Bingham B, Hawke M, Stammberger H (1995) A colour atlas of otorhino laryngology. Dunitz, London

Casselmann JW, Offeciers EF, De Foer B, Govaerts P, Kuhweide R, Somers T (2001) CT and MR imaging of congenital abnormalities of the inner ear and internal auditory canal. Eur J Radiol 40:94–104

Dadas B, Alkan S, Turgut S, Basak T (2001) Primary papillary adenocarcinoma confined to the middle ear and mastoid. Eur Arch Otorhinolaryngol 258:93–95

Doshi SV, Frantz TD, Korol HW (2001) Benign osteoblastoma of the temporal bone: case report and literature review. Am J Otolaryngol 22:211–214

Jäger L, Reiser M (2001) CT and MR imaging of the normal and pathologic conditions of the facial nerve. Eur J Radiol 40:133–146

Kertesz TR, Shelton C, Wiggins RH, Salzman KL, Glastonbury CM, Harnsberger R (2001) Intratemporal facial nerve neuroma: anatomical location and radiological features. Laryngoscope 111:1250–1256

Liliequist B, Thulin A, Tovin D, Wiberg A, Ohmand J (1972) Neurinoma of the labyrinthine portion of the facial nerve. J Neurosurg 37:105–109

Manolidis S, Shohet JA, Jackson CG, Glasscock ME (1999) Malignant glomus tumors. Laryngoscope 109:30–34

Maroldi R, Farina D, Palvarini L, Marconi A, Gadola E, Menni K, Battaglia G (2001) Computed tomography and magnetic resonance imaging of pathologic conditions of the middle ear. Eur J Radiol 40:78–94

Mukherji SK, Albernaz VS, Lo WW, Gattey MJ, Megerian CA, Feghali JG, Brook A, Lewin JS, Lanzieri F (1997) Papillary endolymphatic sac tumors: CT, MR imaging, and angiographic findings in 20 patients. Radiology 202:801–808

Nager GT (1993) Pathology of the ear and temporal bone. Williams and Wilkins, Baltimore

Noujaim SE, Pattekar MA, Cacciarelli A, Sanders WP, Wang AM (2000) Paraganglioma of the temporal bone: role of magnetic resonance imaging versus computed tomography. Top Magn Reson Imaging 11:108–122

Ramirez-Camacho R, Pinilla M, Ramon-y-Cajal S, Garcia-Berrocal JR, Vicente J (1998) Chondrosarcoma of the temporal bone and otosclerosis. ORL J Otorhinolaryngol Relat Spec 60:58–60

Sabnis EV, Mafee MF, Chen R, Alperin N (2000) Magnetic resonance imaging of the normal temporal bone. Top Magn Reson Imaging 11:2–10

Som P, Curtin HD (eds) (1994) Head and neck imaging. Mosby, Baltimore

Swartz JD, Harnsberger HR (1998) Imaging of the temporal bone. Thieme, New York

Tarhan NC, Yologlu Z, Tutar N-U, Coskun M, Agildere AM, Arikan U (2000) Chondromyxoid fibroma of the temporal bone: CT and MRI findings. Eur Radiol 10:1678–1680

Valvassori GE, Mafee MF, Carter BL (1995) Head and neck imaging. Thieme, New York

Van Gilse PHG (1938) Des observations ulterieurs sur la genese des exostosis du conduit externe par l'irritation d'eau froid. Acta Otolaryngol 26:343–348

Wenig BM (1993) Atlas of the head and neck pathology. Saunders, Philadelphia

---

The Clinician's View

I. Dhooge

The complex anatomy of the temporal bone and the different tissue types within makes it host to a large variety of tumoral processes with a broad range of clinical manifestations. Some of them have already been discussed, or will be discussed in other chapters. It is clear that the tumors found in an adult or pediatric population are often of a very different nature.

Computed tomography and MRI studies can help, especially in children, in the differential diagnosis. These studies also provide information regarding tumor size and the proximity and involvement of these tumors with the internal carotid artery, cranial nerves, and intracranial structures. In addition, the presence or absence of bone erosion or destruction can be identified, allowing the surgeon to anticipate the malignant character of the tumor preoperatively.

Imaging can also assist in identifying the ideal location of a biopsy within the temporal bone.

In the follow-up after therapy, imaging can sometimes be helpful in making the difference between fibrotic tissue, recurrence of tumor, or post-radiotherapy swelling.

6 Acute Otomastoiditis and Its Complications

M. LEMMERLING

CONTENTS

6.1
Introduction

The middle ear and mastoid constitute an extension of the upper respiratory tract. Via the aditus ad antrum the mastoid antrum, which is the largest mastoid cell, communicates with the epitympanic portion of the middle ear cavity. The middle ear and adjacent pneumatized portions of the temporal bone are subject to bacterial invasion via the eustachian tube. When a mild infection occurs pain will be present for a short period, the tympanic membrane will be hyperemic and an appropriate therapy leads to healing without functional alterations; however, if an acute infection persists for more than a few days, resorption of the ossicles will occur, as well as of the mastoid, by a process of demineralization and osteoclastic activity. In case of more pronounced disease, the tympanic cavity wall and/or mastoid wall can be destructed and a subperiosteal abscess, Bezold's abscess (break through the mastoid tip), sigmoid sinus thrombosis, or otogenic brain abscess is formed. In rare cases bacterial labyrinthitis can complicate acute infectious middle ear disease. Meningitis is another rare complication of acute infectious

M. LEMMERLING, MD, PhD
Medische Beeldvorming, A.Z. St. Lucas, Groenebriel 1,
9000 Gent, Belgium

otomastoid disease and is most often hematogenous in nature (FRIEDMAN et al. 1990).

The clinical picture of mastoiditis has changed a lot with the advent of antibiotics. A delay is consequently noted in the recognition of the intracranial complications in children and in the institution of appropriate therapy (KUCZKOWSKI and MIKASZEWSKI 2001). Data suggest that the suppurative complications of acute otitis media are increasing due to an increasing incidence of resistant *Streptococcus pneumoniae* (BACH et al. 1998; ZAPALAC et al. 2002). Despite the use of specialized imaging modalities, antibiotics, and microsurgical procedures, the resulting mortality of intracranial otogenic complications is still approximately 10% (KAFTAN and DRAF 2000).

Streptococcus pneumoniae is the most common pathogen causing intracranial-complicating acute otitis media (meningitis, brain abscess, subdural empyema; KAFTAN and DRAF 2000). *Streptococcus pyogenes* is another important pathogen (BAHADORI et al. 2000; DOBBEN et al. 2000). Fungal mastoiditis is almost exclusively seen in immunocompromised patients (SLACK et al. 1999; YATES et al. 1997). Massive granulations and proliferation of fungi can create fistula to the inner ear, mimicking cholesteatoma on imaging studies (OHKI et al. 2001; CHEN et al. 1999). Early surgical débridement followed by antimicrobial therapy may be life preserving in this patient population (CHEN et al. 1999). Other unusual pathogens, such as *Rhodococcus equi*, should be included in the differential diagnosis of the immunocompromised patient with aggressive otitis (IBARRA and JINKINS 1999). Otomastoiditis is a rare but important manifestation of tuberculosis and should be considered if a history of chronic otorrhea resistant to conventional therapy is found in a patient with widespread temporal bone destruction on CT examinations (CAVALLIN and MUREN 2000). Nontuberculous mycobacterial mastoiditis presents in the same manner, but is often resistant to antituberculous agents, so the preferred treatment is mastoidectomy (STEWART et al. 1995).

6.2
Coalescent Mastoiditis and Mastoid Subperiosteal Abscess

The local clinical manifestations of advancing acute mastoiditis are pain and erythema in the mastoid region, tenderness, swelling in the postauricular region with protrusion of the auricle, and edema of the posterosuperior wall of the external auditory canal. All four signs are present in approximately 40% of cases (COHEN-KEREM et al. 1999). Postauricular erythema and protrusion of the auricle are the two most frequent clinical signs of acute mastoiditis for some authors (COHEN-KEREM et al. 1999; BAHADORI et al. 2000), whereas other groups mention that these two specific signs were rare in their population (DHOOGE et al. 1998). In 95% of these patients a concomitant ipsilateral, inflamed, bulging, and immobile eardrum is seen (BAHADORI et al. 2000).

If an acute otomastoid infection persists for more than a few days, resorption of the ossicles and mastoid can occur by a process of demineralization and osteo-clastic activity. In such circumstances mastoid cells will coalesce and the term "coalescent mastoiditis" is used (Fig. 6.1). Recent studies suggest that coalescent mastoiditis has a current incidence of 0.24% patients with suppurative otitis media (SPIEGEL et al. 1998).

Recently, the sensitivity and accuracy of temporal bone CT findings was evaluated for the diagnosis of acute coalescent mastoiditis, by scoring for mastoid bone integrity on three points: the air cell septa; the sigmoid cortical plate; and the lateral cortical wall. Computed tomography turned out to be a valuable technique, and the erosion of the cortical plate that overlies the sigmoid sinus was the most sensitive and specific CT finding for distinguishing coalescent from noncoalescent mastoiditis (ANTONELLI et al. 1999).

Mastoid subperiosteal abscess develops when the process of coalescence of the mastoid cells leads to a breakthrough of the mastoid cortex and a pus collection appears in the postauricular soft tissues. At this moment clinical examinations and imaging studies, CT as well as MR, become very important, since the difference between the periostitis stage and

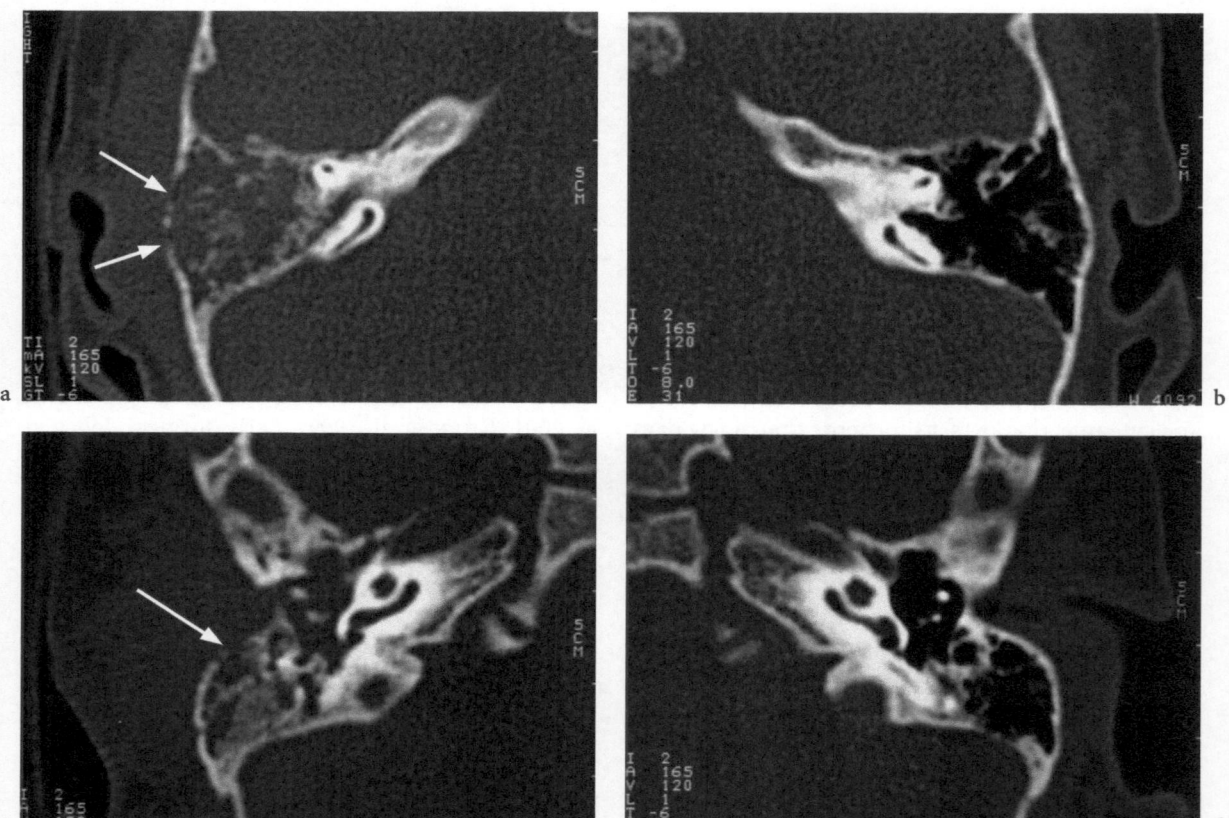

Fig. 6.1. a, c Computed tomography in a patient with coalescent mastoiditis on the right side obviously shows coalescence of the mastoid cells and resorption of the lateral mastoid wall (*arrows*). **b, d** The contralateral normal ear is shown

the abscess stage cannot be deducted from the initial body temperature of the patient, the number of polymorphonuclear cells, or the CRP values (FRANÇOIS et al. 2001). Subperiosteal abscess is seen in nearly 50% of patients diagnosed with coalescent mastoiditis (SPIEGEL et al. 1998). The destructed lateral cortical otomastoid wall is easily visualized on CT examinations, and the images in soft tissue setting will show the present abscess (Fig. 6.2). Magnetic resonance imaging is able to show the same findings.

In a retrospective study of 48 children with postauricular swelling and otoscopic signs of acute otitis media the mastoid pus and the otorrhea were sterile, whereas *Streptococcus pneumoniae* was the most pathogenic (FRANÇOIS et al. 2001). While traditionally in children mastoid subperiosteal abscess required mastoidectomy, the improvement of antibiotic therapy has now changed this approach. It is accepted that uncomplicated acute mastoiditis is treated with myringotomy and intravenous antibiotics (COHEN-KEREM et al. 1999), and that in case of mastoid subperiosteal abscess formation treatment consists of tympanostomy tube insertion, intravenous antibiotics, and postauricular incision with abscess drainage. Such procedure obviates morbidity and complications of mastoid surgery in children (BAUER et al. 2002).

In rare cases the pus escapes the mastoid near the incisura digastrica and tracks along the digastric and sternocleidomastoid muscles into the neck. Such abscesses are classically referred to as Bezold's abscess (SPIEGEL et al. 1998). Reports of Bezold's abscess in children are rare, since their mastoid pneumatization is not yet completed (MARIONO et al. 2001). Most Bezold's abscesses are seen in adults and are associated with a history of cholesteatoma and mastoidectomy (CASTILLO et al. 1998).

6.3
Complications

The clinical course of acute otitis media is often short and the process terminates because of the host's immune system, the infection-resistant properties of the mucosal linings, and the susceptibility of the major organisms to penicillin. Approximately 1–5% of untreated or inadequately treated patients may experience complications. Prior to these complications warning symptoms or signs may be evident: severe earache and/or headache; vertigo; chills and fever; and meningeal symptoms or signs (DOBBEN et al. 2000).

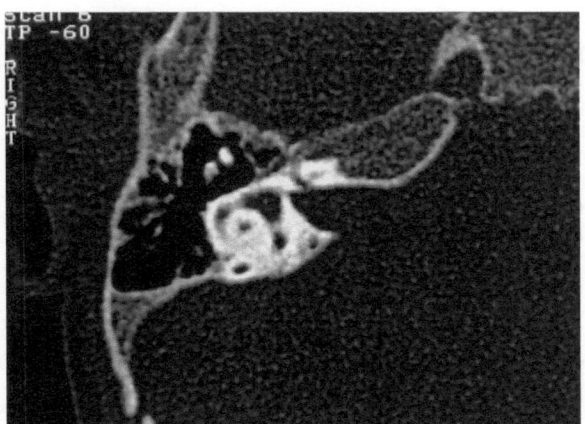

a

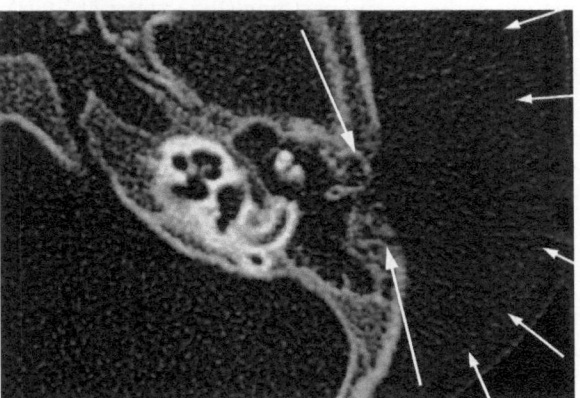

b

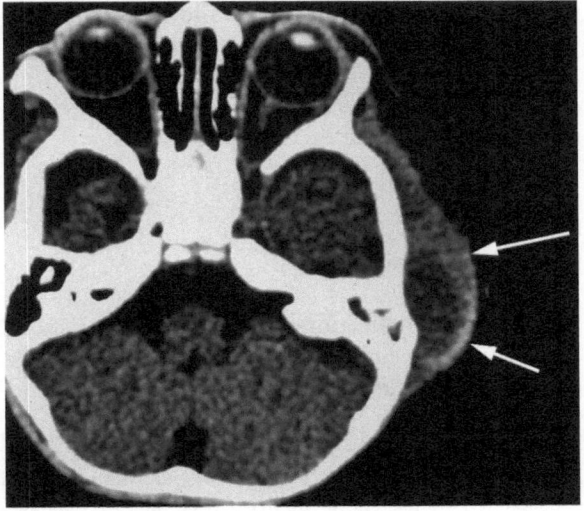

c

Fig. 6.2. Computed tomography of the normal right temporal bone shows **a** a normal lateral otomastoid cortex, whereas on **b** the contralateral side the lateral cortex of the opacified otomastoid is fragmented (*large arrows*) and soft tissue swelling is seen (*small arrows*). **c** This subperiosteal abscess (*arrows*) is best evaluated on images in soft tissue setting

If complications of inflammatory otomastoid disease are suspected, CT permits accurate diagnosis (DOBBEN et al. 2000), but MR is the imaging modality of choice (DOBBEN et al. 2000; MAROLDI et al. 2001)

6.3.1
Otogenic Intracranial Abscess

Increasing temporoparietal headache, near the affected ear, is often the only indication of otogenic brain abscess formation (DOBBEN et al. 2000). Although rarely seen, among all intracranial complications of middle ear disease, epidural abscess formation is the commonest one (BIZAKIS et al. 1998). It is most frequently seen as a severe complication of the untreated cholesteatoma, but is also noted in patients suffering from acute mastoiditis. Its therapy depends on the importance of the abscess formation and ranges from high-dose antibiotics to drainage (KEMPF et al. 1998).

Magnetic resonance is the modality of choice to image these abscesses. In view of imaging characteristics an otogenic intracranial abscess is not different from nonotogenic intracranial abscesses, but its location is typically in the temporal lobe or cerebellum, and the ipsilateral middle ear and mastoid are opacified. The mass generally has a mixed high signal on the T2-weighted images, a mixed low signal on the T1-weighted images, and is surrounded by edema. After intravenous injection of gadolinium, ring enhancement is seen. Hemorrhage may be present in some parts of the abscess (Fig. 6.3).

6.3.2
Sinus Thrombosis

Among all complications of mastoiditis, sigmoid and transverse sinus thrombosis is the least frequent one (ROCHA et al. 2000). It is described to be occasionally complicated by cerebellar venous infarction (NAYAK et al. 1994; RAM et al. 2001). Sinus thrombosis is a difficult entity to diagnose, in the present author's experience, the disease is easiest to recognize on T1-weighted images before intravenous injection of gadolinium, where the thrombus has an increased signal (Fig. 6.4). The MR angiographic techniques with phase contrast are another valuable alternative.

The exact relationship between sinus thrombosis and mastoid disease remains a point of debate in the literature. In many of these thrombosis patients no signs of mastoid infection were present, which is the reason why is it believed that the mastoid changes are likely due to venous congestion as a consequence of the sinus thrombosis and not of mastoiditis (FINK and MCAULEY 2002). In a study of 27 children (of whom 61% were neonates) with cerebral venous thrombosis the most common risk factors were mastoiditis, persistent pulmonary hypertension, cardiac malformation, and dehydration. Many authors suggest to always test these children and young adults for protein-C and antithrombin-III deficiency, since these were the most common coagulopathies found in this population (CARVALHO et al. 2001; RAM et al. 2001).

Sigmoid sinus thrombosis has become increasingly uncommon, whereas in the pre-antibiotic era the condition was mortal in over 90% of the cases. Consequently, a high index of suspicion is actually required to make the diagnosis and opt for early surgical intervention (KEOGH et al. 2001; ROCHA et al. 2000). The presenting signs and symptoms are often subtle or non-specific and not in proportion to the magnitude of the problem, leading to a common delay in diagnosis (FRITSCH et al. 1990; RAM et al. 2001). It suggests that imaging studies be performed in all mastoiditis patients with pain or vertigo that is not rapidly resolving after appropriate antibiotic treatment (KEOGH et al. 2001). Patients may present with otorrhea, otalgia, neck pain, fever, and chills (SEE et al. 2000). The therapeutic strategy is a point of debate, and ranges

---

Fig. 6.3. a In this patient with acute otomastoiditis on the left side the axial T2-weighted image at temporal bone level shows the opacified left otomastoid (*arrows*). **b** The coronal T1-weighted image before injection of gadolinium shows a large hypointense region (*large arrows*) in the temporal lobe of the brain, with some hyperintense (hemorrhagic) components, and the opacified otomastoid is also shown (*small arrows*). **c** On the axial T2-weighted image at temporal lobe level an abscess is visualized (*small arrow*), surrounded by vasogenic edema (*large arrows*). **d** The coronal T2-weighted image shows the continuity between the abscess and its surrounding edema, on one hand (*large arrows*), and the inflammatory/infectious otomastoid disease (*small arrows*), on the other hand. The continuity is realized through an interrupted tegmen tympani. **e** Ring enhancement (*small arrow*) is demonstrated on the T1-weighted image after intravenous injection of gadolinium. The perilesional edema is not enhancing (*large arrows*). **f** The coronal T1-weighted image after gadolinium injection confirms the findings noted on the coronal T2-weighted image, with the enhancing abscess and the non-enhancing edema (*large arrows*) in the temporal lobe region, and the enhancing otomastoid disease (*small arrows*). Note that no linear signal void is present between both enhancing regions, indicating that the normal tegmen tympani is absent

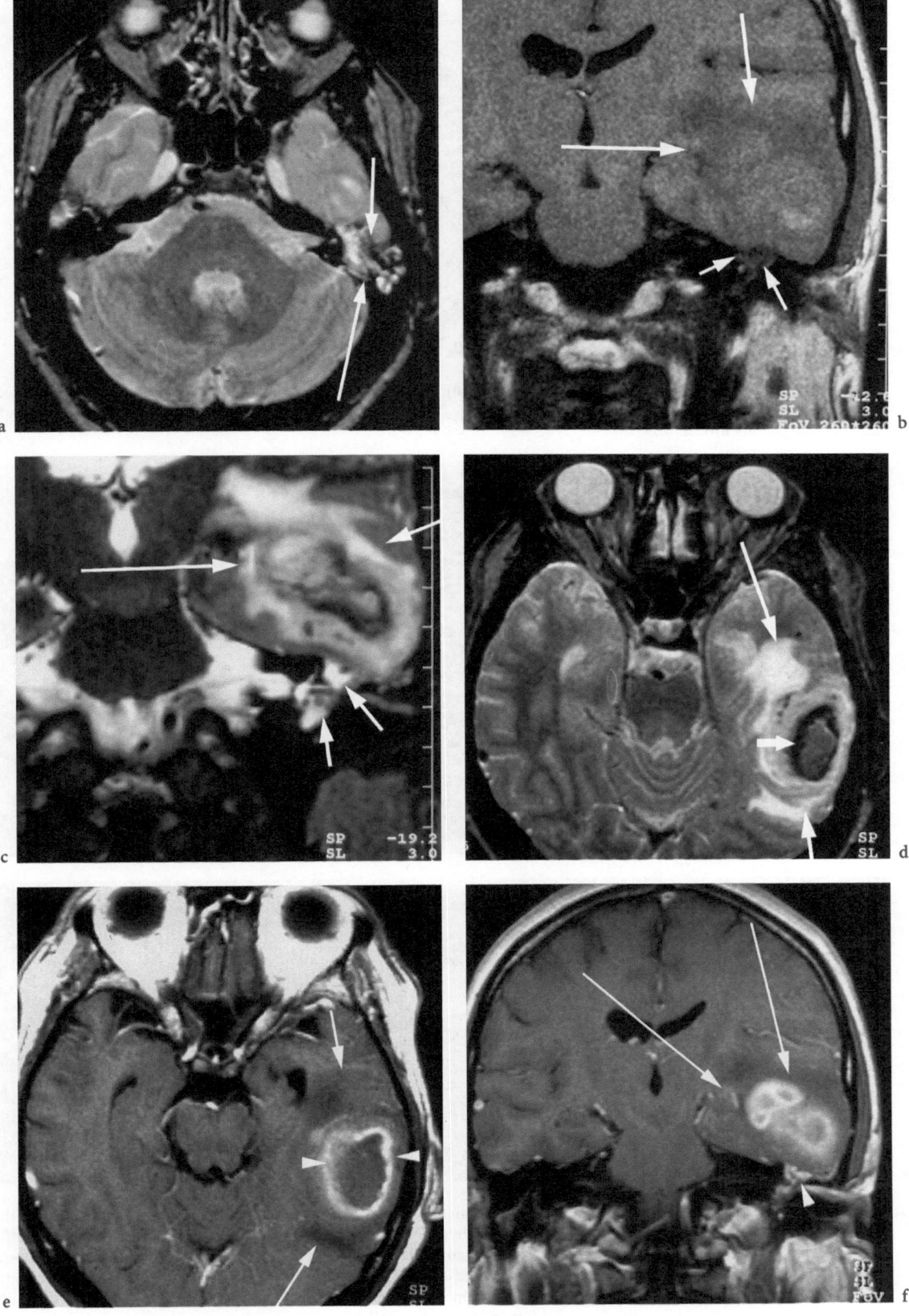

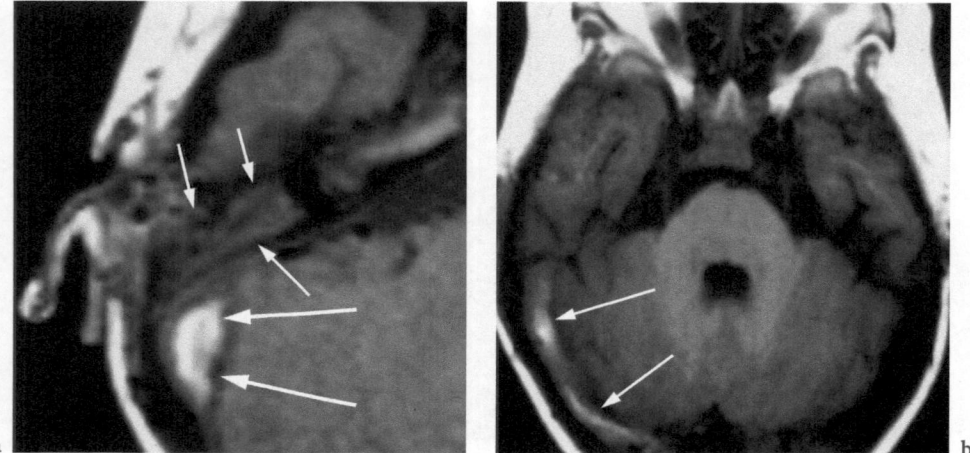

Fig. 6.4. a On the T1-weighted image before gadolinium injection in a patient with right-sided otomastoid opacification (*small arrows*) a high signal is present in the sigmoid sinus (*large arrows*), and is also seen in **b** the transverse sinus (*arrows*). Sigmoid and transverse sinus thrombosis

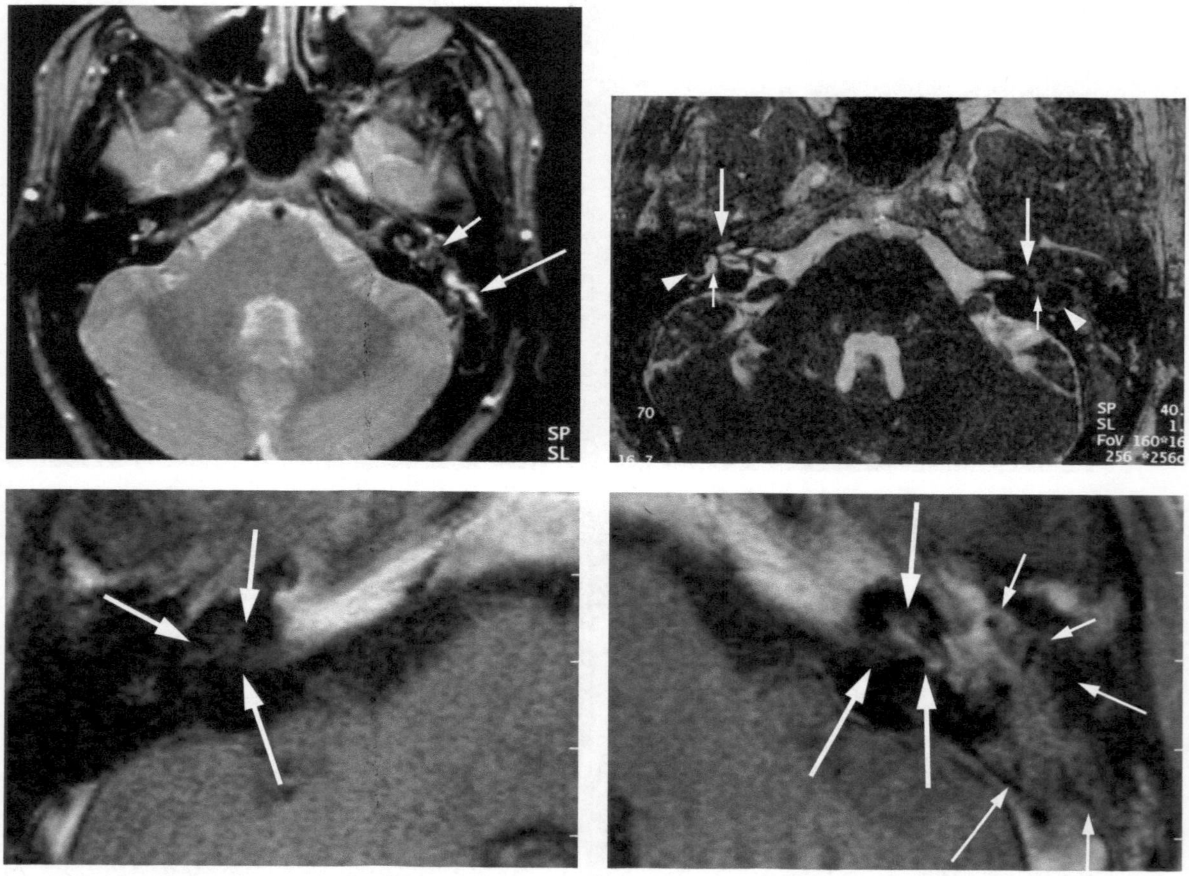

Fig. 6.5. a Axial T2-weighted image in a patient with otomastoiditis shows hyperintense opacification. **b** The 1-mm-thick T2-weighted image through the inner ear shows a normal hyperintense signal on the right side in the vestibule (*small arrow*), cochlea (*large arrow*), and lateral semicircular canal (*arrowhead*), indicating the normal presence of endo- and perilymph. The corresponding contralateral signal intensity is decreased in all these inner ear components. **c** The axial post-gadolinium T1-weighted image on the right side shows a normal signal in the inner ear (*arrows*), whereas **d** the left inner ear enhances strongly (*large arrows*), as well as the opacified left otomastoid (*small arrows*)

from internal jugular vein ligation, over anticoagulant therapy, to the administration of less conventional antibiotic therapy (DALLARI et al. 1997).

6.3.3
Labyrinthitis

Bacterial labyrinthitis that complicates otomastoid disease appears to happen via the round window. More often the involvement of the labyrinth is a reaction to bacterial exotoxins rather than bacterial invasion. This so-called tympanogenic labyrinthitis is unilateral in contrast to meningogenic labyrinthitis. Magnetic resonance imaging is the study of choice and shows that the endo- and perilymphatic spaces are filled with purulent material. The inner ear enhances on the T1-weighted images performed after gadolinium injection (Fig. 6.5).

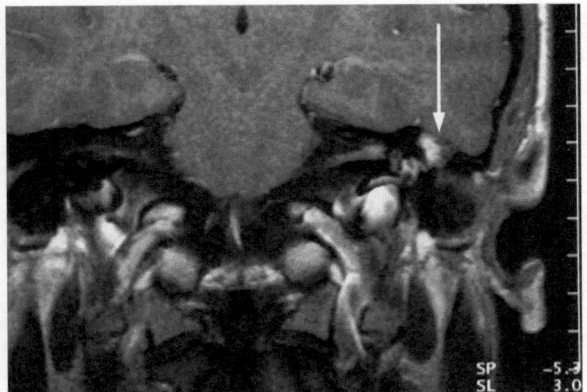

a

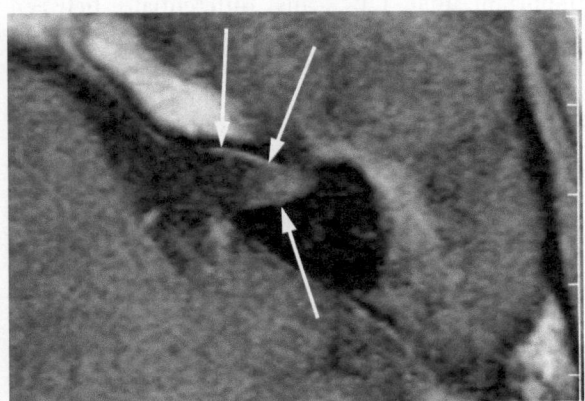

b

Fig. 6.6. a In a patient with acute otomastoiditis the coronal T1-weighted image after gadolinium injection shows the enhancing middle ear cavity and mastoid. **b** The axial T1-weighted image after gadolinium injection in the same patient shows linear enhancement along the walls of the internal auditory meatus, indicating the presence of meningeal thickening and inflammation

6.3.4
Meningitis

Meningitis is another rare complication of acute infectious otomastoid disease and is most often hematogenous in nature (Friedman et al. 1990). The enhancing thickened meningeal structures are best visualized on T1-weighted images after intravenous injection of gadolinium (Fig. 6.6).

References

Antonelli PJ, Garside JA, Mancuso AA, Strickler ST, Kubilis PS (1999) Computed tomography and the diagnosis of coalescent mastoiditis. Otolaryngol Head Neck Surg 120:350–354

Bach KK, Malis DJ, Magit AE, Pransky SM, Kearns DB, Seid AB (1998) Acute coalescent mastoiditis in an infant: an emerging trend? Otolaryngol Head Neck Surg 119:523–525

Bahadori RS, Schwartz RH, Ziai M (2000) Acute mastoiditis in children: an increase in frequency in northern Virginia. Pediatr Infect Dis J 19:212–215

Bauer PW, Brown KR, Jones DT (2002) Mastoid subperiosteal abscess management in children. Int J Pediatr Otorhinolaryngol 63:185–188

Bizakis JG, Velegrakis GA, Papadakis CE, Karampekios SK, Helidonis ES (1998) The silent epidural abscess as a complication of acute otitis media in children. Int J Pediatr Otorhinolaryngol 45:163–166

Carvalho KS, Bodensteiner JB, Connolly PJ, Garg BP (2001) Cerebral venous thrombosis in children. J Child Neurol 16:574–580

Castillo M, Albernaz VS, Mukherji SK, Smith MM, Weissman JL (1998) Imaging of Bezold's abscess. Am J Roentgenol 171:1491–1495

Cavallin L, Muren C (2000) CT findings in tuberculous otomastoiditis. A case report. Acta Radiol 41:49–51

Chen D, Lalwani AK, House JW, Choo D (1999) Aspergillus mastoiditis in acquired immunodeficiency syndrome. Am J Otol 20:561–567

Cohen-Kerem R, Uri N, Rennert H, Peled N, Greenberg E, Efrat M (1999) Acute mastoiditis in children: Is surgical treatment necessary? J Laryngol Otol 113:1081–1085

Dallari S, Zaccarelli SC, Sintini M, Gatti G, Balli R (1997) Acute mastoiditis with complications: a report of two cases. Acta Otorhinolaryngol Belg 51:113–118

Dhooge IJ, Vandenbussche T, Lemmerling M (1998) Value of computed tomography of the temporal bone in acute otomastoiditis. Rev Laryngol Otol Rhino (Bord) 119:91–94

Dobben GD, Raofi B, Mafee MF, Kamel A, Mercurio S (2000) Otogenic intracranial inflammations: role of magnetic resonance imaging. Top Magn Reson Imaging 11:76–86

Fink JN, McAuley DL (2002) Mastoid air sinus abnormalities associated with lateral venous sinus thrombosis: cause or consequence? Stroke 33:290–292

François M, van den Abbeele T, Viala P, Narcy P (2001) Acute external mastoiditis in children: report of a series of 48 cases. Arch Pediatr 8:1050–1054

Friedman EM, McGill TJI, Healy GB (1990) Central nervous system complications associated with acute otitis media in children. Laryngoscope 100:149–151

Fritsch MH, Miyamoto RT, Wood TL (1990) Sigmoid sinus thrombosis diagnosis by contrasted MRI scanning. Otolaryngol Head Neck Surg 103:451–456

Ibarra R, Jinkins JR (1999) Severe otitis and mastoiditis due to *Rhodococcus equi* in a patient with AIDS. Case report. Neuroradiology 41:699–701

Kaftan H, Draf W (2000) Intracranial otogenic complications: in spite of therapeutic progress still a serious problem. Laryngorhinootologie 79:609–615

Kempf HG, Wiel J, Issing PR, Lenarz T (1998) Otogenic brain abscess Laryngorhinootologie 77:462–466

Keogh IJ, Hone SW, Colreavy M, Gaffney R (2001) Sigmoid sinus thrombosis: an old foe revisited. Ir Med J 94:117–118

Kuczkowski J, Mikaszewski B (2001) Intracranial complications of acute and chronic mastoiditis: report of two cases in children. Int J Pediatr Otorhinolaryngol 60:227–237

Marioni G, de Filippis C, Tregnaghi A, Marchese-Ragona R, Staffieri A (2001) Bezold's abscess in children: case report and review of the literature. Int J Pediatr Otorhinolaryngol 61:173–177

Maroldi R, Farina D, Palvarini L, Marconi A, Gadola E, Menni K, Battaglia G (2001) Computed tomography and magnetic resonance imaging of pathologic conditions of the middle ear. Eur J Radiol 40:78–93

Nayak AK, Karnad D, Mahajan MV, Shah A, Meisheri YV (1994) Cerebellar venous infarction in chronic suppurative otitis media. A case report with review of four other cases. Stroke 25:1058–1060

Ohki M, Ito K, Ishimoto S (2001) Fungal mastoiditis in an immunocompetent adult. Eur Arch Otorhinolaryngol 258:106–108

Ram B, Meiklejohn DJ, Nunez DA, Murray A, Watson HG (2001) Combined risk factors contributing to cerebral venous thrombosis in a young woman. J Laryngol Otol 115:307–310

Rocha JL, Kondo W, Gracia CM, Baptista MI, Buchele G, da Cunha CA, Martins LT (2000) Central venous sinus thrombosis following mastoiditis: report of 4 cases and literature review. Braz J Infect Dis 4:307–312

See KC, Leong JL, Tan HK (2000) Otogenic lateral sinus thrombosis: a case report. Ann Acad Med Singapore 29:753–756

Slack CL, Watson DW, Abzug MJ, Shaw C, Chan KH (1999) Fungal mastoiditis in immunocompromised children. Arch Otolaryngol Head Neck Surg 125:73–75

Spiegel JH, Lustig LR, Lee KC, Murr AH, Schindler RA (1998) Contemporary presentation and management of a spectrum of mastoid abscesses. Laryngoscope 108:822–828

Stewart MG, Troendle-Atkins J, Starke JR, Coker NJ (1995) Nontuberculous mycobacterial mastoiditis. Arch Otolaryngol Head Neck Surg 121:225–228

Yates PD, Upile T, Axon PR, de Carpentier J (1997) *Aspergillus* mastoiditis in a patient with acquired immunodeficiency syndrome. J Laryngol Otol 111:560–561

Zapalac JS, Billings KR, Schwade ND, Roland PS (2002) Suppurative complications of acute otitis media in the era of antibiotic resistance. Arch Otolaryngol Head Neck Surg 128:660–663

The Clinician's View

I. DHOOGE

Otitis media is a dynamic disease with a clinical spectrum which may extend from a self-limiting benign condition to a prolonged and sometimes complicated disease. The outcome depends on many different factors. With the advent of broad-spectrum antibiotics, the natural course of middle ear infections has changed significantly. Intracranial and intratemporal complications of infectious ear disease, once common with a high mortality, have become rare. This has led to a generation of ENT specialists and pediatricians trained in atmosphere of complacency in the treatment of otitis media; however, intratemporal and intracranial complications of otitis media are still reported in the literature. The CT scans play a determinant role in confirming the diagnosis and in orienting plans for management. The CT scans allow differentiation between mere opacification of the mastoid system with common acute purulent otitis media and disruption of the cellular system or demineralization of the bone by osteoclastic activity induced through inflammation, indicative for acute mastoiditis.

In deciding the best therapeutic strategy, it is important that CT scans differentiate between partial demineralization of trabeculae (incipience) where adequate conservative treatment is often sufficient (intravenous antibiotics and myringotomy, and coalescence, often combined with extramastoidal spread, necessitating surgery).

Computed tomography scans should also assess in detail the extent of the inflammatory process. Specific attention must be directed toward the integrity of the bony contours of the middle ear and mastoid and possible extratemporal and intracranial involvement should be reported. Indications of extramastoidal spread are signs for performing surgery.

When lateral sinus thrombosis is suspected clinically, MRI is complementarily performed.

7 Otosclerosis

M. Lemmerling

7.1 Etiology and Categories

Otosclerosis is a disorder of the bony labyrinth and exclusively affects human beings. In otosclerosis the ivory-like enchondral bone of the otic capsule is replaced by immature and spongy new bone, and this process of remodeling occurs continuously. The process can become quiescent at any time or may become reactivated, in a way that otosclerotic foci commonly contain both active and inactive regions (Schuknecht 1993a). Unilateral involvement is seen in only approximately 10–15% of the cases and there is a 2:1 female preponderance. The risk to an affected person of having a child who will eventually develop otosclerosis is 1 in 4 (Donnell and Alfi 1980; Shin et al. 2001). In comparison with patients with a sporadic form of otosclerosis, the radiologic lesions are more often detectable, bilateral, and severe in the familial forms (Shin et al. 2001).

Otosclerosis usually has its clinical onset in the third decade, with symptoms of conductive hearing loss due to the impaired movement of the stapes by invasion of the stapediovestibular articulation. Fixation of the stapes by foci located anterior to the oval window – in the so-called region of the fissula ante fenestram – is found in 96% of ears from persons with clinical otosclerosis. In 49% of the cases otosclerotic foci are also present in other locations, of which the most frequent ones are the oval window niche (30%), the cochlear apex (12%), and posterior to the oval window (12%). Round window obliteration is seen in 7% of ears with clini-

cal otosclerosis. Other even rarer sites of involvement are the walls of the internal auditory canal, around the cochlear aqueduct, around the semicircular canals, and within the footplate (Schuknecht and Barber 1985). Incus and malleus invasion each have been reported once, and the internal auditory canal itself is never invaded. Invasion of the labyrinthine spaces rarely occurs (Schuknecht 1993a); however, sensorineural hearing loss can be seen in patients with otosclerosis, and is believed to be caused by the accumulation in the inner ear of products liberated by the growth of the otosclerotic foci that are present in the pericochlear region (Schuknecht 1993a). In patients with pericochlear otosclerotic foci sensorineural hearing loss is present to a higher degree (Guneri et al. 1996).

Two categories of otosclerosis are described on the basis of where the otosclerotic anomalies are seen: fenestral and retrofenestral otosclerosis. As the name suggests (fenestra is the Latin word for window) fenestral otosclerosis affects the lateral labyrinthine wall, including the promontory, facial nerve canal and both the oval and round window niche (Swartz and Harnsberger 1992). Retrofenestral otosclerosis involves the pericochlear otic capsule and is almost always present together with fenestral otosclerosis. For the latter reason it is better to use the term retrofenestral otosclerosis rather than cochlear otosclerosis, another term also in use.

7.2 CT and MRI Appearance

Computed tomography is the tool of choice to investigate for the eventual presence of otosclerotic lesions (Weissman 1996). Both axial and coronal images are performed in order to give a detailed description of the extent and location of the lesions. During the reading of the CT images inspection for contralateral otosclerotic foci is always mandatory, even in case of unilateral clinical findings.

In normal circumstances the bone of the otic capsule is homogeneously dense (Fig. 7.1). The otoscle-

M. Lemmerling, MD, PhD
Medische Beeldvorming, A.Z. St. Lucas, Groenebriel 1,
9000 Gent, Belgium

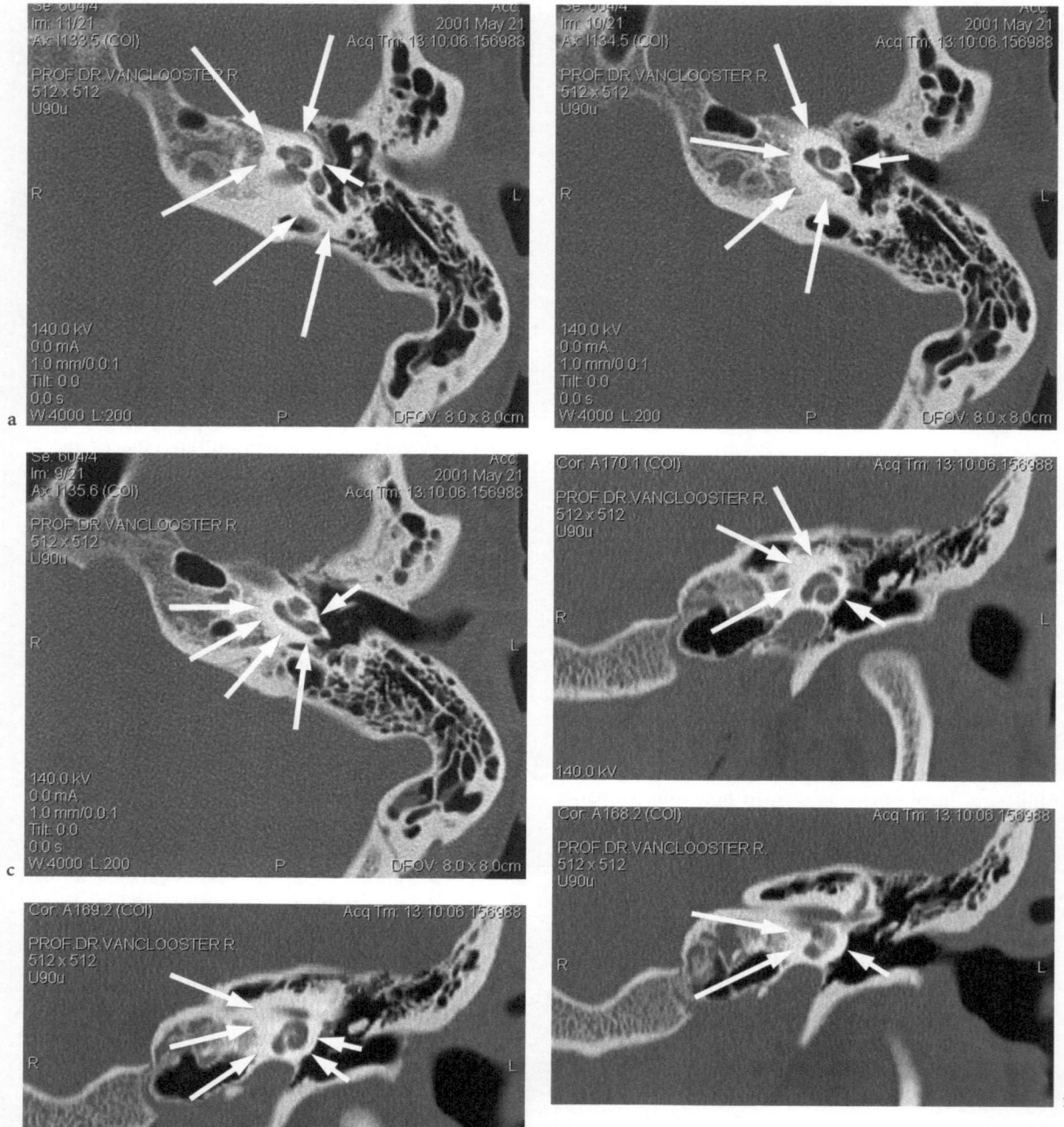

Fig. 7.1. Three consecutive **a–c** axial and **d–f** coronal CT images are shown in a non-otospongiotic ear emphasizing the need for careful inspection of the dense appearance of the normal bone in many regions. It is very important to systematically inspect the region of the fissula ante fenestram on the axial image set, situated just anterior to the oval window and anterior stapes crus, in order to be sure that fenestral otosclerosis is excluded (*small arrows* in **a–c**). The same region can be inspected on the coronal images, too (*small arrows* in **d–f**). An intensely high density must be present in the otic capsule region surrounding the cochlea, in order to be sure that cochlear otosclerosis is excluded (*large arrows* in **a–f**)

rotic foci contain spongy new bone, which appears lucent on CT (Valvassori and Dobben 1985; Miura et al. 1996). These foci are seen in the medial wall of the labyrinth in case of fenestral otosclerosis (Mafee et al. 1985a). It is important to inspect the region of the fissula ante fenestram very carefully, since otosclerotic foci can be very small (Fig. 7.2). Especially the axial images will be helpful in doing so. In some cases footplate thickening is noted (Fig. 7.3; Veillon et al. 2001). Additional foci of retrofenestral otosclerosis can be seen in the otic capsule around the cochlea (Fig. 7.4; Mafee et al. 1985b). It is important to notice round window localizations, since these can obliterate the window and cause problems in inserting a cochlear implant (Fig. 7.5). In extensive cases of retrofenestral otosclerosis a so-called fourth ring of Valvassori has been described (Fig. 7.6).

Magnetic resonance imaging is sporadically used in cases of otosclerosis. Otosclerosis very often leads to severe hearing loss in a chronic progressive manner. Initially, an otospongiotic phase takes place and causes an inflammatory osteolytic process in the otic capsule. During this "active" phase the otospongiotic foci enhance on T1-weighted spin-echo MR images performed after i.v. injection of gadolinium (Ziyeh et al. 1997; Stimmer et al. 2002). On T1-weighted images before gadolinium injection a ring of intermediate signal can be present in the pericochlear and perilabyrinthine regions, and an increased signal may also be seen on the T2-weighted images (Fig. 7.6; Goh et al. 2002). Magnetic resonance imaging has also proven its usefulness in the investigation of complications of stapes surgery performed for otosclerosis. Some of these complications, such as reparative intravestibular granuloma formation, intralabyrinthine hemorrhage, and bacterial labyrinthitis, are detectable with MRI, whereas they pass unrecognized on CT examinations (Rangheard et al. 2001).

7.3
Differential Diagnosis

Osteogenesis imperfecta is a rare disease and is often associated with hearing loss. It is an inherited generalized disorder of type-I collagen synthesis (Zajtchuk and Lindsay 1975; Bergstrom 1981; Berger et al. 1985; Schuknecht 1993b). The classic triad of blue sclerae, spontaneous fractures, and hearing loss is known as the Van der Hoeve and De Kleyn syndrome (Schuknecht 1993b; Czerny and Temmel 1999).

The CT appearance can be indistinguishable from otosclerosis, with lucent bone anterior to the oval window and in the pericochlear otic capsule (Fig. 7.7). On MRI findings have been described similar to those seen in the active phase of otosclerosis: pericochlear soft tissue signal intensities and enhancement after contrast injection (Ziyeh et al. 2000).

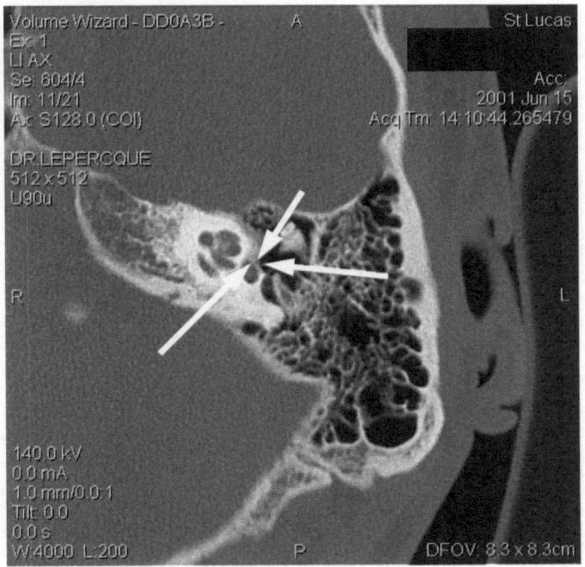

Fig. 7.2. The axial CT image at oval window level shows a hypodense region of otosclerotic origin in the footplate itself, and anterior to the oval window (*arrows*). Note that the footplate is thickened

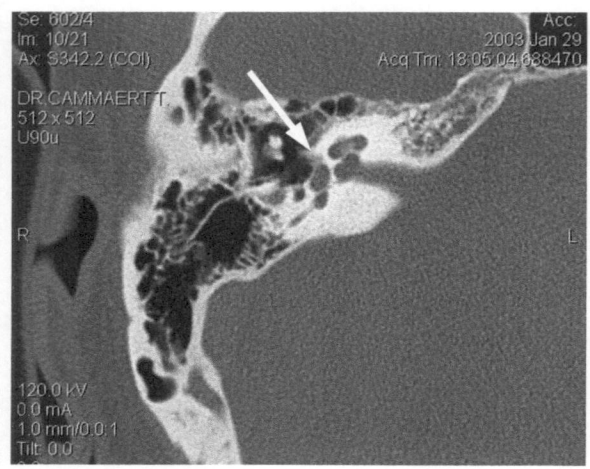

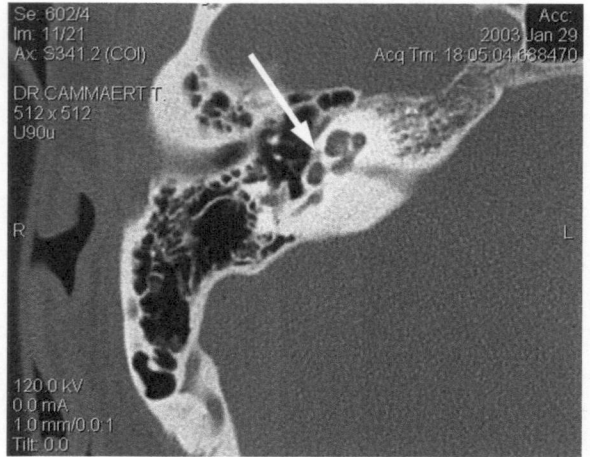

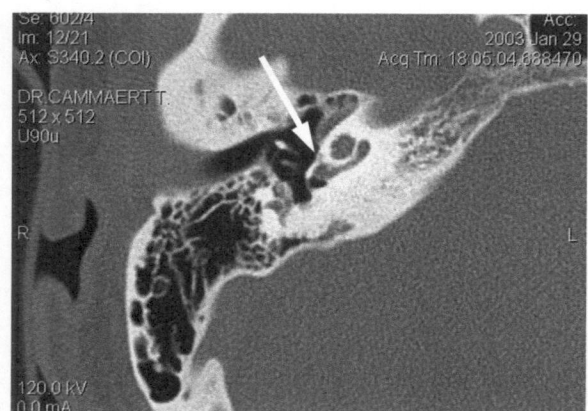

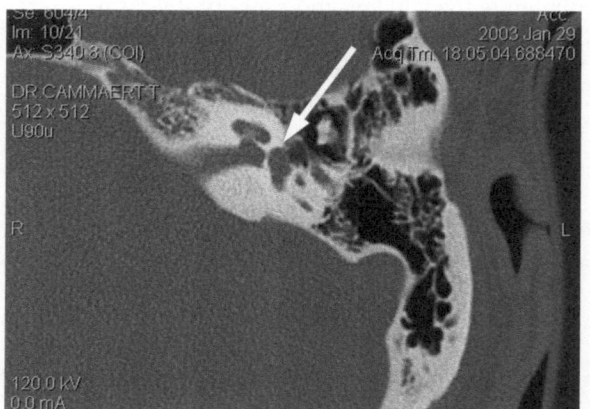

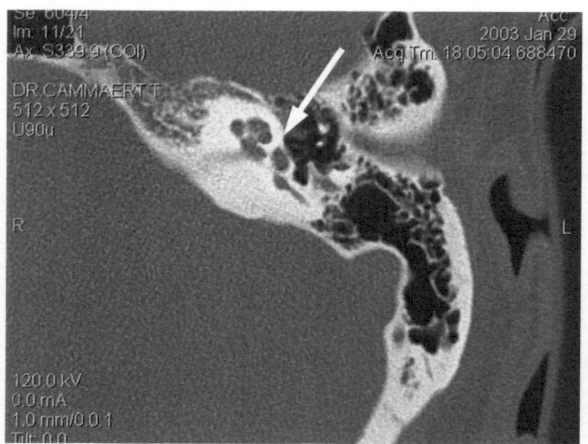

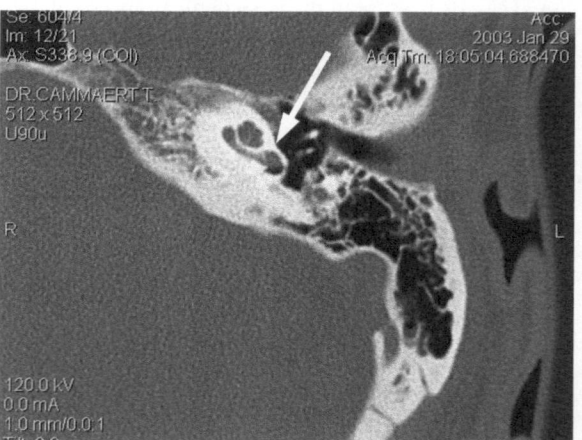

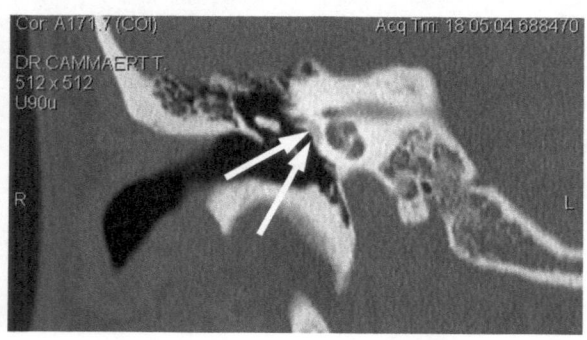

Fig. 7.3. a–c In the right ear three consecutive CT images show a lucent area just anterior to and extending to the oval window: fenestral otosclerosis (*arrow*). In the same patient the normal contralateral ear is shown. **d–f** Note the normal high density anterior to the footplate. **g** In this same patient a coronal reconstruction obviously depicts the otospongiotic focus in the region of the promontory (*arrows*)

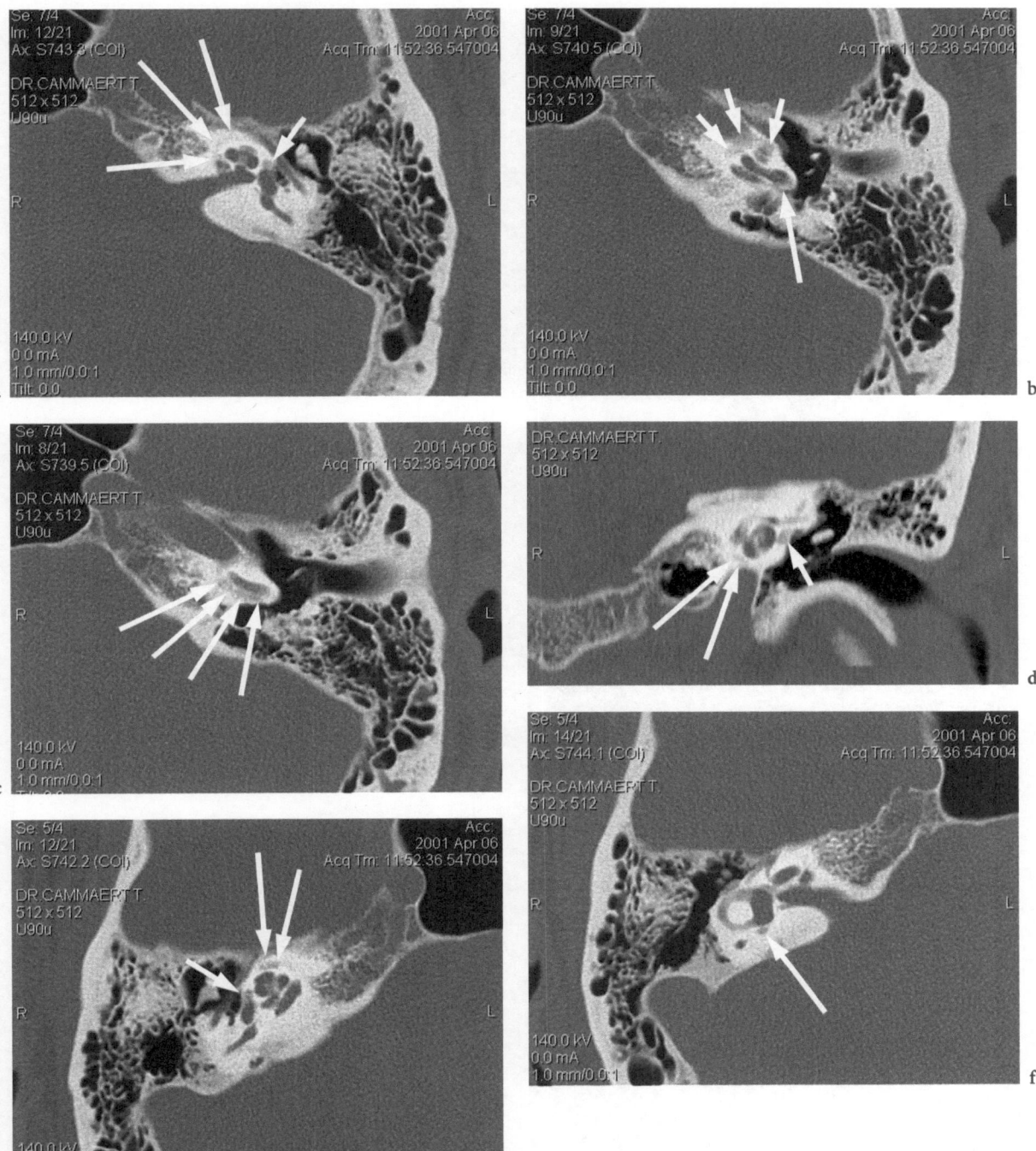

Fig. 7.4a–f. Multiple CT images are shown from a patient with bilateral fenestral and retrofenestral otosclerosis. **a** On the most cranial axial image on the left side lucencies of otosclerotic origin are seen around the cochlea (*large arrows*) and anterior to the oval window (*small arrow*). **b** On the image below cochlear otosclerosis is seen medial to the apical and middle cochlear turns (*small arrows*), but also around the basal cochlear turn, and in the round window region (*large arrows*). **c** On the slice more caudally more otosclerotic foci are obviously present around the basal turn of the cochlea. **d** The coronal image from the same left ear confirms the presence of fenestral (*small arrow*) and retrofenestral (*large arrows*) foci of otosclerosis. **e** In the contralateral right ear the axial image performed at footplate level shows more otosclerotic lucencies at the fissula ante fenestram (*small arrow*) and in the pericochlear otic capsule (*large arrows*). **f** On the slice performed 2 mm more caudally otosclerosis is seen posterior to the vestibule (*arrow*)

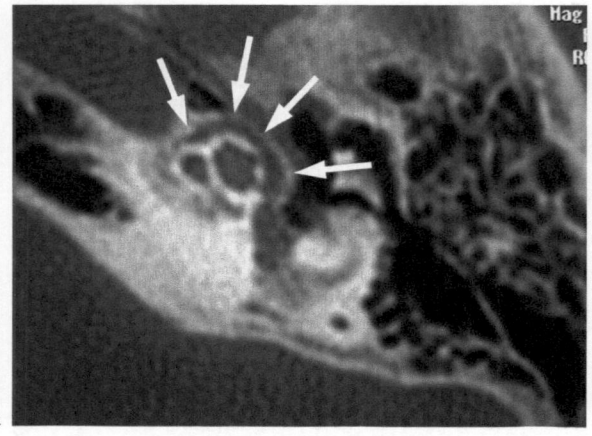

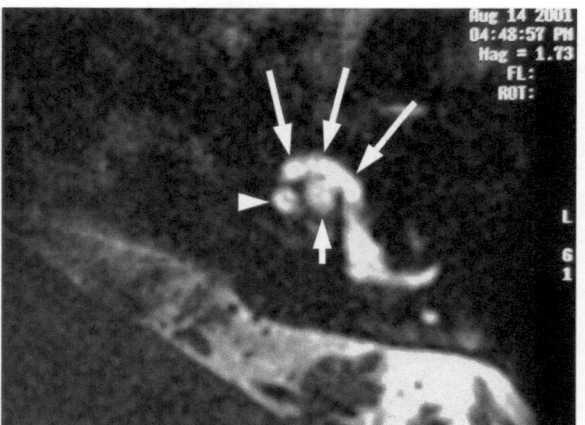

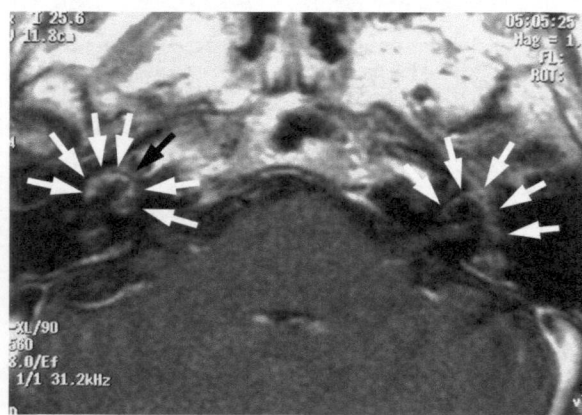

Fig. 7.5. a The axial CT image at the level of the middle and apical turns of the left cochlea shows otosclerotic changes around the cochlea: the so-called fourth ring of Valvassori is seen (*arrows*). **b** The axial 3D fast-spin-echo T2-weigthed image at the same level again demonstrates the fourth ring of Valvassori (*large arrows*), now seen as a semicircular hyperintensity around the middle (*arrowhead*) and apical (*small arrow*) turns of the cochlea. **c** On the axial contrast-enhanced T1-weighted image through both inner ears diffuse semicircular enhancement is noted around the cochlea bilaterally: the diagnosis of bilateral severe retrofenestral otosclerosis in the active phase can be made. (Courtesy of B. De Foer)

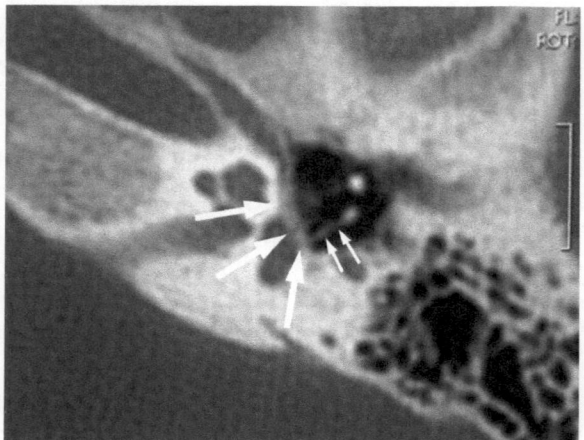

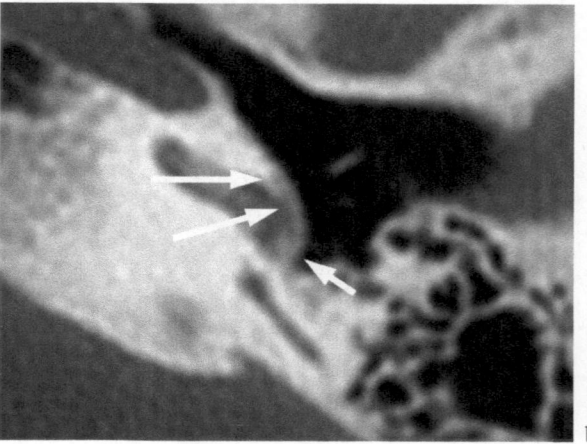

Fig. 7.6. a The axial CT image at the level of the oval window shows an otosclerosis focus at the fissula ante fenestram extending over the oval window, and with diffuse and severe thickening of the footplate (*large arrows*). Note the postoperative status with stapedectomy and replacement by a piston, posteriorly displaced (*small arrows*). **b** The axial CT image at the level of the basal cochlear turn and round window demonstrates the extension of the otosclerotic changes over the promontory toward the round window niche (*large arrows*). There is extension of the otosclerotic changes to the round window with total obliteration of the access to the round window (*small arrow*), thus making a later cochlear implantation virtually impossible. (Courtesy of B. De Foer)

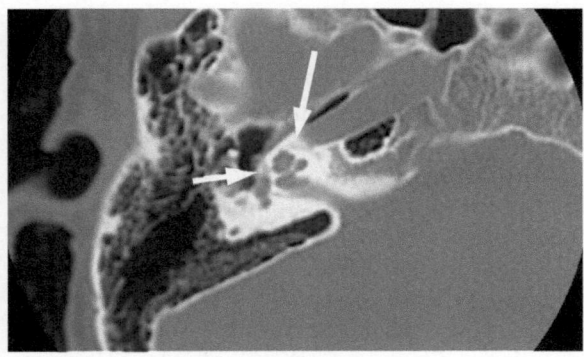
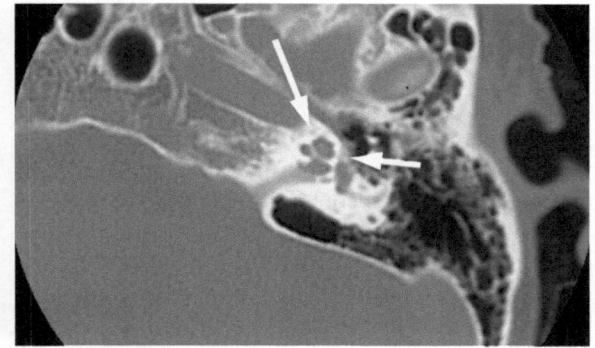

a
b

Fig. 7.7. The axial CT images at footplate level are shown in both temporal bones from a patient with proved osteogenesis imperfecta. Note that the bone in the region of the fissula ante fenestram (*small arrow*) and in the pericochlear region (*large arrow*) has become lucent. The CT findings do not differ from those seen in patients with combined fenestral and retrofenestral otosclerosis. (Courtesy of B. De Foer)

References

Berger G, Hawke M, Johnson A, Proops D (1985) Histopathology of the temporal bone in osteogenesis imperfecta congenita: a report of 5 cases. Laryngoscope 95:193–199

Bergstrom L (1981) Fragile bones and fragile ears. Clin Orthop 159:58–63

Czerny C, Temmel AF (1999) Osteogenesis imperfecta tarda with association of the inner ear also called Van Hoeve-Klein-syndrome. Eur J Radiol 30:162–164

Donnell GN, Alfi OS (1980) Medical genetics for the otorhinolaryngologist. Laryngoscope 90:40–46

Goh JP, Chan LL, Tan TY (2002) MRI of cochlear otosclerosis. Br J Radiol 75:502–505

Guneri E, Ada E, Ceryan K, Guneri A (1996) High-resolution computed tomographic evaluation of the cochlear capsule in otosclerosis: relationscip between densitometry and sensorineural hearing loss. Ann Otol Rhinol Laryngol 105:659–664

Mafee MF, Henrikson GC, Deitch RL, Norouzi P, Kumar A, Kriz R, Valvassori GE (1985a) Use of CT in stapedial otosclerosis. Radiology 156(3):709–714

Mafee MF, Valvassori GE, Deitch RL, Norouzi P, Henrikson GC, Capek V, Applebaum EL (1985b) Use of CT in the evaluation of cochlear otosclerosis. Radiology 156:703–708

Miura M, Naito Y, Takahashi H, Honjo I (1996) Computed tomographic image analysis of ears with otosclerosis. J Otorhinolaryngol Relat Spec 58:200–203

Rangheard AS, Marsot-Dupuch K, Mark AS, Meyer B, Tubiana JM (2001) Postoperative complications in otospongiosis: usefulness of MR imaging. Am J Neuroradiol 22:1171–1178

Schuknecht HF, Barber W (1985) Histologic variants in otosclerosis. Laryngoscope 95:1307–1317

Schuknecht HF (1993a) Disorders of bone. In: Bussy RK (ed) Pathology of the ear, 2nd edn. Lea and Febiger, Philadelphia, pp 365–379

Schuknecht HF (1993b) Disorders of bone. In: Bussy RK (ed) Pathology of the ear, 2nd edn. Lea and Febiger, Philadelphia, pp 390–392

Shin YJ, Calvas P, Deguine O, Charlet JP, Cognard C, Fraysse B (2001) Correlations between computed tomography findings and family history in otosclerotic patients. Otol Neurotol 22:461–464

Stimmer H, Arnold W, Schwaiger M, Laubenacher C (2002) Magnetic resonance imaging and high-resolution computed tomography in the otospongiotic phase of otosclerosis. J Otorhinolaryngol Relat Spec 64:451–453

Swartz JD, Harnsberger HR (eds) (1992) The otic capsule and otodystrophies. Imaging of the temporal bone, 2nd edn. Thieme, New York, pp 227–242

Valvassori GE, Dobben GD (1985) CT densitometry of the cochlear capsule in otosclerosis. Am J Neuroradiol 6:661–667

Veillon F, Riehm S, Emachescu B, Haba D, Roedlich MN, Greget M, Tongio J (2001) Imaging of the windows of the temporal bone. Semin Ultrasound CT MR 22:271–280

Weissman JL (1996) Hearing loss. Radiology 199:593–611

Zajtchuk JT, Lindsay JR (1975) Osteogenesis imperfecta congenital and tarda: a temporal bone report. Ann Otol Rhinol Laryngol 84:350–358

Ziyeh S, Berlis A, Ross UH, Reinhardt MJ, Schumacher M (1997) MRI of active otosclerosis. Neuroradiology 39:453–457

Ziyeh S, Berger R, Reisner K (2000) MRI-visible pericochlear lesions in osteogenesis imperfecta type I. Eur Radiol 10:1675–1677

The Clinician's View

I. Dhooge

The diagnosis of otosclerosis is usually made on the basis of clinical history, physical findings, and audiometric tests. Preoperative imaging may be of some use in ruling out other possible causes of conductive hearing loss and in recognizing obliterative otosclerosis. There are only a few conditions that imitate the triad of conductive hearing loss, normal appearance of the drum membrane, and eventually tinnitus: disruption of the ossicular chain by trauma; congenital malformations of the middle ear; and tympanosclerosis as a sequela of middle ear infections in childhood. Knowledge of the nature and extent of the pathology preoperatively helps the clinician to give the patient realistic expectations for surgical success.

Imaging can be of use postoperatively in the evaluation of cases in which an initial hearing improvement is subsequently lost to visualize a possible dislodging of the prosthesis from the incus or otosclerotic overgrowth at the oval window with fixation of the prosthesis, or the formation of a reparative granuloma. Computed tomography scanning may also be indicated when persistent vertiginous symptoms suggest a prosthesis deep in the vestibule.

8 Imaging of the Congenitally Malformed Temporal Bone

S. S. KOLLIAS

CONTENTS

8.1 Introduction

A distinction should be made between anatomical variations and congenital malformations. Variants are not considered to be anomalies because of their frequent occurrence and their lack of associated functional deficits. Congenital malformations, on the

S. S. KOLLIAS, MD
Chief of MRI, Institute of Neuroradiology, University Hospital of Zurich, Frauenklinikstrasse 10, 8091 Zurich, Switzerland

other hand, are less frequent deviations of normal anatomical development and are frequently associated with functional disorders (GULYA and SCHUKNECHT 1993). Both anatomical variants and congenital malformations, however, are clinically significant for their otological surgeon; the former should be identified for avoiding complications during surgical interventions in the temporal bone and the latter should be precisely diagnosed for patient counseling and for deciding on the appropriate therapeutic procedure. In this respect, imaging probably plays the most essential role, and the accuracy of the information it provides to the surgeon is of utmost importance.

8.2 Imaging Considerations

Optimal identification and characterization of a congenital malformation of the temporal bone in the setting of congenital hearing loss requires high-resolution computed tomography (HRCT) examination with thin sections (<1.5 mm) in axial and coronal plane. The CT remains the modality of choice to examine these patients because it enables simultaneous visualization of both inner ear and middle and external ear malformations. If direct coronal imaging is not possible, overlapping thin-section axial images or a spiral acquisition should be reformatted in the coronal or other oblique planes. Inasmuch as CT is excellent in depicting bony detail, magnetic resonance (MR) imaging is the imaging modality of choice in defining soft tissue structures as well as fluid-containing structures. In the absence of disease, the largest portion of the temporal bone is devoid of MR signal, because air and cortical bone create signal void on both T1- and T2-weighted images due to the absence of mobile protons, and in most cases the pathology is seen as signal where there should be none; therefore, congenital malformations of the middle and external ear are evaluated with HRCT because MRI cannot depict the fine bony detail and variations in pneumatization necessary in the assessment of the middle and external ear.

In patients presenting with sensorineural hearing loss (SNHL) and/or vertigo, MR imaging has become over the past year the primary imaging examination for screening of a congenital inner ear anomaly. The development of phased-array surface coils, which improve the signal-to-noise ratio (S/N) without limiting the size of the field of view (FOV), improvements in the main magnetic field, and gradient strength of MR systems which allow submillimeter-resolution imaging, and the development of several new MR sequences and imaging protocols for high-resolution imaging in clinically acceptable scan times have markedly improved the ability of MR to evaluate the morphology of the human inner ear in vivo. Submillimeter resolution and increased tissue contrast between the cerebrospinal fluid (CSF), intralabyrinthine fluid, cranial nerves and vascular structures in the internal auditory canal, and bone are essential requirements for detailed evaluation of these structures. The natural contrast between fluid, neural structures, and bone is revealed by T2-weighted MR sequences. The hyperintense signal provided by CSF, perilymphatic, and endolymphatic fluids allows the detailed visualization of the osseous fluid-containing structures of the temporal bone. The T1-weighted MR images lack the tissue contrast between fluid, neural structures, and bone, and although postcontrast T1-weighted images remain the most sensitive for the evaluation of tumors and inflammatory changes, anatomic detail is provided only by the heavily T2-weighted images. Three-dimensional (3D) acquisition schemes, such as the 3D Fourier transform constructive interference in steady state (3DFT CISS), true fast imaging with steady precession (true FISP), and 3D fast-spin-echo (3D FSE) provide contiguous high-resolution (spatial resolution 0.4+0.4+0.4 mm) T2-weighted images of the temporal bone and allow high-quality oblique reformations in various planes for the detailed evaluation of inner ear and internal auditory canal (IAC) malformations, and for evaluation of the integrity of the nerves in the IAC as well as the facial nerve in the fallopian canal (SCHMALBROCK et al. 1993, 1995; BROGAN et al. 1991; YING et al. 1995; CASSELMAN et al. 1993, 1997; TIEN et al. 1993; STONE et al. 1998; KOLLIAS et al. 1998). The three-dimensionally complex anatomy of the inner ear structures is difficult to evaluate on routine orthogonal images because these sections display only small portions of the anatomical structures. Oblique reformations achievable with 3D MR sequences, maximum intensity pixel (MIP) projections, and segmentation analysis with surface-rendering postprocessing of the MR data provide more accurate definition of these structures and allow better evaluation of malformations of the otic capsule and the inner ear structures. Planning for cochlear implantation requires both CT and T2-weighted MR high-resolution imaging work-up. Knowledge of the complex regional anatomy and its anatomic variations is mandatory for the evaluation of congenital pathology. Images using advanced data acquisition and post-processing techniques are presently routinely obtained in various centers for the diagnostic work-up of patients with suspected congenital malformations of the temporal bone and are used to illustrate the pathology in this chapter. Volumetric imaging, stereoscopic analysis, and virtual endoscopy using high-resolution MR and/or CT data provide a better understanding of human temporal bone anatomy in vivo and create new possibilities for 3D planning of intervention and quantitative volumetric studies. These techniques are in their formative stages but portend a significant potential that can revolutionize diagnostic and therapeutic procedures in the near future; however, despite amazing progress in imaging resolution over the past years, many small structures, such as Reissner's membrane, the basilar membrane, the saccular and utricular maculae, and the cristae, cannot be identified. Furthermore, a distinction between perilymph and endolymph is not achieved by conventional imaging techniques. Dynamic MR sequences that use oscillating magnetic field gradients phase-locked to an external stimulus have demonstrated in animals the ability to selectively visualize and quantify oscillatory fluid motion of cochlear fluids (DENK et al. 1993). This technique permits detection of displacements far smaller than the spatial resolution and may allow in the future direct visualization of cochlear fluid mechanics noninvasively in humans.

8.3
Pinna, External Auditory Canal, Tympanic Membrane, and Ring

8.3.1
Embryology

The first signs of auricular development appear in the fourth week of gestation at the first ectodermal branchial groove as tissue condensations of the mandibular (first) and hyoid (second) branchial arches. By the sixth gestational week these condensations form three ridges on each side of the branchial groove, known as the hillocks of His, the differential growth and fusion of which will eventually form the different parts of the auricle. Several theories are proposed regarding the specific contribution of the arches to the formation of the tragus and the helix (for discussion see GULYA and SCHUKNECHT 1993). The most plausible theory (WOOD-JONES and WEN 1934) favors that the hillocks of the first branchial arch form the tragus, and the hillocks of the second branchial arch give rise to the helix (Fig. 8.1). By the second month of development the first branchial groove grows inward and the hillocks fuse to form an anterior and a posterior fold on each side of this cleft. The folds eventually fuse in the upper portion of the first branchial groove to form the pinna. By the end of the second month, cartilage develops from the mesenchyma of the folds. The pinna reaches adult configuration by the 20th gestational week; however, it continues to grow until 9 years of age.

During the fourth and fifth gestational weeks the ectoderm of the first branchial groove is in contact with the endoderm of the first pharyngeal pouch. This contact is interrupted by the sixth week through ingrowth of mesoderm. At the eighth week, the inward extension of the groove towards the middle ear forms a funnel-shaped depression between the first and the second branchial arches forming a primitive canal from which the fibrocartilaginous external auditory canal will eventually develop. During the ninth week of gestation, a solid cord of ectoderm, known as the meatal plug, grows inward from the fundus of the primitive external auditory canal towards the middle ear (Fig. 8.2). The mesenchyma between the medial portion of the meatal plug and the middle ear forms the central fibrous portion of the tympanic membrane. The first of four small ossification centers of the bony tympanic ring appears at approximately the same time. By the seventh gestational month the central cells of the solid meatal plug start disintegrating, beginning in its deepest portion near the tympanic

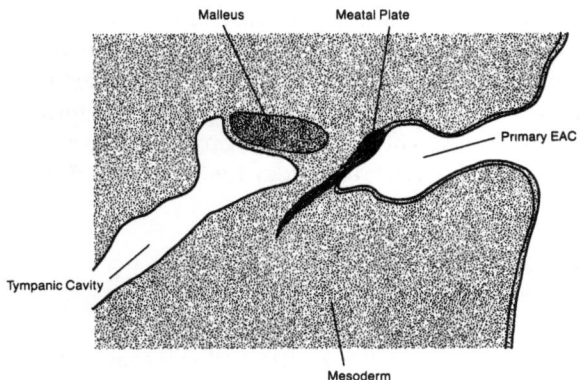

Fig. 8.2. The embryological development of the external auditory canal. The external auditory canal forms from an inward extension of the first branchial groove towards the middle ear. The meatal plug is a solid cord of ectoderm that grows inward from the fundus of the external auditory canal that after disintegration and canalization will become the bony external auditory canal and the superficial layer of the tympanic membrane. The central fibrous portion of the tympanic membrane is formed by the mesenchyma located between the meatal plate and the tympanic cavity. (From GULYA and SCHUKNECHT 1993)

membrane. The ectodermal plate becomes the inner bony part of the external auditory canal, whereas the remaining cells after the central disintegration of the meatal plug become the epithelial lining of the bony canal and the superficial layer of the tympanic membrane. The inner mucosal layer of the tympanic membrane derives from endodermal tissue of the tympanic cavity. The tympanic membrane is nearly horizontal during early life, compared with the adult orientation of 50–60° from the horizontal plane. The tympanic ring forms from the fusion of the ossification centers and it is fully developed by the 16th gestational week. The ring starts becoming fixed to the otic capsule by the 34th week and this fusion is not complete until birth. The connective tissue around the tympanic membrane continues to ossify up to 3 years after birth forming the sides and

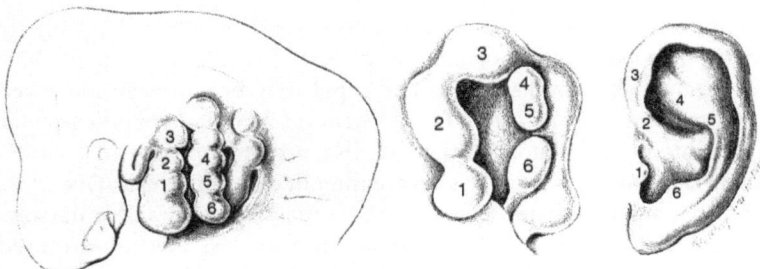

Fig. 8.1. The embryological development of the auricle from the first and second branchial arches. The hillocks of the first branchial arch form the tragus, and the hillocks of the second branchial arch give rise to the helix. (From GULYA and SCHUKNECHT 1993)

inferior wall of the bony external auditory canal. The superior wall is formed by the horizontal plate of the temporal squama. The walls of the outer cartilaginous part of the external auditory canal are formed by an extension of the auricular cartilage (GULYA and SCHUKNECHT 1993; BELLUCCI 1981; DAYAL 1973)

8.3.2
Congenital Malformations

Malformations of the auricle and external auditory canal include microtia, external auditory canal stenosis or atresia, and external auditory canal duplication anomalies (type I and type II branchial cleft cysts).

8.3.2.1
Microtia

Microtia is a deformity of the ear denoting a smaller-than-normal auricle with a large variability of expression. It is generally seen as an isolated malformation, although some consider it to be a manifestation of the oculoauriculovertebral spectrum (OAVS) where, in addition, there are other facial-, vertebral-, and renal-associated anomalies. This association requires that patients with microtia be subjected to intensive studies and physical examinations searching for associated malformations in order to provide adequate genetic counseling and management (LLANO RIVAS et al. 1999). Microtia is divided into three grades:
1. Grade I represents a minor deformity with the auricle being smaller than normal but with all parts discernible.
2. In grade II the auricle is a curving or vertical ridge of tissue.
3. Grade III represents the most severe malformation where only a rudimentary soft tissue structure is present without any resemblance to the normal auricle (MARX 1926; LAMBERT and DODSON 1996).

A variety of external, middle, and, less frequently, inner ear malformations are associated with microtia, which necessitate an extended diagnostic protocol including otological and audiological evaluation, clinical genetics, and high-resolution neuroradiological imaging from the neonatal period (CALZOLARI et al. 1999). One large series reported bilateral deformities in 23% of the patients with microtia and a marked direct correlation between the severity of auricular deformity and that of the middle ear and external auditory canal. In cases of minor microtia, stenosis of the external auditory canal was the most common

abnormality, whereas in those with major microtia, atresia was predominant. Middle ear malformations depended also on the severity of the auricular anomalies. Ossicular dysplasias occurred in 98% of cases. Inner ear malformations were found in 13% of cases, emphasizing that the inner ear should also be carefully examined in cases of microtia (MAYER 1997).

8.3.2.2
Stenosis and Atresia of the External Auditory Canal

The external auditory canal is composed of a medial, bony portion (approximately half to two-thirds of the total length of the canal) and a lateral, cartilaginous portion. The bony canal is usually narrower than the cartilaginous portion and is directed medially, anteriorly, and slightly inferiorly exhibiting a wide variation in size and configuration. The bone forming the anterior wall of the canal separating it from the temporomandibular joint (TMJ) is approximately 1.5 mm thick, varying from 0.2 to 4 mm (HASSO et al. 1995).

Stenosis or atresia of the external auditory canal is caused by failure of development of the first branchial groove either due to lack of formation of the primitive auditory canal or failure of canalization of the meatal plug. Failure of normal meatal and tympanic ring development affects the normal growth of the middle ear and the TMJ.

The incidence of congenital aural atresia is 1 in 10,000–20,000 live births. Bilateral involvement is noted in approximately 29% of cases with variable degree of deformities on each side (JAFEK et al. 1975). Although its occurrence is sporadic, genetic transmission occurs in many syndromes associated with aural atresia such as branchiootorenal syndrome, Crouzon's disease, Treacher Collins syndrome, hemifacial microsomia, Klippel-Feil syndrome, mandibulofacial dysostosis, oculoauriculovertebral dysplasia, Apert's syndrome, Pfeiffer's syndrome, frontometaphyseal dysplasia, and Möbius Syndrome (HASSO et al. 1995).

A stenotic external auditory canal is defined as such when its diameter is 4 mm or less or when the ear speculum that fits is more than two sizes smaller than normal for age (COLE and JARSDOERFER 1990; JAFFE 1977). The canal may be diffusely narrowed or may be focally stenotic. Middle ear and ossicular abnormalities are also present in cases of stenosis but are less severe than in cases of atresia. Over 90% of adolescence with a bony stenosis and a narrowing of the canal to 2 mm or less develop acquired cholesteatoma of the external auditory canal due to entrapment of epithelial debris in the medial end of the canal with potential perforation of the tympanic membrane and associated bone destruction. This has also been reported in children with a less severe stenosis of 3–4 mm (COLE and JARSDOERFER 1990; BENTON and BELLET 1997).

Atresia of the external auditory canal can be membranous (fibrous) or bony. Membranous atresia is usually associated with stenosis of the bony canal, and it is characterized by the presence of a soft tissue mass where the tympanic membrane is usually located (Fig. 8.3; HANAFEE and BERGSTROM 1980). It is associated with less severe deformities of the middle ear and the ossicles. In bony atresia the normal tympanic membrane is replaced by a bony plate, which extents at variable thickness across the external auditory canal forming the lateral wall of the mesotympanum (BELLUCCI 1981). Occasionally, there may be a short segment of the external auditory canal medial to the atretic plate, which may become the site of development of a cholesteatoma (HOENK et al. 1969).

Complete bony atresia is associated with severe middle ear, ossicular, mandibular, and facial nerve abnormalities (Fig. 8.4). Adjacent skull base structures tend to migrate toward the area usually occupied by the external auditory canal (BENTON and BELLET 2000). The condylar fossa is higher than usual and displaced posteriorly, whereas the mastoid process is displaced anteriorly. The glenoid fossa may be markedly flattened or even absent. The mandibular condyle may be close to the mastoid process and directly lateral to the middle ear affecting the ability of the surgeon to reconstruct the external auditory canal. The most severe, but also rare, associated malformation is absence of the ascending ramus of the mandible. The jugular bulb may be high and the tegmen low. Facial nerve anomalies are common. Dehiscence and inferior displacement of the tympanic segment and anterior and lateral displacement of the mastoid segment are expected in most severe malformations. The most frequent abnormal course of the facial nerve

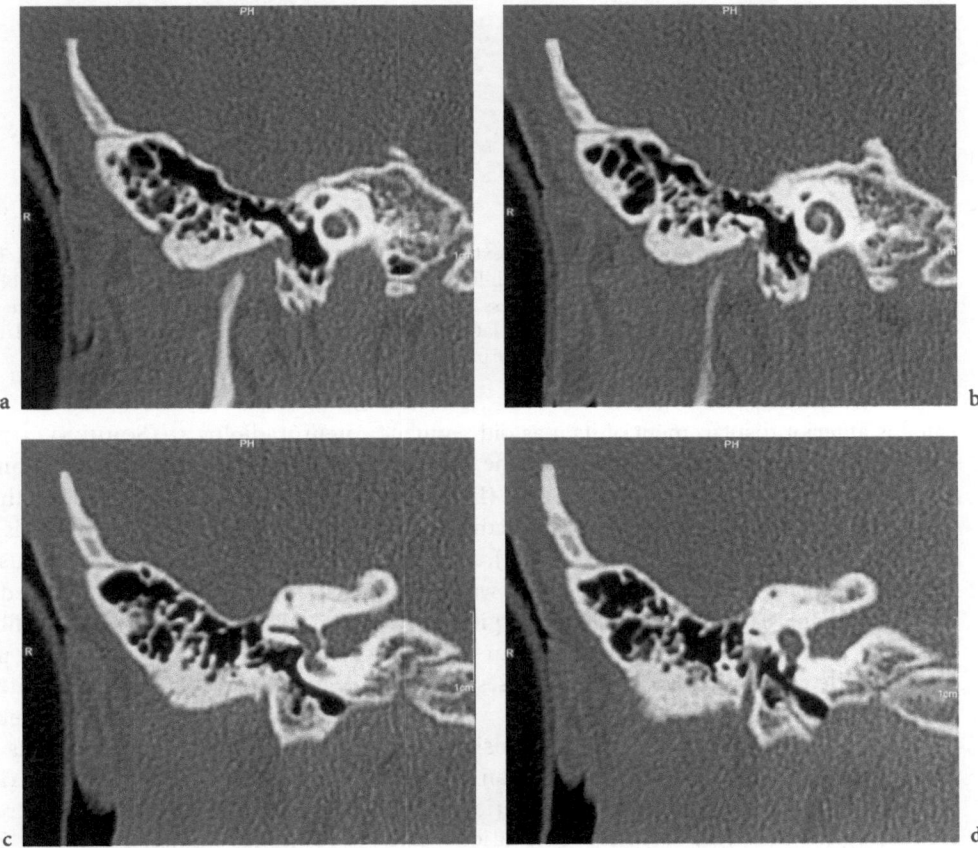

Fig. 8.3a–d. Membranous atresia of the external auditory canal. Coronal CT scans. The external auditory canal is absent and is replaced by a soft tissue that is attached to the tympanic membrane. **a, b** The ossicles in the middle ear are underdeveloped. The mastoid process is displaced posteriorly and the mandibular condyle is directly lateral to the middle ear cavity. **c, d** The mastoid segment of the facial nerve canal is displaced anteriorly. The inner ear structures are normal

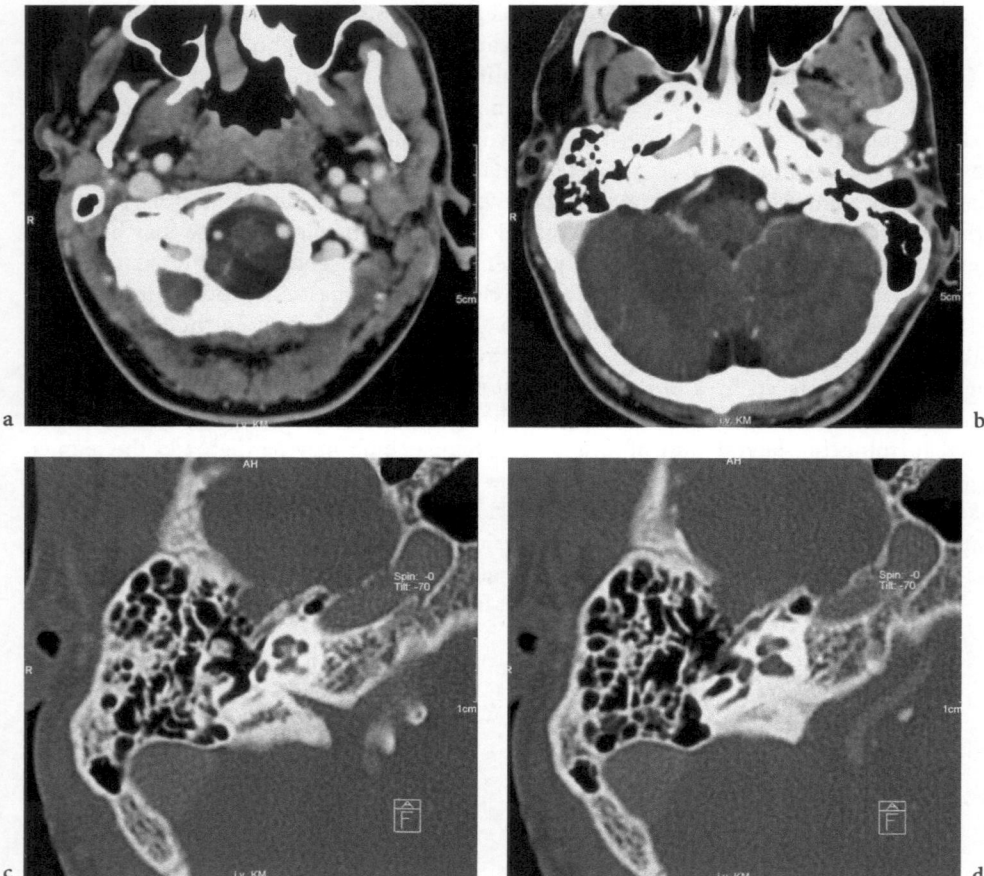

Fig. 8.4a–d. Complete bony atresia of the right external auditory canal (type C). Axial CT scans. **a** There is severe microtia with a small tag representing the outer ear, which lies inferiorly. The horizontal ramus of the mandible is hypoplastic and the ascending ramus is absent. **b** The mastoid process has migrated anteriorly due to the absence of the external auditory canal. **c** The ossicles in the middle ear are fused in the lateral wall of the cavity to the bony atresia plate. **d** The posterior portion of the tympanic segment of the facial nerve and the posterior genu lie directly in the tympanic cavity

canal is anterior displacement of its mastoid segment covering the round window and limiting the access of the surgeon to the to the middle ear space (LAMBERT and DODSON 1996). A significantly reduced distance is found between the facial canal and the TMJ, as well as between the facial canal and the posterior wall of the cavum tympani (SAVIC et al. 1989). In a surgical series the facial nerve was found to emerge from the skull base into the condylar fossa in 25% of cases (JAHRS-DOERFER and LAMBERT 1998).

Several classifications of the stenosis/atresia spectrum have been proposed based on various parameters including clinical examination, neuroradiological findings, surgical observations, and histopathological studies. The author prefers the Schuknecht classification as slightly modified by BENTON and BELLET because of its simplicity and clinical utility to both the otological surgeon and the neuroradiologist (SCHUKNECHT 1989; BENTON and BELLET 2000). This classification is as follows:

- Type A (meatal) atresia: the lateral fibrocartilaginous part of the canal is stenotic. (The term atresia is permissible because stenosis is at one end of the continuum related to total atresia.)
- Type B (partial) atresia: the fibrocartilaginous and bony parts of the canal are narrowed and sometimes tortuous. The tympanic membrane is small. The manubrium of the malleus is frequently short and curved and the malleus may be fixed to the epitympanum or tympanic ring.
- Type C (total) atresia: there is absence of the external auditory canal, a partial or complete bony atresia plate, and a well-developed middle ear cavity. The malleus and incus are deformed and fused. The malleus neck is fused to the atretic bone (Fig. 8.4).

- Type D (hypopneumatic total) atresia: in addition to the abnormalities present in type C, the middle ear cavity is underdeveloped, and there is little or no mastoid pneumatization. The facial nerve is often aberrant (Fig. 8.5).

The evaluation of patients with atresia of the external auditory canal requires an early and rigorous assessment for possible surgical repair that would maximize the chance of hearing recovery and minimize the potential of surgical complications.

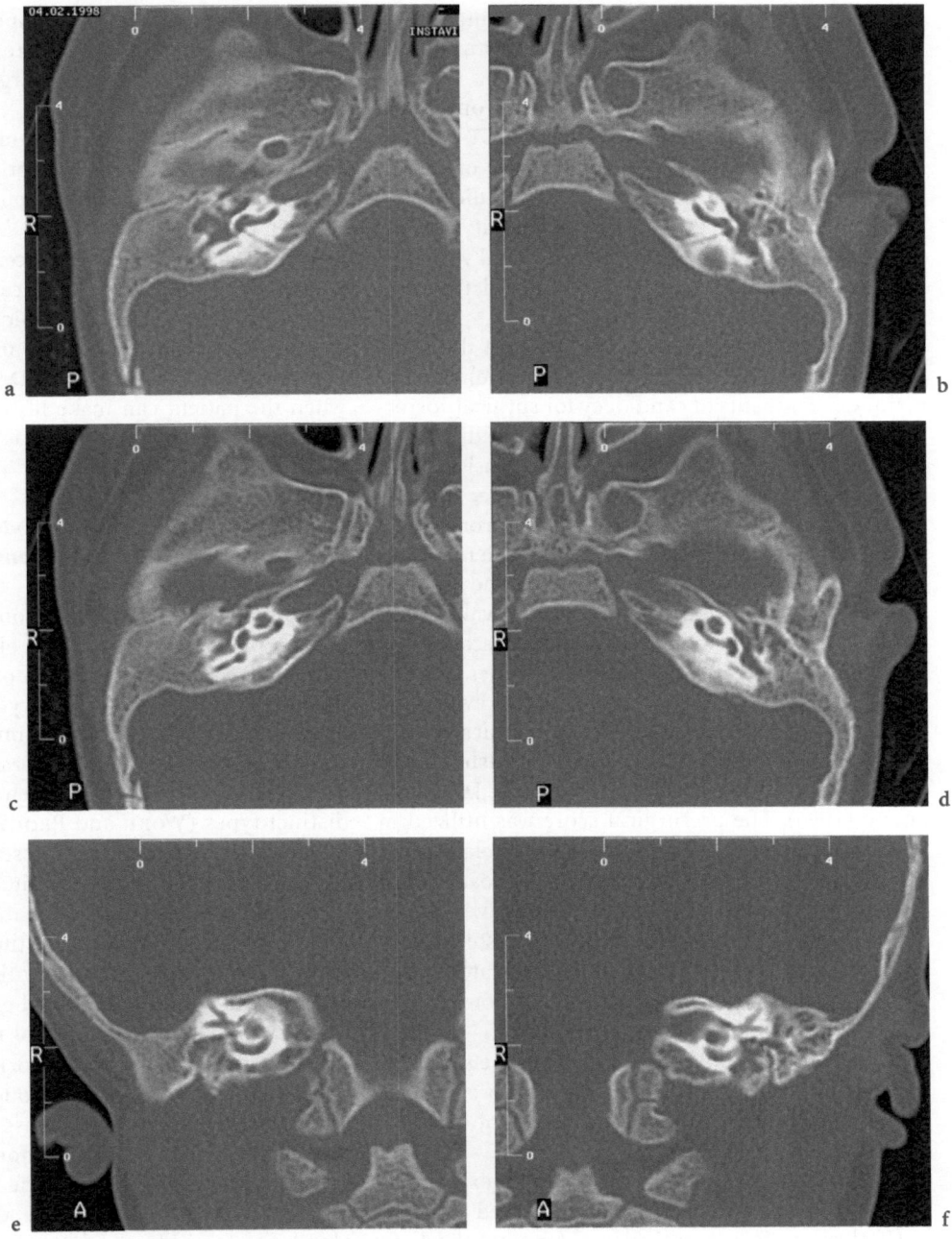

Fig. 8.5a–f. Severe bilateral atresia of the external auditory canal with underdeveloped middle ear cavity (type D). **a–d** On the axial CT scans the external auditory canal is replaced bilaterally by a bony atresia plate and the mastoid process is displaced anteriorly and abnormally under-pneumatized (particularly on the right side). The middle ear cavities are underdeveloped and there is no evidence of middle ear ossicles. **e, f** On the coronal CT images the facial nerve canal is abnormal bilaterally, with the posterior genu being located in the middle of the under-pneumatized middle ear cavity and its mastoid segment being anteriorly displaced and shortened

Essential to this evaluation are the physical examination, audiometric assessment, and detailed, high-resolution imaging of the temporal bone using CT for staging of the abnormality. It is also recommended in case of an infant with aural atresia to consult, at an early stage, with other medical specialists including a plastic surgeon, geneticists, or developmental pediatrician, who will be playing a role in the management of the child (LAMBERT and DODSON 1996).

Surgery for congenital aural atresia is one of the most challenging ear operations. The CT appearance of the malformation, including type of atresia, pneumatization and size of the tympanic cavity, pneumatization of the mastoid, integrity of the middle ear ossicles and the oval and round windows, and the course of the facial nerve (particularly its relationship to the to the oval window – anterior displacement of the mastoidal segment of the nerve restricts access to the middle ear space) are the major determinants of candidacy for surgical correction, avoidance of complications, and prediction of postoperative hearing results. It is emphasized that, although the development of the auricle, external auditory canal, and middle ear is distinct from that of the inner, patients with severe aural atresia may have associated inner ear malformations and the cochlear and vestibular labyrinth should be also evaluated in these children. A ten-point surgical rating scale based on HRCT of the temporal bone that provides the neuroradiologists with a stepwise method of evaluating these scans and allows them to communicate these findings to otological surgeons in a consistent fashion has been proposed by YEAKLEY and JAHRSDOERFER (1996). The presurgical score was utilized in selecting surgical candidates and was correlated with the intraoperative findings as well as the postsurgical results by comparing pre- and postoperative speech-reception threshold. According to this system, there are eight critical areas of temporal bone anatomy, and each receives one rating scale point as follows:

1. Open and not stenotic oval window
2. Width of the middle ear cavity from the promontory to the atresia plate of 3 mm or more
3. Course of the facial nerve that does not interfere with the surgical approach
4. Presence of the malleus–incus complex even if there is tympanic fixation of the fused ossicles. (If there is severe ossicular deformity, the long process of the incus is absent, or there is ossicular dissociation between the malleus–incus and the stapes the point is not awarded.)
5. Presence of mastoid pneumatization
6. Visible incudostapedial articulation
7. Present and not stenotic round window
8. Normal appearance of the external ear. An additional two points are awarded if the stapes suprastructure is present and normal. Patients with a presurgical rating less than or equal to five points are not considered surgical candidates. Normality of the inner ear structures and the IAC, as well as present cochlear function, are absolute conditions that must be satisfied for surgery.

Surgery for bilateral congenital aural atresia is performed after the age of 5 or 6 years as the child approaches school age and when accurate audiometric test results have been obtained, temporal bone pneumatization is well advanced, and children are cooperative with postoperative care. The same time is also optimal for repair of the microtia (LAMBERT and DODSON 1996). The timing for surgery in cases of unilateral atresia is controversial. Delay until adulthood, when the patient can make his or her own decision based on the risks and benefits, is recommended.

8.3.2.3
Duplication Anomalies of the External Auditory Canal (First Branchial Cleft Anomalies)

These malformations result from a failure of obliteration of the ventral portion of the first branchial cleft and represent a spectrum of congenital defects including sinuses, fistulas, and cysts (MUKHERJI 1993; OLSEN et al. 1980). They are uncommon and only sporadically reported in the literature (LAMBERT and DODSON 1996). They have been classified into two distinct types (WORK and PROCTOR 1963). Type I is of ectodermal origin and represents a duplication of the membranous external auditory canal. It appears as a cystic mass behind the ear, posterior, inferior, and medial to the conchal cartilage and pinna, and with the sinus tract paralleling the external canal. It may also lie within the parotid gland, in which case it is usually lateral to the facial nerve. Type II is of ectodermal and mesodermal origin and represents a duplication of the cartilaginous and membranous external canal. It appears as mass in the anterolateral neck, anterior to the sternocleidomastoid muscle and superior to the hyoid bone. The sinus tract courses over the angle of the mandible, through the parotid gland, passing in front of or behind the facial nerve, and ends at the bony-cartilaginous junction of the external auditory canal or, rarely, it may extend to the middle ear (LAMBERT and DODSON 1996; MUKHERJI 1993; OLSEN et al. 1980). The most common clinical presentation is recurrent periauricular abscess formation or sinus tract drainage presenting as otor-rhea or peri-auricular drainage. Commonly, they are inadequately treated with incision and drainage procedures to combat infection followed by scar tissue formation. Years may elapse before definitive diagnosis and treatment. High-resolution CT is essential to determine the cystic nature of the lesion and to delineate the bony detail. Fistulography facilitates visualization of the entire length of the sinus or the fistula. Definitive treatment is complete surgical excision, which should include facilities to achieve ear surgery and superficial parotidectomy including facial nerve exposure because of the variable relation of the fistula to the facial nerve (LAMBERT and DODSON 1996; WITTEKINDT et al. 2001).

8.4
Middle Ear and Eustachian Tube

8.4.1
Embryology

The middle ear cavity communicates through the Eustachian tube with the epipharynx and through the aditus ad antrum with the mastoid air cells. The tympanic cavity and the auditory tube form from an outward expansion of the endoderm-lined first (and perhaps the second) pharyngeal pouch. This outpouching of the foregut appears during the third gestational week and grows dorsally towards the area between the primitive external auditory canal and the otic capsule forming the tubotympanic recess. The anterior portion of this recess will develop into the Eustachian (auditory) tube, whereas the dorsal portion will become the tympanic cavity. By the fourth week of gestation the blind dorsal end of the recess comes in contact with the overlying ectoderm of the first branchial groove, which later deepens to form the external auditory meatus. This contact is soon lost by interposition of mesoderm from which the inner layer of the tympanic membrane and part of the ossicles will eventually develop (Fig. 8.2). By the end of 8 weeks the mesenchyma surrounding the primary middle ear cavity undergoes progressive resorption allowing for progressive cavitation and expansion of the tympanic cavity. This process first appears in the lower part of the cavity, the hypotympanic recess, while the atrium and the epitympanic recess are still mesenchymatous. Concomitantly, growth of the fetal head results to the narrowing and elongation of the medial aspect of the tubotympanic recess leading to

the formation of the Eustachian tube. Resorption of the mesenchyma of the middle ear progresses to eventually reach the epitympanic recess. The atrium and the epitympanic recess form between the tenth and thirteenth weeks, the aditus ad antrum at the end of the fifth month, the mastoid antrum at the end of the sixth month, and the mastoid cells at the eighth gestational month. In this process the mesenchymal tissue becomes less cellular and then is absorbed into the mucoperiosteal membrane, which covers the middle ear cavity and the developing ossicles. Remnants of this mesenchyma become the supporting ligaments of the auditory ossicles. By the time of birth, the antrum of the infant is nearly as large as that of an adult, whereas the mastoid continues to develop for 5–10 years after birth. The Eustachian tube continues to lengthen between the fourth and fifth months of gestation and areas of chondrification arise in the surrounding mesoderm forming the fibrocartilaginous part of the tube.

The rest of the middle ear structures (e.g., ossicles, muscles, tendons) form from mesoderm of the first and second branchial arches. Each brachial arch possesses a neurovascular pedicle and is reinforced by condensed mesenchymal tissue, the so-called visceral bars (the mandibular visceral bar for the first branchial arch and hyoid visceral bar for the second). The Meckel's and Reichert's cartilages are formed in the ventromedial portions of the respective visceral bars and will eventually become bone forming the middle ear ossicles. The manubrium of the malleus and the long process of the incus derive from the hyoid visceral bar, whereas the head of the malleus and the body of the incus develop from the mandibular visceral bar. The anterior process of the malleus forms from intramembranous ossification distinct from the visceral bars. The capitulum, crura and tympanic (lateral) surface of the footplate of the stapes develop from the hyoid visceral bar, whereas the vestibular (medial) surface of the footplate develops from the cartilaginous otic capsule. The mandibular nerve, the nerve of the first arch, innervates the tensor tympani muscle, whereas the stapedius muscle is innervated by the facial nerve, the nerve of the second branchial arch. A condensation of the mesenchyma of the second branchial arch, representing the rudiment of the stapes, appears by the end of the fourth week of gestation. During the fifth and sixth weeks this blastemal mass develops a ring-like configuration around the stapedial artery, which explains the annular shape configuration of the stapes. During the seventh week, the stapedial ring enlarges to approach the otic capsule at the region of the future oval widow and the mesenchymal tissue differentiates into cartilage. By the 16th week, the area of fusion between the otic capsule and the stapes differentiates to dense fibrous tissue giving rise to the vestibular (medial) surface of the stapes footplate. An oval-shaped zone, the future annular ligament, indicates the separation of the stapes from the otic capsule, which undergoes cartilaginous differentiation. At approximately the same time ossification is initiated and terminates by the sixth fetal month, although some modifications continue until the second half of the ninth month. The blastemae of the malleus and the incus appear also at the fourth gestational week. Progressive ossicular growths occur as cartilaginous models until the fifteenth gestational week when they reach adult morphology and the process of ossification is initiated. By the 27th week ossification is finished and the ossicles are surrounded by mucous membrane, which connects them to the walls of the tympanic cavity and provides the support for the ligaments and the blood supply to the ossicles (GULYA and SCHUKNECHT 1993; AREY and REA 1974; WILLIAMS 1992; DELVERT and LAFON 1986).

8.4.2
Congenital Malformations

Congenital anomalies of the middle ear may affect the normal development of the tympanic cavity or malformations of the ossicles and form a continuum with varying degrees of involvement. They result from an anomalous development of the first and/or second branchial arches or may be associated with an abnormal tympanic ring in which case later they are invariably associated with variable degrees of a malformed external auditory canal (HASSO et al. 1995). Conductive hearing loss, the presence of other anomalies, such as microtia and external auditory canal stenosis or atresia, as well as otoscopic detection of a retrotympanic mass in a young child, should raise the suspicion of a middle ear malformation.

8.4.2.1
Middle Ear Malformations Associated
with External Auditory Canal Deformities

The spectrum of middle ear anomalies in cases of tympanic ring dysplasia or aplasia ranges from mild forms that include a normal tympanic cavity with morphologically normal ossicles partially fused to each other or to the lateral wall of the attic, to severe forms where the middle ear cavity is very hypoplastic and the ossicles are severely deformed and fused or may even be completely absent. The most common finding in the first case is fusion of the malleus to the atretic plate (Fig. 8.4). The anterior (short) process of the malleus forms from intramembranous ossification of the tympanic ring distinct from the visceral bars. When the tympanic ring is not normally formed, the neck of the malleus is fused to the atretic plate. The severe forms are related with advanced stenosis or atresia of the external auditory canal and with variable degrees of associated facial nerve canal and TMJ deformities, as described in the previous section of external auditory canal atresia (Figs. 8.5, 8.6; KASEEF and JARDIN 1986; JAHRSDOERFER 1980; PHELPS and LLOYD 1983; HASSO et al. 1995; GULYA and SCHUKNECHT 1993).

8.4.2.2
Isolated Ossicular Deformities

Isolated ossicular deformities are not rare and they are caused by dysplasia of the first and/or second branchial arches. They have been seen in 38% of cases with congenital deformities of the external and/or middle ear and they were bilateral in 50% of these cases (SWARTZ and FAERBER 1985). The child usually presents with a 40- to 60-dB conductive hearing loss and a normal external auditory canal, and the main differential diagnosis is that of fenestral otosclerosis, infection, or trauma (KASEEF and JARDIN 1986). The first branchial arch (Meckel's cartilage) forms most of the malleus and part of the incus (see Embryology section above). In cases of first branchial arch dysplasia, the malleus may be fused to the epitympanic wall and the handle of the malleus may be thickened or absent. Mandibular malformations may also be present because the mandible is also formed by the cartilage of the first branchial arch (HASSO et al. 1995). Isolated maldevelopment of the second branchial arch (Reichert's cartilage) leads to congenital malformations of the capitulum, crura, and tympanic (lateral) surface of the footplate of the stapes, the long process of the incus, the facial nerve canal, and the styloid process which all develop from the same embryonic primordium. In isolated ossicular deformities, the stapes is the most commonly affected ossicle ranging from complete absence to various crural deformities (SWARTZ and FAERBER 1985). The long process of the incus may be absent, hypoplastic, or may be replaced by fibrous tissue, and the incudostapedial articulation may be dislocated. Thorough neuroimaging is essential in patients suspected for ossicular

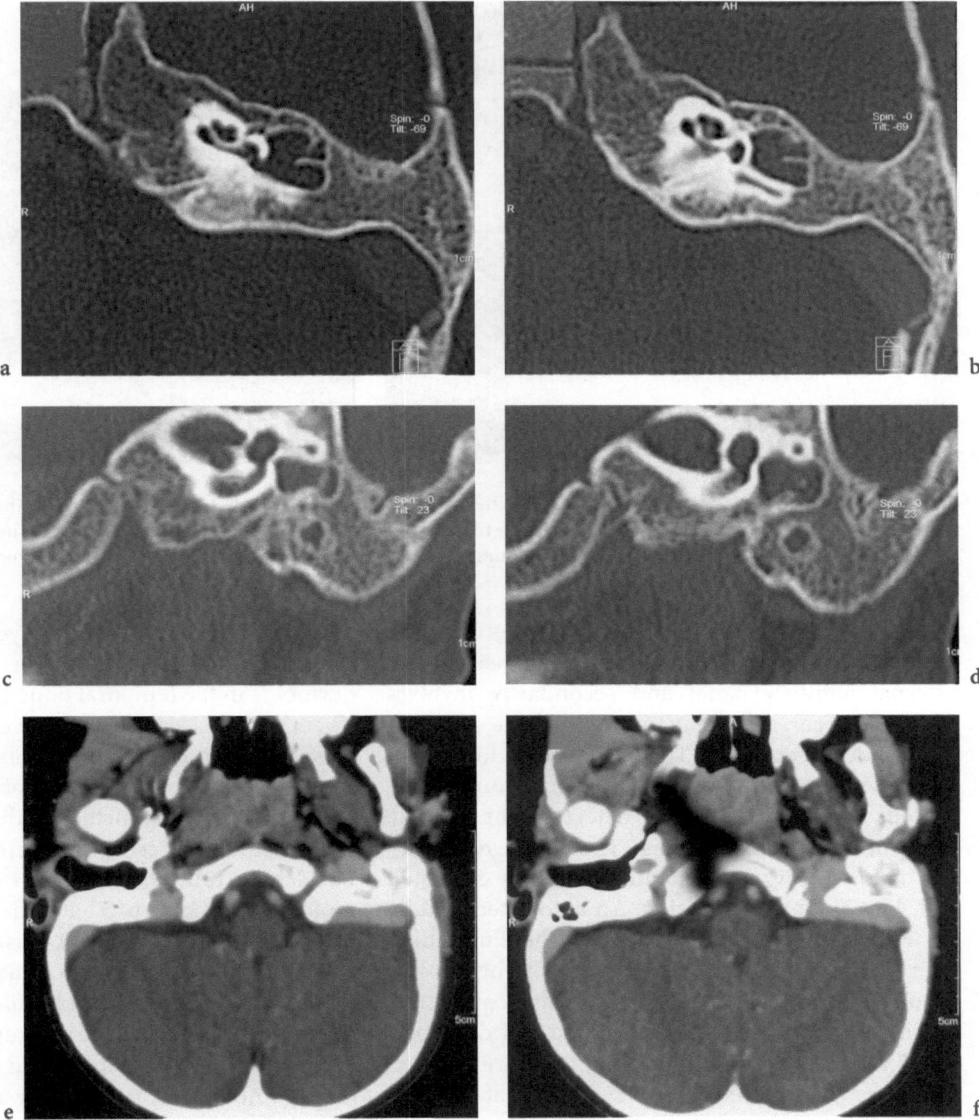

Fig. 8.6a–f. Severe middle ear anomalies associated with external auditory canal atresia. **a, b** Axial and **c, d** coronal CT images demonstrate left-sided external auditory canal atresia associated with severe underdevelopment of the middle ear cavity and complete absence of the ossicular chain. Severe mandibular, temporomandibular (TM) joint, and facial nerve canal anomalies were also present. **e, f** Axial CT scan shows the hypoplastic mandible and the absence TM on the left side

malformation and should be focused not only in the evaluation of the ossicles but should also include assessment of the tympanic cavity, oval window, and location of the facial nerve canal for planning and performing the appropriate surgical intervention. Abnormalities of the facial nerve canal caused by dysplasias of the second branchial arch may include aberrant course of the facial nerve (as described in the cases of external auditory canal atresia), bony dehiscences due to incomplete bony development of the canal, and anomalous duplication or triplication

of the nerve. A bifid facial nerve can be detected with high-resolution T2-weighted MR imaging and shows a splitting of the mastoid segment into two canals that reunite at the level of the stylomastoid foramen (Fig. 8.7).

8.4.2.3
Congenital Cholesteatoma of the Middle Ear

Presence of embryonic debris in the tympanic cavity and the mastoid air cells may give rise to a congenital

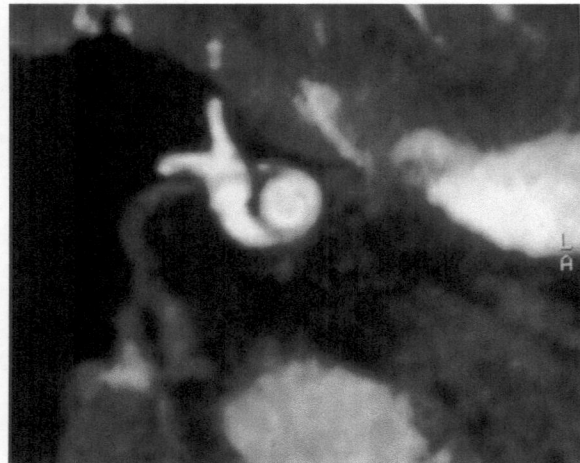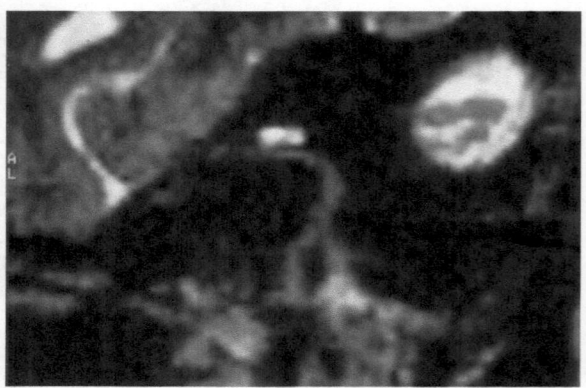

a   b

Fig. 8.7a, b. Bipartite facial nerve demonstrated with high-resolution T2-weighted MR imaging. **a** Maximum intensity projection and **b** T2-weighted oblique parasagittal MR images reformatted along the mastoid segment of the facial nerve demonstrate a splitting of the nerve into two trunks in its vertical course that reunite at the level of the stylomastoid foramen

middle ear cholesteatoma. In this case, as opposed to a cholesteatoma arising from a stenosis of the external auditory canal and secondarily involves the middle ear, the tympanic membrane is intact (LEVENSON et al. 1989). They are usually located in the mesotympanum close to the manubrium of the malleus and they are usually detected otoscopically as a white retrotympanic mass. The middle ear cavity and the ossicular chain should be carefully evaluated with HRCT for bony erosion. An associated middle ear effusion, from obstruction of the Eustachian tube may obscure the visualization of the cholesteatoma. Children usually present with conductive hearing loss. The mean age at the time of diagnosis is 4–5 years and boys are three times more affected than girls (LEVENSON et al. 1989; McGill et al. 1991; FRIEDBERG 1994).

8.4.2.4
Congenital Dermoids

Congenital dermoids are benign developmental anomalies rather than true neoplasms, and various terms have been used to describe these lesions including dermoid cyst, teratoid tumor, hamartoma, and hairy polyp. They are composed of a disorganized conglomeration of mesodermal and ectodermal derivatives and originate during early embryogenesis, around the fourth week of gestation, when the endodermal lining of the first pharyngeal pouch comes in contact with the overlying ectoderm of the first branchial groove. An inclusion of ectoderm into the endodermal lining during this short period

of contact between the two layers is believed to be the underlying mechanism for the development of dermoids in the temporal bone (KOLLIAS et al. 1995). Twenty-four cases of dermoids of the temporal bone have been reported in the otolaryngological literature describing multiple sites of involvement within the temporal bone, including the middle ear cavity, the mastoid air cells, the petrous apex, and the Eustachian tube. In cases of Eustachian tube dermoids, the patients present with a history of chronic ear drainage and recurrent episodes of otitis media which is resistant to antimicrobial therapy. Tympanic membrane perforation and inflammatory polyps or granulation tissue may be accompanied findings. The age at the time of presentation is usually during early infancy. Adequate preoperative imaging is essential for planning the approach for complete surgical removal of the lesion. They are well-defined, nonenhancing masses of fatty consistency, surrounded by a smooth capsule corresponding to the skin covering. They produce expansion and occasionally erosion of the bone. The extent of the lesion to the nasopharynx, and middle ear cavity, and the potential involvement of the ossicular chain should be accurately evaluated. The ectodermal and mesodermal origin of these tumors differentiate them histologically from cholesteatomas, which are only of ectodermal origin and from teratomas composed of all three germinal layers. In imaging, the typical findings of a well-defined, non-enhancing tumor of fatty consistency differentiate them from cholesteatomas, and the lack of calcification and heterogeneity from the teratomas (Fig. 8.8; KOLLIAS et al. 1995).

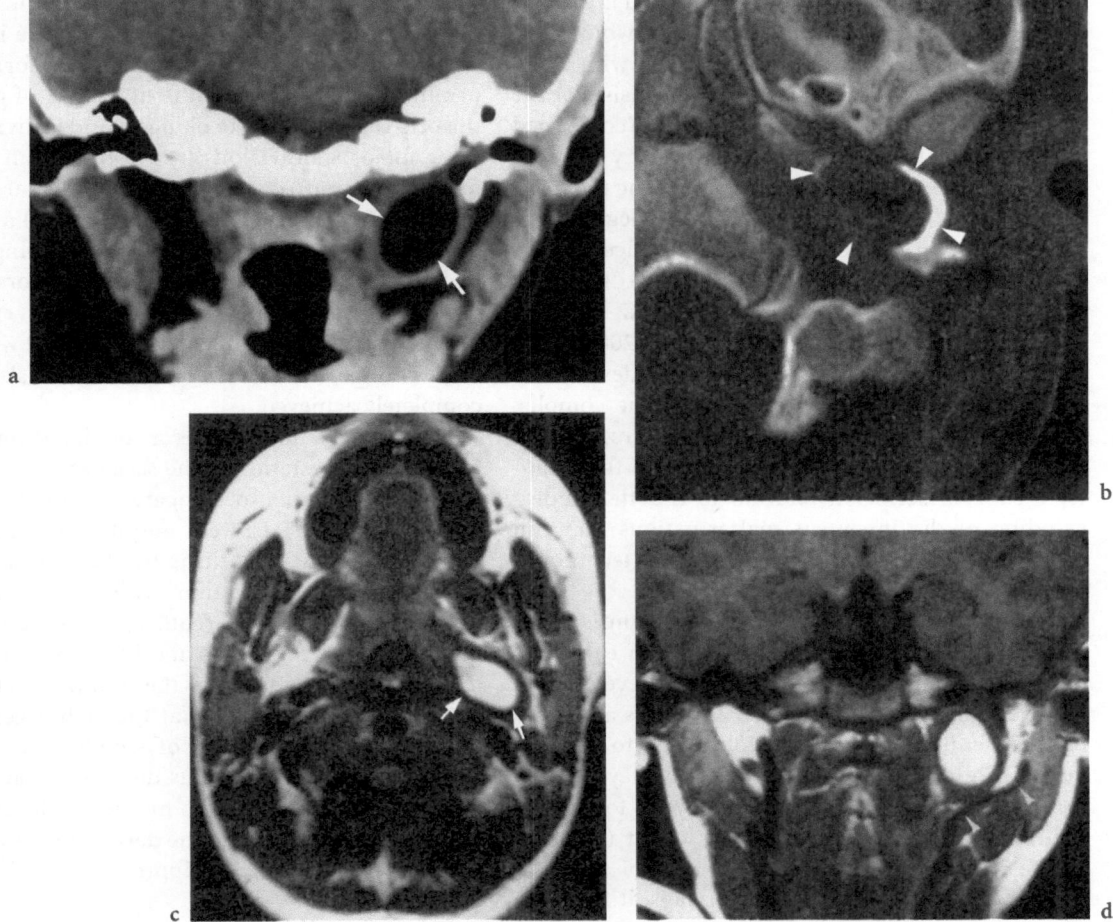

Fig. 8.8a–d. Congenital dermoid of the Eustachian tube. **a** Coronal CT scan shows a low-attenuation mass surrounded by a soft tissue capsule (*white arrows*) extending along the left Eustachian tube canal from the middle ear cavity to the left parapharyngeal space. **b** Bone-algorithm axial CT scan shows the expansion of the Eustachian tube canal by the mass. **c** Axial and **c** coronal T1-weighted images show the homogeneous high-signal intensity matrix of the lesion

8.5
Inner Ear and Internal Auditory Canal

8.5.1
Embryology

The inner ear is defined as the osseous labyrinth, a complex series of cavities in the petrous temporal bone, and the contained membranous labyrinth, a corresponding complex set of interconnected membranous sacs and ducts. The osseous labyrinth consists of the bony edifice for the vestibule, cochlea, semicircular canals, vestibular aqueduct, and cochlear aqueduct. The membranous labyrinth consists of the utricle and saccule (located within the bony vestibule), the semicircular ducts (located within the bony semicircular canals), the cochlear duct (located within the bony cochlea), and the endolymphatic duct and sac (located partly within the bony vestibular aqueduct). The membranous labyrinth contains endolymph, a fluid rich in potassium and low in sodium similar to intracellular fluids, and represents the endolymphatic space. The fluid-filled spaces interposed between the membranous labyrinth and the bony labyrinth contain perilymph, a clear fluid similar to cerebrospinal and other extracellular tissue fluid, and represent the perilymphatic space. The cochlear aqueduct is the only structure of the osseous labyrinth that does not contain a corresponding membranous structure, and forms part of the perilymphatic system. Ontogenetically and phylogenetically, the membranous labyrinth is the most ancient part of the auditory apparatus and is divided into two portions: (a) a sensory portion, which contains the cochlear labyrinth (concerned with hearing) and the vestibular labyrinth that consists of the utricle, saccule, and semicircular ducts (concerned with equilibrium); and (b) a non-sensory element formed by the endolymphatic duct and sac the main function of which is believed to be the degradation and absorption of the endolymph produced in the sensory labyrinth (GULYA and SCHUKNECHT 1993; WILLIAMS et al. 1990; SWARTZ et al. 1996a; DANIELS et al. 1996; KOLLIAS 1997; NAIDICH et al. 2000).

An excellent source for a detailed description on the embryological development of the complex inner ear structures is provided by GULYA and SCHUKNECHT (1993). For the purposes of this chapter a short description relevant to a better understanding of the inner ear malformations that can be detected with current neuroimaging techniques is provided.

The *membranous labyrinth* derives from surface ectoderm near the rhombencephalon on each side of the developing head. It begins its development at the end of the third gestational week as a plaque-like thickening of the neural fold distal to the first branchial groove, which in the next few days invaginates into the underlying mesenchyma to form a sac-like structure, the auditory (otic) pit (Fig. 8.9). In the fourth gestational week, fusion of tissue at the outer edges of the otic pit separates it from the surface, creating the otic vesicle, or otocyst, which migrates inwards closer to the neural tube towards the developing skull base. Already at this early stage, the endolymphatic appendage can be identified in the dorsomedial aspect of the otic vesicle. The future semicircular ducts appear as two protuberances in

the dorsal aspect of the otocyst. At the same time, the mesenchyma surrounding the otic vesicle increases in cell density developing in precartilage forming the primitive otic capsule. At the fifth week of gestation the otic vesicle begins to elongate and is divided into three major subdivisions by the formation of three folds: (a) a ventromedial projection demarcates the developing saccule and cochlear duct; (b) a dorsally directed pouch demarcates the developing utricle and its semicircular ducts; and (c) a dorsomedial projection demarcates the developing endolymphatic duct and sac. Between 10 and 12 weeks the adult configuration of the membranous labyrinth is completely achieved.

The *cochlear duct* forms a tubular diverticulum at 6 weeks of gestation in the saccular portion of the otocyst and begins to elongate spirally completing one turn by the sixth week and its entire two and a half to three-quarters turns by the eighth to tenth week. The communication with the saccule narrows to form the ductus reuniens of Hensen. Further growth of the duct occurs in caliber only and attains its final triangular shape by the 16th week. The organ of Corti first appears also at the eighth gestational week from differentiation of simple epithelium of the wall of the membranous duct and attains maximum size by midterm. The modiolus, the tympanic and vestibular scalae, and the developing otic capsule begin to differentiate at approximately the eighth gestational week.

The primordial *semicircular ducts* appear at the sixth week of gestation as two flattened sacs. The lateral semicircular duct arises independently, whereas the superior and posterior ducts arise from a common outpouching which accounts for their common opening into the utricle. The central portions of these

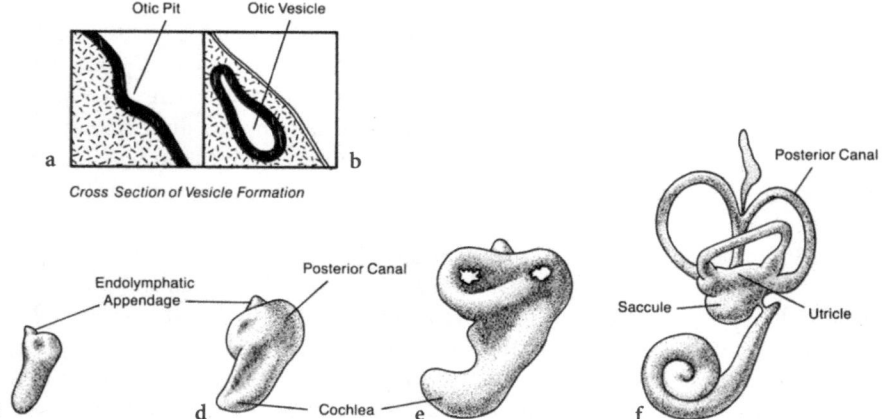

Fig. 8.9a–c. The embryological development of the membranous labyrinth from the **a, b** 3 weeks to **c** 9 weeks of gestation. (From GULYA and SCHUKNECHT 1993)

rudiments undergo partial obliteration retaining patent only the peripheral portion thereby creating the semicircular ducts. The three ducts progress to a position in three planes perpendicular to each other. One of their ends, which open into the utricle, dilates to form the membranous ampulla of the semicircular ducts. The morphogenesis of the superior semicircular duct is completed by approximately 20 weeks of gestation being followed by the posterior and lastly by the lateral duct.

The *endolymphatic duct* appears as a small append-age in the dorsomedial aspect of the otic vesicle at the sixth week of gestation. It is narrow proximally at the connection with the vestibule and progressively widens distally assuming by the eighth week a fusi-form, sac-like configuration representing the endo-lymphatic sac. By midterm the endolymphatic duct bends caudally and runs parallel to the posteromedial aspect of the common crus. The endolymphatic sac lies in the posterior fossa, adjacent to the sigmoid sinus, and it continues to grow as the posterior fossa expands to triple or even quadruple the size it was at midterm.

The *otic capsule (osseous labyrinth)* develops from cartilaginous differentiation of the mesenchyma that encompasses the inner ear and eventually forms the petrous portion of the temporal bone. This differen-tiation occurs everywhere around the membranous labyrinth except in the region of the developing endolymphatic duct and a small area in the medial wall, which marks the future location of the internal auditory canal. Between the sixth and eighth gesta-tional weeks the precartilage differentiates into true cartilage. Eventually, perichondrium starts forming in the twelfth week and proceeds to the beginning of ossification of the cartilage by the sixteenth week. Ossification involves 14 centers that fuse with each other to form a single protective capsule around the membranous labyrinth and the perilymphatic space. Ossification appears at approximately 16 weeks and is completed shortly before birth. The otic capsule consists of compact lamellar bone and is the densest bone in the body. The ossification of the otic capsule is intimately related with that of the fundus and the adjacent walls of the IAC.

The primordial *cochlear aqueduct* appears as a rarefaction of the otic capsular precartilage at the seventh gestation week and extends from the medial wall of the basal turn of the cochlea to the posterior cranial fossa. It provides the route of communication between the scala tympani (perilymphatic space) and the subarachnoid space of the posterior fossa. A progressive elongation of the cochlear aqueduct occurs by 32 weeks and by the 40th week arachnoid tissue has grown into the aqueduct to form a mem-brane lining.

The *perilymphatic labyrinth* occupies the space between the membranous labyrinth and inner peri-osteal layer of the otic capsule. This space arises from the mesodermal tissue surrounding the membranous labyrinth by retrogressive change in precartilage, but instead of differentiating into mature cartilage (as with development of the otic capsule) it differentiates into a loose vascular reticulum. The process of forma-tion of the perilymphatic space involves progressive vacuolation of the periotic mesenchyma resulting in an uninterrupted space, except of scattered tra-beculae extending between the membranous and the bony labyrinths that provide support and conduits for vascular supply. At the level of the cochlea, the perilymphatic spaces are separated by the cochlear duct into two spaces, the scala vestibuli and the scala tympani, which only communicate at the tip of the cochlea, the helicotrema. The formation of the peri-lymphatic labyrinth begins at the eighth gestational week and occurs rapidly around the cochlear, cana-licular, and vestibular portions of the membranous labyrinth being completed at approximately the 24th gestational week.

As a general remark relevant to the imaging evaluation of the malformed temporal bone, it is emphasized that the embryological development of the inner ear is independent from the development of the external and middle ear. This means that con-genital malformations of the inner ear usually occur in the presence of a normal middle and external ear, and vice versa; however, there is a certain percentage (approximately 10–15%) of cases with concomitant involvement of all three ear compartments. These cases are explained by the fact that mesenchyma is involved in the development of all portions of the ear and both genetic and nongenetic teratogenic factors may influence normal development of mesenchyma at critical developmental stages, thus leading to com-bined malformations (HASSO et al. 1995).

8.5.2
Congenital Malformations

Detailed neuroradiological evaluation of the inner ear structures for potential malformations in children with congenital deafness is of utmost importance for determining the appropriate auditory training pro-gram, for planning the appropriate potential surgical treatment, and because surgery for middle or external ear malformations would never be performed without complete assessment of cochlear function.

Congenital malformations of the inner ear may involve the membranous labyrinth, the perilymphatic space, and the otic capsule. They may manifest as isolated deformities of the cochlea, vestibule, semicircular canals, and vestibular aqueduct, or they may involve to a variable degree several inner ear structures depending on the induction time of the malformation during embryological development. At the present stage of development, imaging can only identify deformities of the bony labyrinth. It is emphasized, however, that malformations of the otic capsule may not reflect microscopic abnormalities of the membranous labyrinth or the perilymphatic space. Despite recent progress of MRI technology with the development of high-resolution, heavily T2-weighted sequences for the detailed depiction of the fluid-filled inner ear, minute structures of the membranous labyrinth, such as the organ of Corti, or the spiral ganglia, and the labyrinthine membranes separating the endolymphatic from the perilymphatic spaces, still escape in vivo imaging detection in humans; however, common inherited causes of sensorineural hearing loss, such as the Alexander, Siedenmann-Bing, and Scheibe deformities, involve portions of the membranous labyrinth and manifest normally formed otic capsules escaping imaging detection because the osseous labyrinth is normal. Only 20% of patients with congenital sensorineural hearing loss (SNHL) have radiographic correlates of their inner ear anomaly (JACKLER et al. 1987).

Several classification schemes have been advanced to describe these malformations. For practical purposes, in this chapter a descriptive anatomical classification follows emphasizing the aspects that can be detected by modern neuroimaging techniques used in human studies (i.e., High- resolution CT and MRI). Although the IAC is not part of the inner ear and its embryological development is distinct from that of the labyrinth, congenital anomalies of this structure are included herein because several IAC dysplasias can be associated with malformations of the inner ear structures.

8.5.2.1
Malformations of the Vestibule

The vestibule is the central chamber of the osseous labyrinth measuring approximately 4 mm in diameter. It lies medial to the tympanic cavity, and has discrete openings in its bony walls for the cochlea anteriorly, the semicircular canals posteriorly, and

the cribriform or cribrose area medially, which represents clustered tiny openings for the bundles of the vestibular and cochlear nerves (Fig. 8.10a–d). The vestibular aqueduct opens into the posteroinferior aspect of the vestibule (GULYA and SCHUKNECHT 1993; SWARTZ et al. 1996b; KOLLIAS 1997).

Malformations of the vestibule rarely occur isolated being more commonly associated with anomalies of other inner ear structures particularly of the semicircular canals. The most common situation is that of a dilated vestibule with partial or complete assimilation of the semicircular canals, particularly the lateral semicircular canal (Fig. 8.10e–g; JACKLER et al. 1987; LAGUNDOYE et al. 1975). The vestibule itself may rarely be isolated enlarged. Bilateral deformities of the vestibule have been associated with thalidomide-induced embryopathy in association with other malformations of the cochlea, IAC, and middle ear (LAGUNDOYE et al. 1975). This combination is rare without the history of thalidomide administration during the first trimester of pregnancy.

8.5.2.2
Malformations of the Semicircular Canals

The osseous semicircular canals are located posterosuperior relative to the vestibule and measure approximately 0.8 mm in diameter, but they expand to double their diameter at the osseous ampulla. The canals are orthogonal related to each other and contain the three semicircular membranous ducts which communicate with the membranous utricle in the same manner the bony canals communicate with the vestibule (Fig. 8.10a–d; GULYA and SCHUKNECHT 1993; DANIELS et al. 1996; KOLLIAS 1997).

Malformations of the semicircular canals are the most common of the inner ear congenital anomalies (Fig. 8.10e–g). The lateral semicircular canal is the last single structure to be formed during embryogenesis of the inner ear and its malformation can be found as an isolated anomaly, in which case it is not usually associated with severe hearing loss and may not be clinically significant (PETASNICK 1973; KASEEF and JARDIN 1986; JACKLER et al. 1987). Malformations of the superior and posterior semicircular canals are commonly associated with a dysplastic lateral semicircular canal and are usually associated with profound deafness. The canals may be narrow but most commonly are short and wide and in severe malformations may be completely absent or appear as small protrusions in the dilated vestibular cavity. Aplasia or congenital obliteration of the canals may occasionally be difficult to differentiate from labyrinthitis ossificans. Congenital absence of the superior

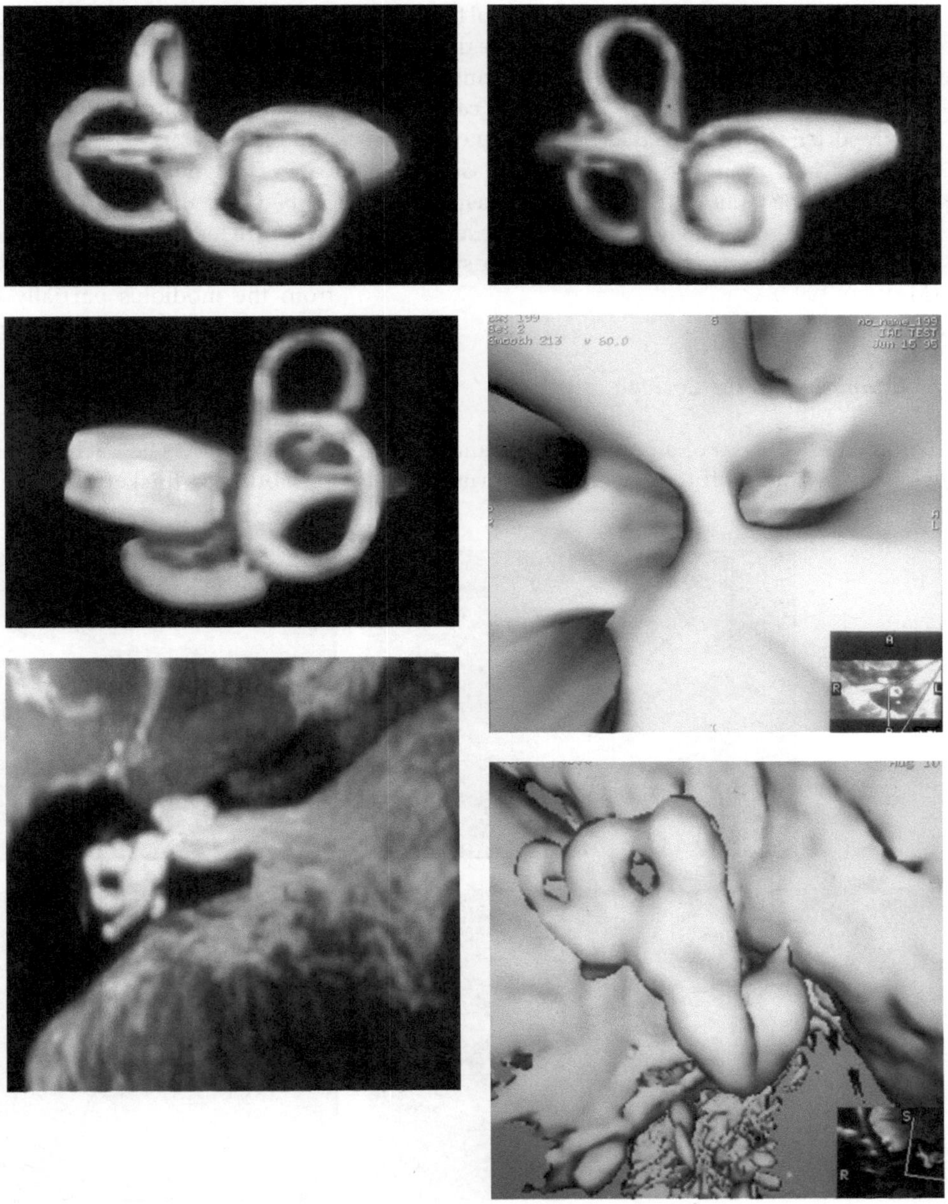

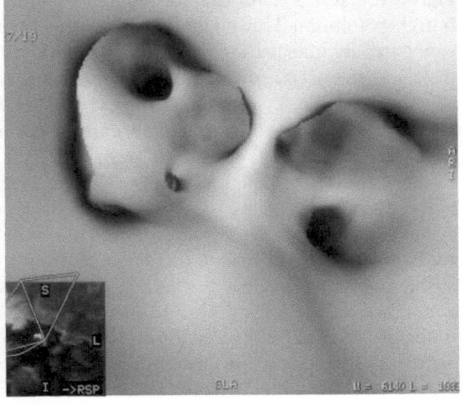

Fig. 8.10a–g. Three-dimensional images of the **a–d** normal and **e** congenitally malformed (vestibule and semicircular canals). **a–c** Surface-rendered
MR images of the inner ear structures and the internal auditory canal. The
vestibule is the central chamber of the labyrinth communicating anteriorly
with the cochlea, posteriorly with the semicircular canals, and medially
with the internal auditory canal. **b** Anterior and **c** posterior views of the
semicircular canals show their orthogonal relation to each other and the
common crus formed by the fusion of the posterior fusion of the superior
and posterior semicircular canal. **d** Endoscopic view towards the posterior vestibule shows five openings through which the semicircular canals
communicate with the bony vestibule. **e** Maximum intensity pixel (MIP)
projection, and **f** surface-rendered MR images show a globular-appearing
vestibule and a short and wide lateral semicircular canal. **g** The virtual otoscopic MR image from within the vestibule shows the partial assimilation
of the semicircular canals in the dilated vestibule

semicircular canal is associated with a typical flattening in the superior aspect of the temporal bone due to the absence of the arcuate eminence (KASEEF and JARDIN 1986). Absence of all three semicircular canals has been reported in CHARGE association (MUROFUSHI et al. 1997), KALLMAN (HILL et al. 1992), and Goldenhar syndromes (LEMMERLING et al. 2000). Absence of the common crus with a single posterosuperior semicircular canal has been also found in Goldenhar syndrome (MANFRE 1997).

8.5.2.3
Malformations of the Cochlea

The cochlea consists of a 32-mm spiral canal, which winds two-and-a-half to three-quarter turns around a central bony axis, the modiolus. Its height is approximately 5 mm and its apex points inferiorly, laterally, and anteriorly. At the junction of the IAC and the modiolus of the cochlea, the cochlear nerve and blood vessels create a central bony defect in the core of the modiolus. The modiolus is an hourglass-shaped, rectangular, triangular, or trapezoidal bony structure located along the central axis of cochlea. A delicate bony projection, the spiral lamina, projects from the modiolus partially dividing the cochlear canal into the scala vestibuli anteriorly and the scala tympani posteriorly (Fig. 11a, b). The osseous spiral lamina of the cochlea supports the organ of Corti and the termination of the neurovascular supply to this organ. The cochlear turns are separated by each other by thicker partitions that do not transmit

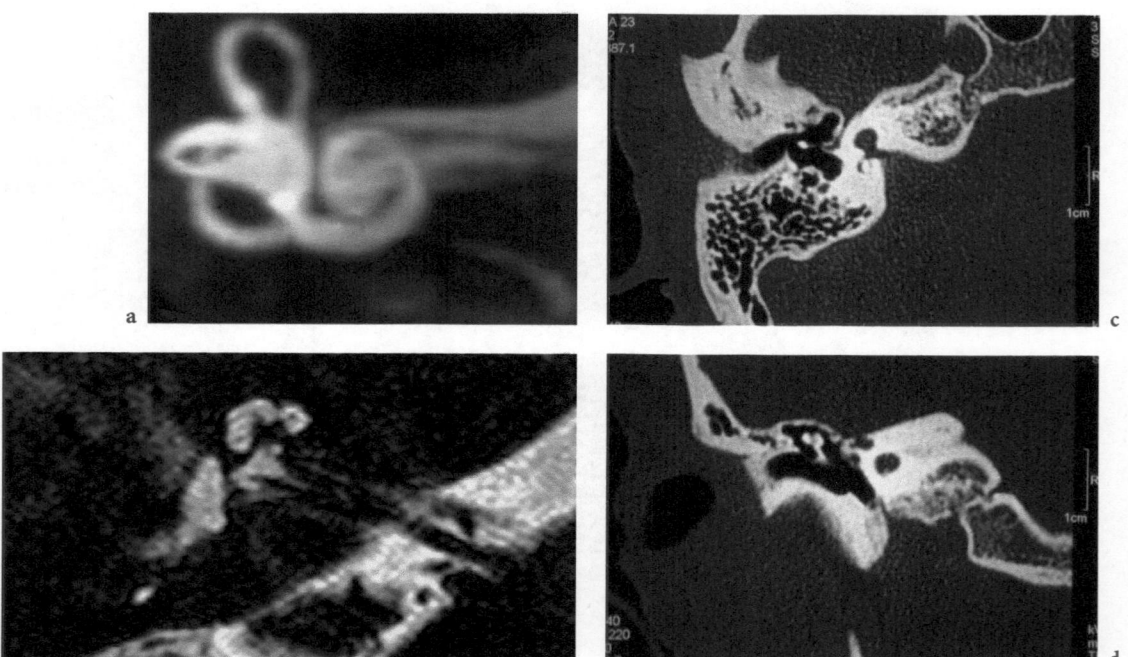

Fig. 8.11. a, b Images of the normal and **c–j** congenitally malformed cochlea. **a** Maximum intensity pixel (MIP) projection and ▷ **b** high-resolution T2-weighted MR images obtained with 3-T MR system demonstrate the spiral morphology of the cochlear canal and its internal architecture with the modiolus, the spiral lamina, and the interscalar septa. The membranous cochlear duct and the organ of Corti are beyond the spatial resolution of in vivo MR examinations in humans. **c** Axial and **d** coronal CT images depict a common cavity type of malformation representing a developmental arrest of the labyrinthine structures at an early stage with complete absence of differentiated inner ear structures. **e** Reformatted T2-weighted MR image reveals a case of cochlear agenesis with associated aplasia of the cochlear nerve. A cystic fluid-filled cavity is present medial to the internal auditory canal. **f** Axial T2-weighted image shows a case of cochlear hypoplasia resulting from a developmental arrest before the sixth gestational week, the time of formation of the basal turn of the cochlea. The cochlea is represented by a small cystic cavity devoid of any internal architecture. The MIP projection MR images in the **g** axial and **h** coronal planes and **j** 3D surface-rendered reconstructions demonstrate a case of unilateral incomplete partition (classical Mondini malformation). The cochlea on the left side is flat and cystic dilated with absent partition between the middle and apical turns. It connects with an abnormally dilated vestibule and the semicircular canals are also widened and shortened. **k** The MIP projection and **l** surface-rendered MR images in Mondini's malformation show the normal development of the basal cochlear turn and the absence of differential development of the middle and apical turns which are replaced by a single ovoid cavity communicating with the basal turn. The lateral semicircular canal is also abnormal

neurovascular elements, the interscalar septa that are seen connecting the inner wall of the cochlea to the modiolus. The cochlea contains the cochlear duct or scala media, which is part of the membranous labyrinth containing endolymph and should not be confused with the cochlear aqueduct, which makes part of the perilymphatic system and contains CSF. Defects in the interscalar septum between the middle and apical turns are a common variation of no functional significance (GULYA and SCHUKNECHT 1993).

A broad spectrum of anomalous cochlear patterns have been described, most of which have been categorized together under the term "Mondini's dysplasia." JACKLER et al. (1987), based on a review of 63 patients with 98 congenitally malformed ears, have been able to recognize a number of distinct anatomic patterns

from their radiographic appearance and found a remarkable similarity between these morphologies and the appearance of the inner ear at various stages of embryogenesis. They proposed a classification system based on the theory that these deformities result from an arrest of development during varying stages of inner ear organogenesis (Fig. 8.12; JACKLER et al. 1987). These stages comprise a spectrum ranging from complete labyrinthine aplasia (classic Michel's deformity), where there is no inner ear development and the inner ear is represented by a small single cystic cavity or several small cavities, to incomplete partition (classic Mondini's malformation) representing a small cochlea with incomplete or no interscalar septa (Fig. 8.11); thus, according to this classification, the histopathological description of Michel's

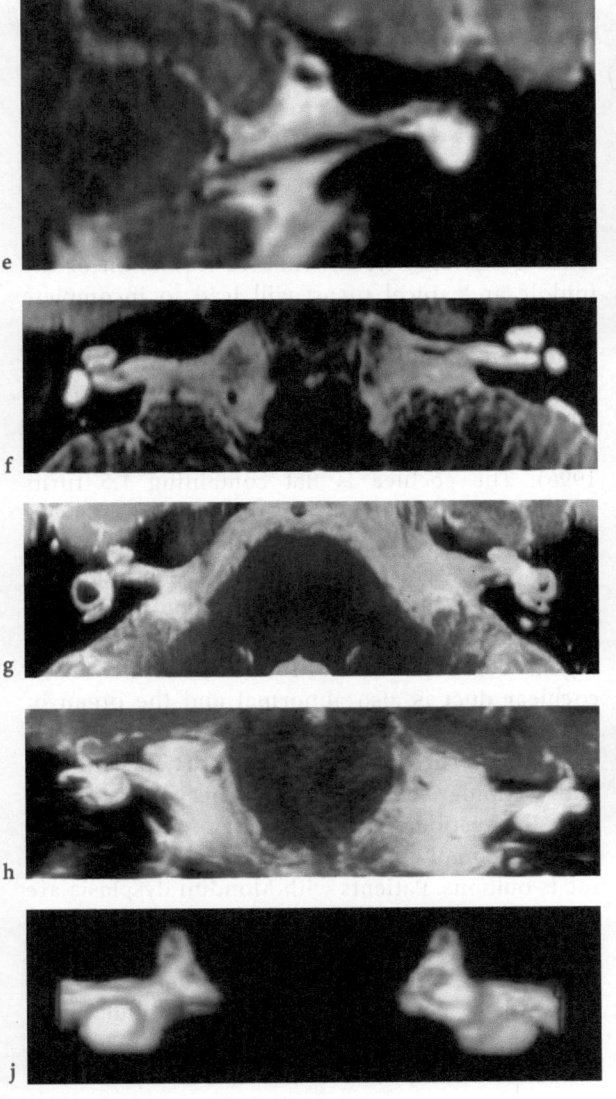

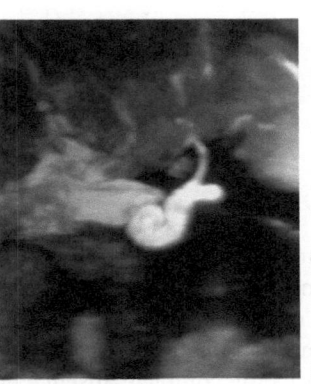

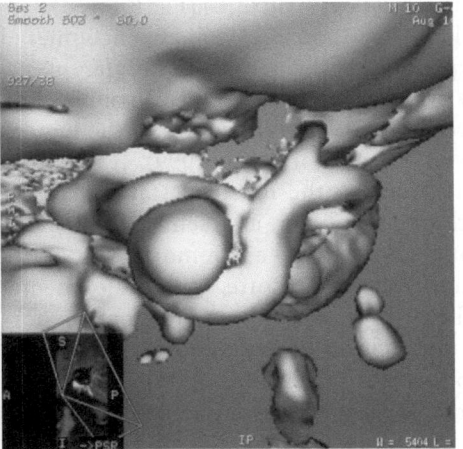

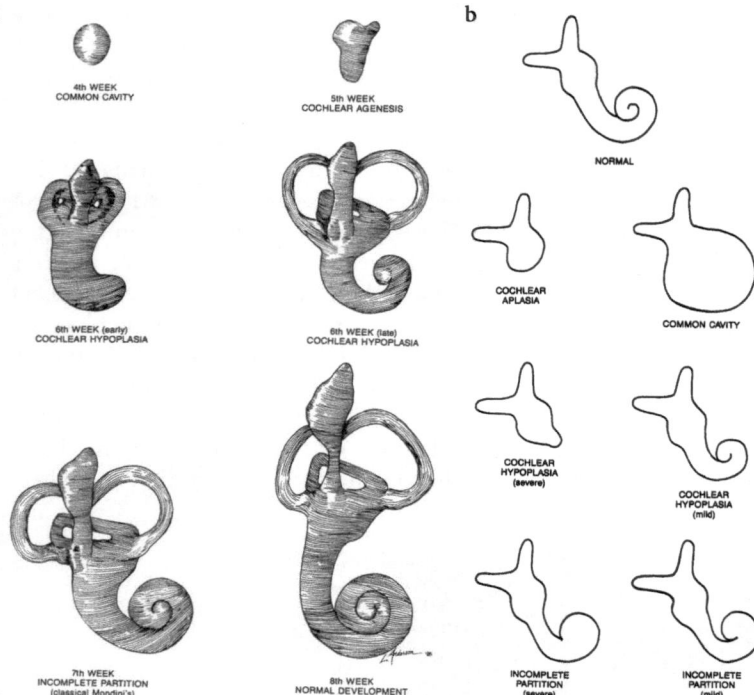

Fig. 8.12. Representations of the **a** embryogenesis of cochlear malformations and **b** their corresponding radiographic patterns. (From JACKLER et al. 1987)

deformity corresponds to the morphological pattern of inner ear development during the third gestation week and therefore this malformation occurs due to a developmental arrest at the otic placode (ectodermal) stage. Imaging reveals the complete absence of differentiated inner ear structures (Fig. 8.11c, d).

Other skull base anomalies that are encountered include hypoplasia of the petrous bone, platyplasia, anomalies of the stapes, the cochleovestibular and facial nerves, and an aberrant course of the jugular veins (MARSOT-DUPUCH et al. 1999). A developmental arrest during the fourth gestational week, before cochlear, vestibular, and semicircular canal differentiation, will lead to a common cystic cavity without internal architecture. A developmental arrest at the fifth gestational week, before the formation of the cochlear diverticulum in the otocyst, will lead to cochlear aplasia (Fig. 8.11e). The cochlea fails to form and appears as a rudimentary single cavity. The vestibule and semicircular canals are also commonly malformed. An arrest of cochlear development in the sixth gestational week, at the time of formation of the basal cochlear turn, will lead to variable degrees of cochlear hypoplasia. It manifests as a small cochlea with absent middle and apical turns that may be associated with malformed or normal vestibule and semicircular canals (Fig. 8.11f).

A developmental arrest between the eighth and tenth gestational weeks, time of formation of the middle and apical turns, will lead to incomplete partition of the cochlea, the classic Mondini malformation. Mondini first described this malformation histologically in 1791 in association with a large vestibule, malformed semicircular canals, and immature sensorineural structures (MONDINI 1996). The cochlea is flat containing 1.5 turns instead of the normal 2.75. On imaging, the basal turn is normally formed and connects to a single ovoid cavity, which has replaced the middle and apical turns (Fig. 8.11g–j). It is the most common major cochlear malformation observed with imaging studies (MAFEE et al. 1984). The membranous cochlear duct is also abnormal and the organ of Corti may be normal or may be underdeveloped or incomplete. The cochlear duct is short, the auditory and vestibular sense organs and nerves are immature, the vestibule is large, the semicircular canals are wide, small or missing, and the endolymphatic sac is bulbous. Patients with Mondini dysplasia are predisposed to developing CSF leak and meningitis (BARR and WERSALL 1965; CARTER et al. 1975). Incomplete expressions of the disorder may occur with little or no loss of auditory or vestibular dysfunction, whereas severe forms show no hearing or vestibular response. The disorder may occur in association with anomalies in other organs, such as in Klippel-Feil syndrome, Pendred's syndrome, trisomy syndrome, and DiGeorge's syndrome, or it may occur in isolation. It may unilateral or may involve both ears. In some cases the footplate of the stapes is partly or totally replaced by a thin membrane that may rupture and lead to spontaneous CSF otorrhea and meningitis (SCHUKNECHT 1980; PAPARELLA 1980).

8.5.2.4
Malformations of the Vestibular Aqueduct

The bony vestibular aqueduct is a channel that contains one or more small veins, the membranous endolymphatic duct, and part of the endolymphatic sac as it passes from the vestibule to the posterior surface of the petrous pyramid. The endolymphatic duct is a short single-lumen tubule, whereas the endolymphatic sac is a much larger and highly complex structure of interconnecting tubules and cisterns which are not surrounded by perilymph like the rest of the membranous labyrinth but instead by abundant stroma. The sac is accommodated partially within the expanded bony vestibular aqueduct and partially between layers of dura matter outside the vestibular aqueduct. The distal end of the sac overlaps the sigmoid sinus in as many as 40% of cases (GULYA and SCHUKNECHT 1993; LO et al. 1997; KOLLIAS 1997). On axial images it is seen coursing parallel to the posterior semicircular canal towards the vestibule. This structure is more accurately defined on T2-weighted MR images, reformatted along the long axis of the aqueduct revealing its conical shape with the narrow part pointing towards the vestibular orifice and the base at the posterior surface of the temporal bone (Fig. 8.13a–e; OEHLER et al. 1995). Measurement of the diameter at the mid-portion of the aqueduct is considered abnormal if it measures more than 1.5 mm. Non-visibility need not be pathological. The aqueduct is not visualized in 25% of cases on T2-weighted images (DAHLEN et al. 1997). The length of the aqueduct is variable and determined by the degree of perilabyrinthine and infralabyrinthine pneumatization.

Two types of malformative syndromes have been described which appear to be associated with different patterns of pathological and clinical manifestations: the "narrow vestibular aqueduct syndrome", characterized by an abnormally small vestibular aqueduct, and the "large vestibular aqueduct syndrome" characterized by an abnormally large vestibular aqueduct (VALVASSORI and WILBRAND

1986) (Fig. 8.13f–m). A totally obliterated or filiform aqueduct has been associated with Meniere's disease (TANIOKA et al. 1997). The large vestibular aqueduct syndrome with large endolymphatic duct and sac was described as a distinct clinical entity in 1978 by VALVASSORI and CLEMIS (1978) using polytomographic images. In 3700 consecutive cases referred for inner ear tomography they found 50 cases (1.5%) with a large aqueduct ranging from 1.5 to 8 mm in the anteroposterior diameter. It was bilateral in 72% of cases. In addition to the enlarged aqueduct, other associated inner ear anomalies of the vestibule, semicircular canals, and cochlea were identified in 60% of this population. Bilateral involvement was twice as common as unilateral with a female-to-male predominance of 3:2. Most cases were associated with congenital hearing losses. They suggested that a large aqueduct presumably represents an arrested phase of inner ear development common to all 50 cases. The malformation itself was first described by MONDINI in 1791 and presently has come to be recognized as the most common imaging abnormality associated with congenital sensorineural hearing loss (MAFEE et al. 1992). ANTONELLI et al. (1998) graded the severity of the malformation by assessing the width of the aqueduct and the configuration of the widening close to vestibule into five grades of increasing severity, which they found to correlate with the degree of hearing impairment. The evolution of newer imaging techniques has also allowed better assessment of the frequency and type of associated abnormalities which is of paramount importance for the prognosis and therapeutic planning of patients with a large vestibular aqueduct. In an MR study of 63 patients, DAVIDSON et al. (1999) found cochlear anomalies in 76% of cases manifesting as modiolar deficiency, dysmorphism, and scalar asymmetry, vestibular abnormalities in 40% of cases and abnormal semicircular canal in 13% of cases. Several mechanisms have been proposed to explain the progressive SNHL in patients with enlarged vestibular aqueduct including cochlear injury caused by pressure effects, physiological endolymph dysfunction, and susceptibility to minor trauma (JACKLER and DE LA CRUZ 1989). Modiolar deficiency is the most frequent cochlear finding and has been reported to occur in 100% of ears with a large vestibular aqueduct examined by HRCT (LEMMERLING et al. 1997). This association suggests that a large vestibular aqueduct may be only occasionally, if ever, an isolated developmental anomaly of the inner ear, and that the modiolar deficiencies seen in these patients may contribute to the progressive sensorineural hearing loss.

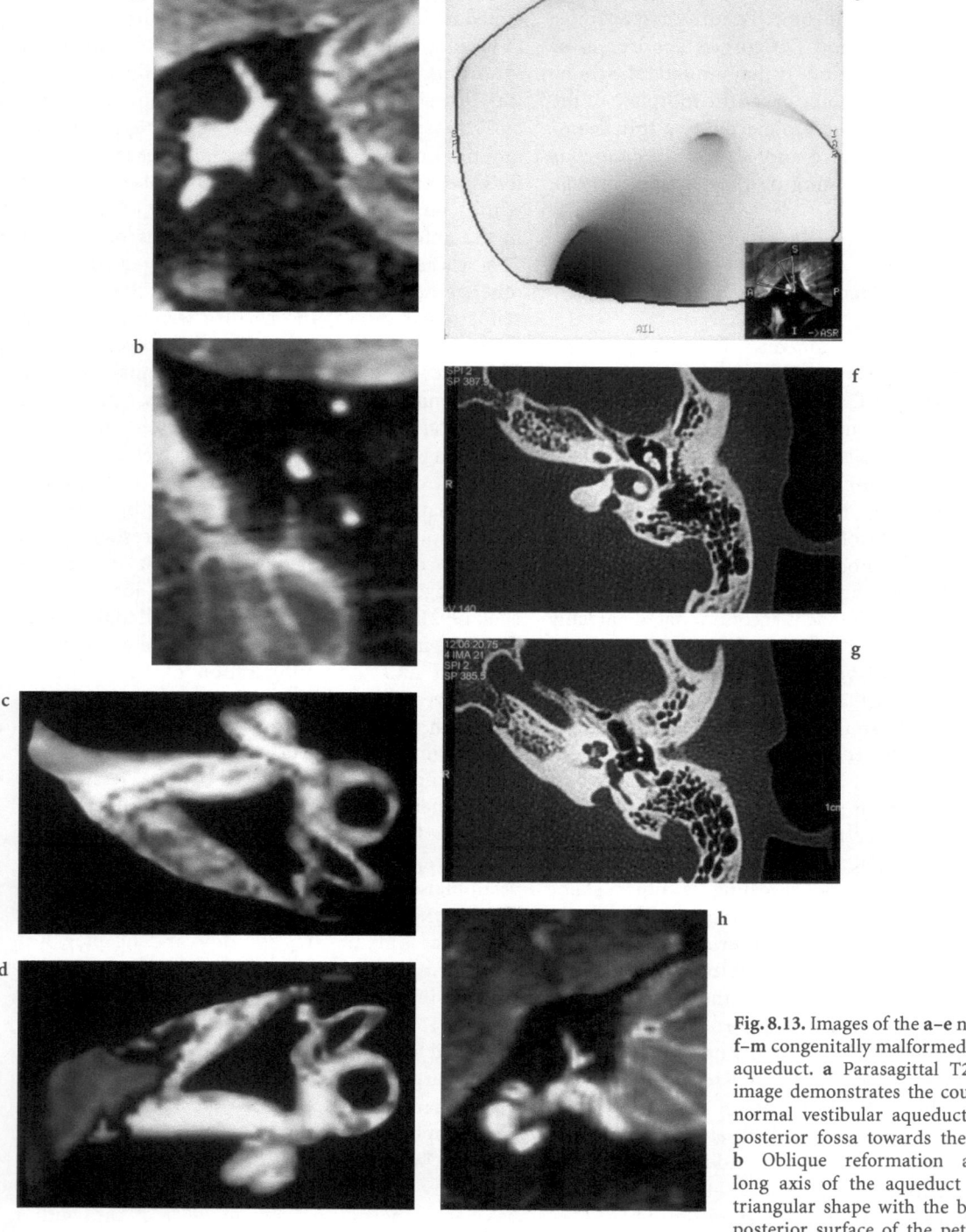

Fig. 8.13. Images of the **a–e** normal and **f–m** congenitally malformed vestibular aqueduct. **a** Parasagittal T2-weighted image demonstrates the course of the normal vestibular aqueduct from the posterior fossa towards the vestibule. **b** Oblique reformation along the long axis of the aqueduct shows its triangular shape with the base in the posterior surface of the petrous bone and the apex pointing to the common crus. **c, d** The 3D surface-rendered MR images demonstrate the irregular shape of the endolymphatic sac and the small endolymphatic duct entering the posteroinferior aspect of the vestibule. **e** Virtual otoscopic MR image from within the vestibule shows the small opening of the vestibular orifice for the entrance of the endolymphatic duct into the osseous vestibule. **f, g** Axial CT images reveal a large vestibular aqueduct in the posterior surface of the temporal bone running parallel to the posterior semicircular canal. **h** Reformatted T2-weighted and **j** MIP projection MR images demonstrate the dilated endolymphatic sac extending outside the bony vestibular aqueduct in the posterior fossa covered by dura. **k–m** Surface-rendered MR images give a better impression for the extent of pathology demonstrating the dilatation of the endolymphatic sac and duct in their entire length

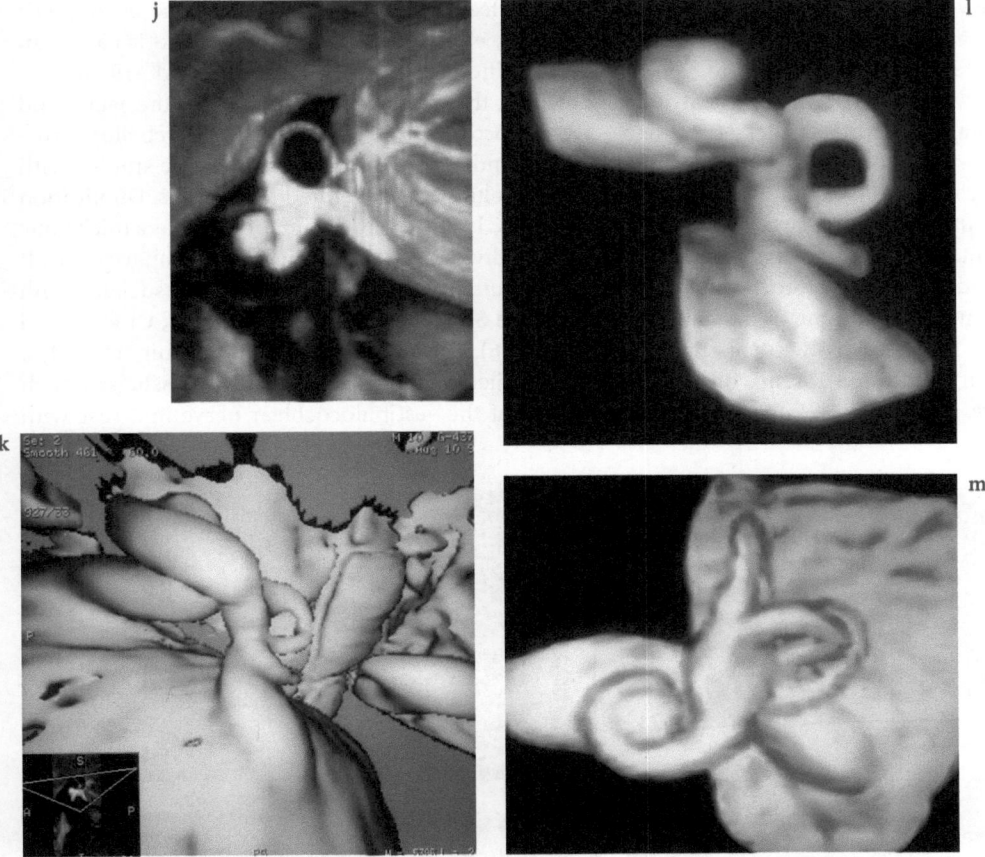

8.5.2.5
Malformations of the Cochlear Aqueduct

The cochlear aqueduct is a bony canal that traverses the petrous pyramid from the scala tympani of the basal turn of the cochlea, close to round window, to an external, funnel-shaped aperture on the inferior surface of the petrous pyramid at the anterior division of the jugular foramen. It connects the scala tympani with the subarachnoid space of the posterior fossa. The cranial aperture of the cochlear aqueduct is a flattened funnel that is anatomically adjacent to the trunk of the glossopharyngeal nerve. Large variations in the length of the aqueduct ranging from 6.2 to 12.9 mm and the diameter of its external aperture ranging from 0.8 to 6.7 mm have been reported (GULYA and SCHUKNECHT 1993; KOLLIAS 1997).

The cochlear aqueduct is considered abnormally dilated when it shows a uniform caliber of over 0.5 mm through its entire course, rather than tapering into a minute structure close to the round window (KASEEF and JARDIN 1986). Abnormal cochlear aqueduct is found in 15% of patients with congenital ear malformations and increases the risk of cerebrospinal otorrhea and meningeal infection following stapedectomies (TOMURA et al. 1995).

8.5.2.6
Malformations of the Internal Auditory Canal

The IAC is a bony neurovascular channel providing a conduit for the facial, cochlear, and vestibular nerves, the nervus intermedius, and the labyrinthine artery and vein from the posterior cranial fossa into the temporal bone. There are large variations in the size, shape, and orientation of the canal, which reflect variations in the size and the degree of pneumatization of the temporal bone. The canal is usually uniformly cylindrical, but funnel-shaped canals with a smaller diameter at either its medial or lateral aspects, central hourglass-like narrowing, or localized areas of widening (cupping) in its anterior wall are common anatomic variants and should not be interpreted as abnormal. Although small interaural differences may occur, there is a relative constancy in the diameter of the paired IACs in the same individual which reflects the constancy of the volume of the contained neuro-vascular bundle for a particular individual (GULYA and SCHUKNECHT 1993; PORTMANN et al. 1975). High-resolution, T2-weighted MR images identify in great detail the contained neurovascular structures and their anatomic relationships within the canal (Fig. 8.14a–e; RUBINSTEIN et al. 1996).

Malformations of the IAC include extreme narrowing, duplication anomalies, and abnormal orientation (Fig. 8.14f–o). Marked dilatation of the canal is of questionable significance except in neurofibromatosis (KASEEF and JARDIN 1986). A narrow canal <2.5 mm in diameter implies an associated absence of the vestibulocochlear nerve and this is a contraindication

for cochlear implantation (CASSELMAN et al. 1997; SHELTON et al. 1989). An atretic or stenotic canal can be identified on high-resolution CT and MR images; however, the associated anomalies of the facial and vestibulocochlear nerves in the cerebellopontine cistern and within the canal can only be studied with high-resolution T2-weighted MR images. Duplication of the IAC is a rare anomaly manifesting as a thick bony septum dividing the canal into two compartments. It may be unilateral or bilateral and is associated with complete SNHL (WEISSMAN et al. 1991; CURTIN and MAY 1986). The author had the opportunity to study a case of bilateral duplication of the IAC associated with aplasia of the vestibulocochlear nerve in a case with

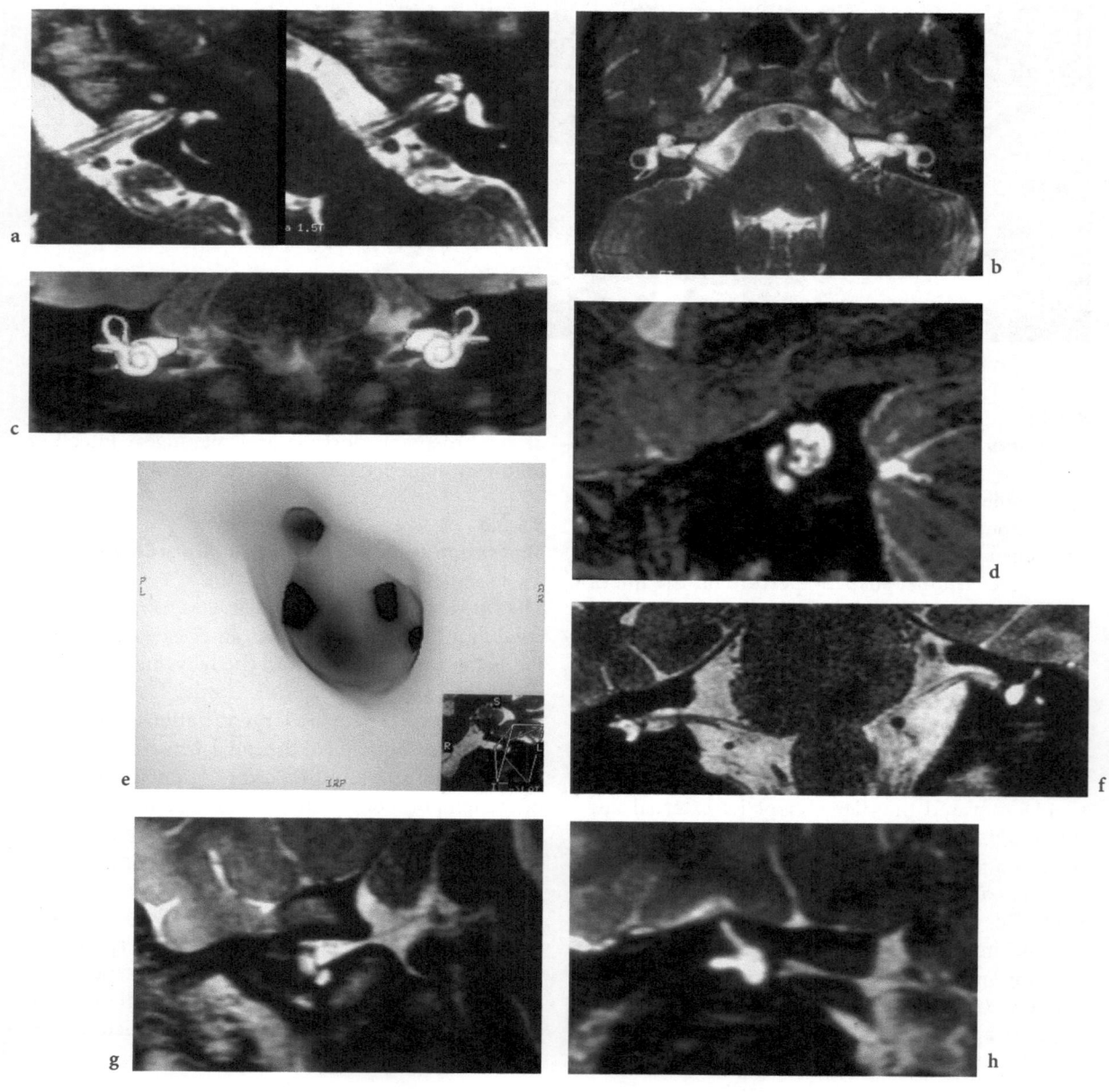

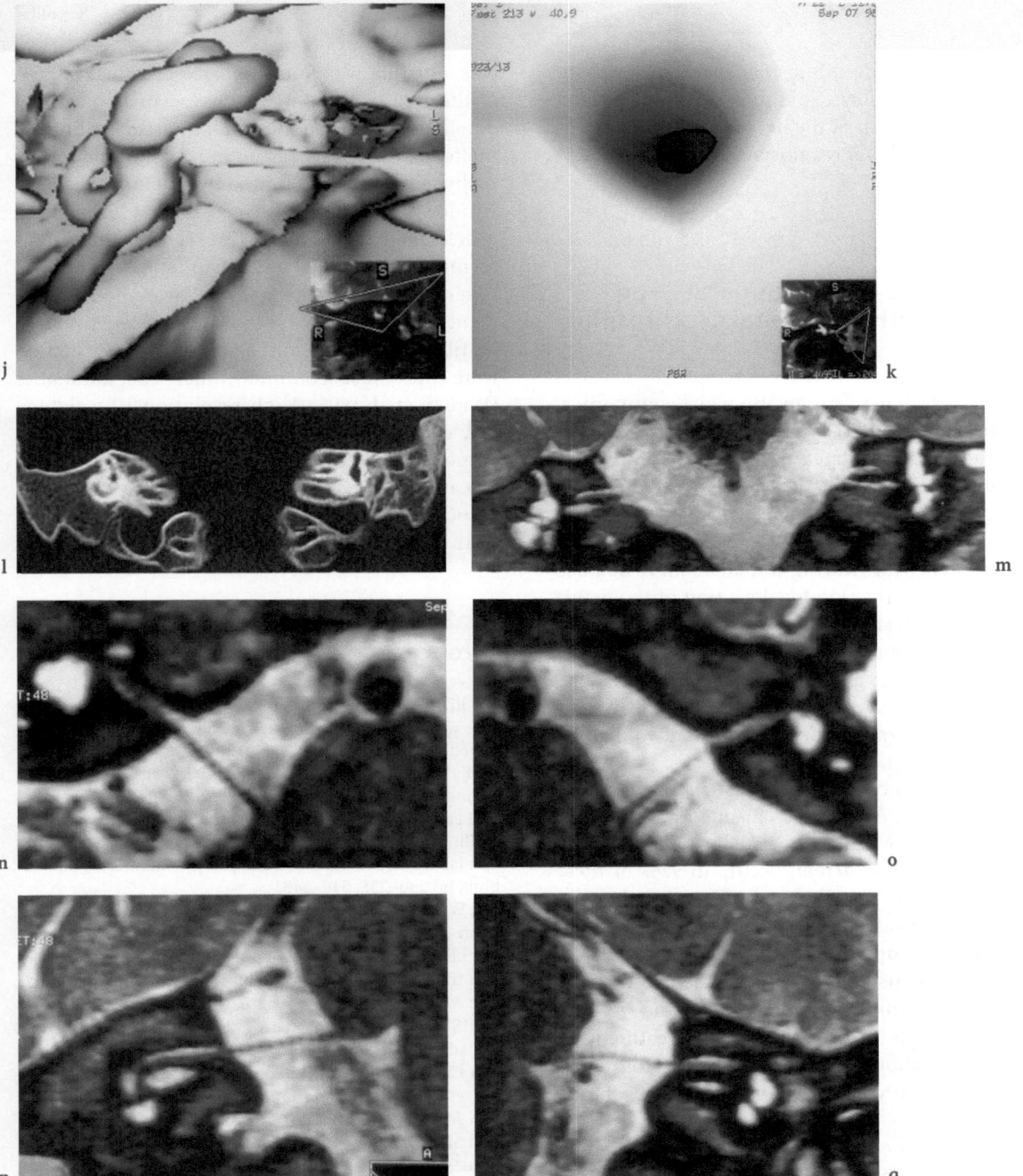

◁ **Fig. 8.14. a–e** Images of the normal and **f–o** congenitally malformed internal auditory canal. **a** Axial high-resolution T2-weighted images and **b** surface-rendered images in axial and **c** coronal projections demonstrate the normal shape and orientation of the canal and the presence of its contained neurovascular structures. **d** Sagittal T2-weighted and **e** virtual otoscopic images at the level of the fundus reveal four nerves in an ordered arrangement with the facial and cochlear nerves located anteriorly (the facial being always superior to the cochlear) and the superior and inferior branches of the vestibular nerve posteriorly. **f** Coronal T2-weighted image in a child with craniosynostosis reveals an abnormally shaped and oriented canal on the left with the inferior lip of the internal acoustic meatus pointing upwards and compressing the facial and vestibulocochlear nerves. **g** Coronal T2-weighted MR image shows an abnormally narrow internal auditory canal associated with aplasia of the cochlear nerve. A very thin nerve, representing the facial nerve, is seen coursing in CPA cistern and the superior portion of the canal. **j** T2-weighted, **k** surface-rendered, and **l** virtual otoscopic MR images reveal a severe stenosis of the internal auditory canal. The vestibulocochlear nerve is absent and a single opening from the facial nerve is present in the virtual otoscopic reconstruction. The osseous labyrinthine structures are normally formed. **l** Coronal CT and **m** coronal, **n, o** axial, and **p, q** oblique reformatted T2-weighted MR images in a patient with Goldenhar syndrome reveal a bilateral duplication of the internal auditory through a horizontal bony septum into a superior and inferior compartment. The facial nerve can be identified on the high-resolution images coursing in the superior compartment of the canal, but the vestibulocochlear nerve is aplastic on the right side and severely hypoplastic on the left

Goldenhar syndrome. Abnormal orientation of the canal, most commonly exhibiting an upward pointing with compression of the nerve structures, may be associated with several craniosynostosis syndromes.

8.6
Malformations of the Temporal Bone Associated with Congenital Cerebrospinal Fluid Fistula

A congenital CSF fistula is an abnormal communication between the subarachnoid space and the middle ear cavity, which is related to a congenital anomaly of the temporal bone. The possibility of a congenital fistula should always be suspected in patients with repeated episodes of meningitis, particularly if they are associated with hearing impairment. A detailed radiological investigation for detection of the fistula and for demonstration of an associated abnormality of the temporal bone is necessary (APPEL and VIGN-AUD 1986; HASSO et al. 1995).

Spontaneous CSF otorrhea is rare. WETMORE et al. (1987) in a literature review reported two distinct subtypes:

1. The childhood type which is associated with congenital defects of the otic capsule and occurs in 72% of cases. Meningitis, usually pneumococcal and frequently recurrent, occurs in 92% of these cases. The child usually has unilateral and sometimes bilateral absence of cochlear and vestibular function and commonly exhibits a Mondini deformity. The CSF usually enters the inner ear through a dural defect in the lateral aspect of the IAC and exists through the oval window. Treatment in these cases should consist of stapedectomy and packing of the vestibule with muscle or subtotal petrosectomy.

2. The adult type representing 28% of cases of spontaneous CSF otorrhea is characterized by bony dehiscences, most commonly of the tegmen tympani or tegmen mastoideum and less commonly of the posterior fossa plate. The meningeal defects are either meningoencephaloceles or simply holes in the dura. Therapy in these cases should consist of a mastoidectomy in conjunction with a transtemporal supralabyrinthine (middle fossa) approach if a meningoencephalocele of the tegmen is found. In a retrospective study of 94 pediatric patients who underwent exploratory tympanotomy for perilymphatic fistula due to unexplained progressive or fluctuating hearing loss, a fistula was found in 81% of cases. In 86% of these cases there was an associated congenital deformity of the middle ear, inner ear, or both. A malformed stapes was the most common abnormality seen (60%), followed by a deformed round window (30.8%), a deformed incus (16.9%), and a deformed promontory (3%). Often these malformations coexisted amongst themselves or with inner ear abnormalities. Inner ear malformations identified on CT were seen in 32% of cases. A large vestibular aqueduct and a Mondini malformation were the most common inner ear anomalies (WEBER et al. 1993). High-resolution T2-weighted MR cisternography and CT cisternography can demonstrate the presence and site of the fistula in cases with active CSF leakage, and screen for associated malformations of the temporal bone (SHETTY et al. 1997).

References

Antonelli PJ, Nall AV, Lemmerling MM et al. (1998) Hearing loss with cochlear modiolar defects and large vestibular aqueducts. Am J Otol 19:306–312

Appel B, Vignaud J (1986) Cerebrospinal fluid fistulae due to a congenital defect of the petrous bone. In: Vignaud J (ed) The ear. Masson, Paris, pp 126–133

Arey LB, Real RL (1974) Developmental anatomy: a textbook and laboratory manual of embryology. Saunders, Philadelphia, pp 236–238, 546–548

Barr B, Wersall J (1965) Cerebrospinal otorrhea with meningitis in congenital deafness. Arch Otolaryngol 81:26–28

Bellucci RJ (1981) Congenital aural malformations: diagnosis and treatment. Otolaryngol Clin North Am 14:95–124

Benton C, Bellet PS (1997) The ear and temporal bone. In: Ball SW (ed) Pediatric neuroradiology. Lippincott-Raven, Philadelphia, pp 607–669

Benton C, Bellet PS (2000) Imaging of congenital anomalies of the temporal bone. Neuroimaging Clin North Am 10:35–53

Brogan M, Chakeres DW, Schmalbrock P (1991) High resolution 3DFT MR imaging of the endolymphatic duct and soft tissues of the otic capsule AJNR 12:1–11

Calzolari F, Garani G, Sensi A, Martini A (1999) Clinical and radiological evaluation in children with microtia. Br J Audiol 33:3003–3012

Carter BL, Wolport SM, Karmody CS (1975) Reccurent meningitis associated with an anomaly of the inner ear. Neuroradiology 9:55–61

Casselman JW, Kuhweide R, Deimling M et al. (1993) Constructive interference in steady state-3DFT MR imaging of the inner ear and cerebellopontine angle. Am J Neuroradiol 14:47–57

Casselman W, Offeciers FE, Govaerts PJ et al. (1997) Aplasia and hypoplasia of the vestibulocochlear nerve: diagnosis with MR imaging. Radiology 202:773–781

Cole RR, Jahrsdoerfer RA (1990) The risk of cholesteatoma in congenital aural stenosis. Laryngoscope 100:576–578

Curtin HD, May M (1986) Double internal auditory canal associated with progressive facial weakness. Am J Otol 7: 275–281

Dahlen RT, Harnsberger R, Gray SD et al. (1997) Overlapping thin-section fast spin-echo MR of the large vestibular aqueduct syndrome. AJNR 18:67–75

Daniels DL, Swartz JD, Harnsberger HR et al. (1996) Anatomic moment. Hearing I: the cochlea. Am J Neuroradiol 17:1237–1241

Davidson HC, Harnsberger HR, Lemmerling MM et al. (1999) MR evaluation of vestibulocochlear anomalies associated with large endolymphatic duct and sac. AJNR 20: 1435–1441

Dayal VS (1973) Embryology of the ear. Can J Otolaryngol 2: 136

Delvert JP, Lafon J (1986) Embryology of the temporal bone. In: Vignaud J (ed) The ear. Masson, Paris, pp 1–7

Denk W, Keolian RM, Ogawa S, Jelinski LW (1993) Oscillatory flow in the cochlea visualized by a magnetic resonance imaging technique. Proc Natl Acad Sci USA 90:1595–1598

Friedberg J (1994) Congenital cholesteatoma. Laryngoscope 104:1–24

Gulya AJ, Schuknecht HF (1993) Anatomy of the temporal bone with surgical implications. Parthenon, New York, pp 129–160, 235–288

Hanafee WN, Bergstrom L (1980) Radiology of congenital deformities of the ear. Head Neck Surg 2:213–221

Hasso A, Casselman JW, Broadwell RA (1995) Temporal bone congenital anomalies. In: Som PM, Curtin HD (eds) Head and neck imaging, 3rd edn, vol 2. Mosby, St. Louis, pp 1351–1390

Hill J, Elliott C, Colquhoun I (1992) Audiological, vestibular and radiological abnormalities in Kallman's syndrome. J Laryngol Otol 106:530–534

Hoenk BE, McCabe BF, Anson BJ (1969) Cholesteatoma auris behind a bony atresia plate. Arch Otolaryngol 89:470–477

Jackler RK, Cruz A de la (1989) The large vestibular aqueduct syndrome. Laryngoscope 99:1238–1243

Jackler RK, Luxford WM, House WF (1987) Congenital malformations of the inner ear. Laryngoscope 97:2–14

Jafek BW, Nager GT, Strife J et al. (1975) Congenital aural atresia: an analysis of 311 cases. Trans Am Acad Ophthalmol Otolaryngol 98:807–812

Jaffe BF (1977) Hearing loss in children: a comprehensive text. University Park Press, Baltimore

Jahrsdoerfer R (1980) Congenital malformations of the ear: analysis of 94 operations. Ann Otol 89:348–352

Jahrsdoerfer RA, Lambert PR (1998) Facial nerve injury in congenital aural atresia surgery. Am J Otol 19:283–2877

Kaseef LG, Jardin C (1986) Malformations: the radiological examination of ear malformations. In: Vignaud J (ed) The ear. Masson, Paris, pp 104–125

Kollias SS, Ball WS, Prenger EC, Myers CM III (1995) Dermoids of the Eustachian tube: CT and MR findings with histologic correlation. Am J Neuroradiol 16:663–668

Kollias SS (1997) Normal MRI of the temporal bone with variants and pitfalls. Proc Int Congr Head and Neck Radiology, Strasbourg, 15–18 October, pp 130–150

Kollias SS, Valavanis A, Linder T, Fisch U (1998) High resolution T2 weighted magnetic resonance (MR) imaging of the facial nerve. In: Yanagihara N, Murakami S (eds) New horizons in facial nerve research and facial expression. Kugler, Hague, The Netherlands, pp 151–157

Lagundoye SB, Martinson FD, Fajemisin AA (1975) The syndrome of enlarged vestibule and dysplasia of the lateral semicircular canal in congenital deafness. Radiology 115: 377–378

Lambert PR, Dodson E (1996) Congenital malformations of the external auditory canal. Otolaryngol Clin North Am 29:741–760

Lemmerling MM, Mancuso AA, Antonelli PJ, Kubilis PS (1997) Normal modiolus: CT appearance in patients with a large vestibular aqueduct. Radiology 204:213–219

Lemmerling MM, Vanzieleghem BD, Mortier GR et al. (2000) Unilateral semicircular canal aplasia in Goldenhar's syndrome. AJNR 21:1334–1336

Levenson MJ, Michaels L, Parisier SC (1989) Congenital cholesteatomas of the middle ear in children: origin and management. Otolaryngol Clin North Am 22:941–954

Llano Rivas I, Gonzalez-del-Angel A, del Castillo V et al. (1999) Microtia: a clinical and genetic study at the National Institute of Pediatrics in Mexico City. Arch Med Res 30:120–124

Lo WW, Daniels DL, Chakeres DW et al. (1997) The endolymphatic duct and sac. Am J Neuroradiol 18:881–887

Mafee MF, Selis JE, Yannias DA et al. (1984) Congenital sensorineural hearing loss. Radiology 150:427–434

Mafee MF, Charletta D, Kumar A, Belmont H (1992) Large vestibular aqueduct and congenital SNHL. AJNR 13:805–819

Manfre L, Genuardi P, Tortorici M, Lagalla R (1997) Absence of the common crus in Goldenhar syndrome. AJNR 18: 773–775

Marsot-Dupuch K, Dominguez-Brito A, Ghasli K, Chouard C-H (1999) CT and MR findings of Michel anomaly: inner ear aplasia. AJNR 20:281–284

Marx H (1926) Die Missbildungen des Ohres. In: Denker W, Kahler H (ed) Handbuch der Hals-Nasen-Ohrenkunde. Springer, Berlin Heidelberg New York

Mayer TE, Brueckmann H, Siegert R, Witt A, Weerda H (1997) High resolution CT of the temporal bone in dysplasia of the auricle and external auditory canal. Am J Neuroradiol 18:53–65

McGill TJ, Merchant S, Healy GB et al. (1991) Congenital cholesteatoma of the middle ear in children: a clinical and histopathological report. Laryngoscope 1001:606–613

Mondini C (1996) Minor works of Carlo Mondini: the anatomical section of a boy born deaf. Am J Otol 18:288–293

Mukherji SK, Tart RP, Slattery WH, Stringer SP, Benson MT, Mancuso AA (1993) Evaluation of first branchial anomalies by CT and MR. J Comput Assist Tomogr 17:576–581

Murofushi T, Ouvrier RA, Parker GD et al. (1997) Vestibular abnormalities in CHARGE association. Ann Otol Rhinol Laryngol 106:129–134

Naidich TP, Mann SS, Som PM (2000) Imaging of the osseous, membranous, and perilymphatic labyrinths. Neuroimaging Clin North Am 10:23–34

Oehler MC, Chakeres DW, Scmalbrock P (1995) Reformatted planar "Christmas tree" MR appearance of the endolymphatic sac. AJNR 16:1525–1528

Olsen KD, Maragos NE, Weiland LH (1980) First branchial cleft anomalies. Laryngoscope 90:423–436

Paparella MM (1980) Mondini's deafness: a review of histopathology. Ann Otol Rhinol Laryngol Suppl 89:1–10

Petasnick JP (1973) Congenital malformations of the ear. Otolaryng Clin North Am 6:413–428

Phelps PD, Lioyd GAS (1983) Radiology of the ear. Blackwell, Oxford, pp 22–48

Portmann M, Steckers JM, Charachon R, Chuard C (1975) The internal auditory meatus: anatomy, pathology, and surgery. Churchill Livingston, New York

Rubinstein D, Sandberg EJ, Cajade-Law AG (1996) Anatomy of the facial and vestibulocochlear nerves in the internal auditory canal. AJNR 17:1099–1105

Savic D, Jasovic A, Djeric D (1989) The relations of the mastoid segment of the facial cnal to surrounding structures in congenital middle ear malformations. Int J Pediatr Otorrhinolaryngol 18:13–19

Schmalbrock P, Brogan MA, Chakeres et al. (1993) Optimization of submillimeter resolution MR imaging methods for the inner ear. J Magn Reson Imaging 3:451–459

Schmalbrock P, Pruski J, Sun L et al. (1995) Phased array RF coils for high resolution MRI of the inner ear and brainstem. J Comput Assist Tomogr 19:8–14

Schuknecht HF (1980) Mondini dysplasia: a clinical and pathological study. Ann Otol Rhinol Laryngol 89:1–23

Schuknecht HF (1989) Congenital aural atresia. Laryngoscope 99:908–917

Shelton C, Luxford WM, Tonokawa LL (1989) The narrow internal auditory canal in children: a contraindicaion to cochlear implants. Otolaryngol Head Neck Surg 100:227–231

Shetty PG, Shroff MM, Kirtane MV, Karmarkar SS (1997) Cerebrospinal fluid otorhinorrhea in patients with defects through the lamina cribrosa of the internal auditory canal. Am J Neuroradiol 18:478–481

Stone JA, Chakeres DW, Schmalbrock P (1998) High resolution imaging of the auditory pathway. MRI Clin North Am 6: 195–217

Swartz JD, Faerber EN (1985) Congenital malformations of the external and middle ear: high resolution CT findings of surgical importance. AJR 144:501–506

Swartz JD, Daniels DL, Harnsberger HR et al. (1996a) The temporal bone. Am J Neuroradiol 17:201–204

Swartz JD, Daniels DL, Harnsberger HR et al. (1996b) Balance and equilibrium I. The vestibule and semicircular canals. Am J Neuroradiol 17:17–21

Tanioka H, Kaga K, Araki H, Sasaki Y (1997) MR of the endolymphatic duct and sac: findings in Meniere disease. AJNR 18:45–51

Tien RD, Felsberg GJ, Macfall J (1993) Three-dimensional MR gradient recalled echo imaging of the inner ear: comparison of FID and echo imaging techniques. Magn Reson Imaging 11:429–435

Tomura N, Sashi R, Kobayashi M et al. (1995) Normal variations of the temporal bone on high-resolution CT: their incidence and clinical significance. Clin Radiol 50: 144–148

Valvassori GE, Clemis JD (1978) The large vestibular aqueduct syndrome. Laryngoscope 88:723–728

Valvassori GE, Wilbrand HF (1986) Vestibular and cochlear aqueduct. In: Vignaud J (ed) The ear. Masson, Paris, pp 304–311

Weber PC, Perez BA, Bluestone CD (1993) Congenital perilymphatic fistula and associated middle ear abnormalities. Laryngoscope 103:160–164

Weissman JL, Arriaga M, Crtin HD, Hirsch B (1991) Duplication anomaly of the internal auditory canal. AJNR 12: 867–869

Wetmore SJ, Herrmann P, Fisch U (1987) Spontaneous cerebrospinal fluid otorrhea. Am J Otol 8:96–102

Williams GH (1992) Developmental anatomy of the ear. In: English GM (ed) Otolaryngology. Lippincott, Philadelphia, pp 1–67

Williams PL, Warwick R, Dyson M, Bannister LH (eds) (1990) Gray's anatomy, 37th edn. Churrchill-Livingstone, Edinburgh

Wittekindt C, Schondorf J, Stennert E, Jungehulsing M (2001) Duplication of the external auditory canal: a report of three cases. Int J Pediatr Otorhinolaryngol 58:179–184

Wood-Jones F, Wen I-C (1934) Development of the external ear. J Anat 68:525

Work WP, Proctor CA (1963) The otologist and first branchial cleft anomalies. Ann Otol Rhinol Laryngol 72:584

Yeakley JW, Jahrsdoerfer RA (1996) CT evaluation of congenital aural atresia: what the radiologist and surgeon need to know. J Comput Assist Tomogr 20:724–731

Ying K, Schmalbrock P, Clymer B (1995) Echo-time reduction for submillimeter resolution imaging with 3D phase encoded time reduced acquisition method. Magn Reson Med 33:82–87

The Clinician's View

I. Dhooge

Probably the most fascinating embryological phenomenon in the ENT domain is the ontogenetic development of the external, middle, and inner ear. The pinna grows from three of the six auricular humps, the ossicles and middle ear muscles derive from the first and second branchial arch, the middle ear space derives from an extension of the first pharyngeal pouch, and the inner ear originates from the ectodermal neural crest. The ontogenic development explains the fact that external and middle ear anomalies are often associated and can be associated with facial, cervical, and skeletal dysplasias. Inner ear anomalies are often isolated. When in a child a malformation occurs of the outer and/or middle ear, it is often noticed shortly after birth and the child is referred for evaluation. With the advent of early screening programs for hearing loss, ENT doctors are also increasingly more confronted with infants with uni- or bilateral neurosensory hearing loss without outer or middle ear or craniofacial malformations. In all cases it is necessary to determine the child's usable residual hearing and the need for amplification as soon as possible after birth. Although radiographic studies at an early age are rarely applicable to immediate rehabilitative plans, they may be important in providing information on the extent of malformations (outer-, middle-, inner ear, and/or nervous structures) and the possible etiology (isolated or syndromal). Counseling of the patient and determining the best therapy plan is based on an understanding of the extent of the defect. Radiology is also important to rule out the possibility of congenital cholesteatoma.

When surgery is considered, radio-imaging of the temporal bone is necessary in all patients to determine the patients' candidacy for surgical correction of hearing. Jahrsdoefer et al. developed a grading system based on pre-operative temporal bone CT and auricular appearance to aid in patient selection for surgical correction of hearing. This grading system correlates well with the degree of hearing improvement achieved. Proper selection of patients maximizes the opportunity for hearing recovery and minimizes the potential for surgical complications.

9 Tumors of Cerebellopontine Angle, Internal Auditory Canal, and Inner Ear

B. De Foer

Contents

9.1
Introduction

This chapter focuses on the main features of tumoral lesions of the cerebellopontine angle, internal auditory canal, and inner ear. It highlights imaging techniques and the most important imaging characteristics of these lesions. A small overview of less common lesions is also given.

9.2
Tumors of Cerebellopontine Angle

9.2.1
Introduction

Tumors of the cerebellopontine angle (CPA) are frequent. They represent approximately 6–10% of all

intracranial tumors. Vestibulocochlear schwannomas and meningiomas are the two most frequent lesions accounting for approximately 85–90% of all CPA tumors. The CPA is outlined by the meninges of the cerebellopontine cistern. In addition to cerebrospinal fluid (CSF), the CPA contains nerves, arteries, and possibly embryologic remnants. The fifth through eighth cranial nerves are in the upper part of the CPA cistern, and the lower portion contains the ninth, tenth, and eleventh cranial nerves (Smirniotopoulos et al. 1993).

Each of these structures can be the site of origin of CPA lesions. Furthermore, lesions can also originate in the surrounding structures such as temporal bone, skull base, or brain stem, and they can also extend into the CPA (Bonneville et al. 2001).

9.2.2
Symptoms and Signs of CPA Tumors

A great variety of symptoms and signs of CPA tumors can be found. None of these symptoms can be linked to a single type of lesion; therefore, these symptoms and signs are highly non-specific. Moreover, lesions of the internal auditory canal and membranous labyrinth can present with the same scala of signs and symptoms as smaller CPA lesions. Masses arising in the CPA typically manifest by either cranial neuropathies or signs of posterior fossa mass effect (Smirniotopoulos et al. 1993).

Although only 1–10% of adults with sensorineural hearing loss have a vestibulocochlear schwannoma, 95% of patients with vestibulocochlear schwannoma have hearing loss. Most cases manifest as progressive unilateral sensorineural hearing loss, but 20% present with sudden hearing loss (Heier et al.1997; Swartz 1998). Often, tinnitus is an accompanying symptom. Symptoms and signs of vestibular dysfunction are a less common presenting symptom possibly due to a better accommodation of the central nervous system to unilateral vestibular dysfunction compared with unilateral cochlear denervation (Swartz 1998).

B. De Foer, MD
Department of Radiology, A.Z. Sint-Augustinus, Oosterveld-laan 24, 2610 Antwerp (Wilrijk), Belgium

Facial motor dysfunction (cranial nerve VII), facial sensory dysfunction (cranial nerve V), and taste disturbance (chorda tympani) are all possible and non-specific symptoms of CPA lesions. Headache, nausea, vomiting, and disorders of gait and balance are usually non-lateralizing signs of a posterior fossa mass (SMIRNIOTOPOULOS et al. 1993).

9.2.3
Vestibulocochlear Schwannoma

Acoustic schwannoma (acoustic nerve neuroma or neurinoma) actually arises from the vestibulocochlear nerve and is probably more accurately termed vestibulocochlear schwannoma. It is by far the most common neoplasm of the CPA cistern, accounting for 85% of all CPA tumors. Approximately 95% of diagnosed vestibulocochlear schwannomas are unilateral, whereas less than 5% are bilateral and associated with neurofibromatosis type II (Fig. 9.1). Type-II neurofibromatosis is an inherited autosomal-dominant syndrome characterized by a propensity for developing multiple schwannomas, meningiomas, and gliomas of ependymal derivation (SMIRNIOTOPOULOS et al. 1993; SWARTZ 1998).

Schwannomas are encapsulated, benign, slowly growing neoplasms arising from the Schwann cells

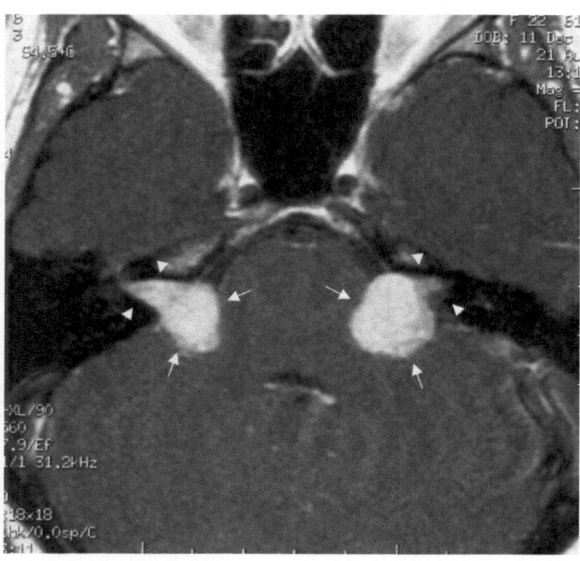

Fig. 9.1. Bilateral vestibulocochlear schwannoma: neurofibromatosis, type 2. Axial enhanced T1-weighted MR image: bilateral uniform enhancing mass lesion with a canalicular (*arrowheads*) and cisternal (*arrows*) component: bilateral vestibulocochlear schwannoma highly suggestive of neurofibromatosis, type 2

of the cranial, spinal, and peripheral nerves. Primary intracranial nerve sheath neoplasms are nearly always schwannomas and they do not have malignant potential. Grossly, a vestibulocochlear schwannoma is usually firm and encapsulated; however, regions of hemorrhage, edema, and cyst formation may be found. Two types of tissues are found in schwannomas. Antoni-A-type tissue is compact, whereas type-B tissue is characterized by loose texture, often with cyst formation. Usually type-A tissue predominates in vestibulocochlear schwannomas (SWARTZ 1998).

It is known that vestibulocochlear schwannomas probably arise inside the internal auditory canal or near its mouth but then secondarily grow into the fluid-filled CPA cistern. The reason for this is that the portion of the eighth cranial nerve traversing the CSF of the CPA cistern does not have Schwann cells but rather oligodendrocytes; however, at the opening of the internal auditory canal there is a transition zone at which the myelin production switches from the oligodendrocytes to the Schwann cells. Schwannomas can also originate in the region of the vestibular (Scarpa's) ganglion, near the fundus of the internal auditory canal (SMIRNIOTOPOULOS et al. 1993; SWARTZ 1998).

Although originating in the internal auditory canal, in larger schwannomas the greatest portion of the tumor is usually in the CPA. The growth rate of vestibulocochlear schwannomas is unpredictable (SMIRNIOTOPOULOS et al. 1993; SWARTZ 1998).

On imaging, the mass is roughly spherical and almost invariably there is a funnel-shaped component that extends into the internal auditory canal ("ice cream cone" appearance; Fig. 9.2). When large, it has a dominant CPA component compressing the adjacent middle cerebellar peduncle and the brain stem. Occasionally, a vestibulocochlear schwannoma may entirely be within the CPA cistern without an intracanalicular component.

The primary imaging tool for evaluation of CPA tumors is MRI. As mentioned, the clinical suspicion of a vestibulocochlear schwannoma is based on a large scala of non-specific symptoms; therefore, in the appropriate clinical setting, there is no role for enhanced CT in the radiologic evaluation of patients clinically suspected of having an acoustic schwannoma (SWARTZ 1998). Unenhanced CT can be used in the preoperative anatomic evaluation of the temporal bone and posterior fossa.

On MR images, the schwannoma is a spherical mass that forms acute angles with the petrous bone.

For T1-weighted imaging, thin-slice (2–3 mm) fast-spin-echo (FSE) T1-weighted images are required in order to diminish volume averaging.

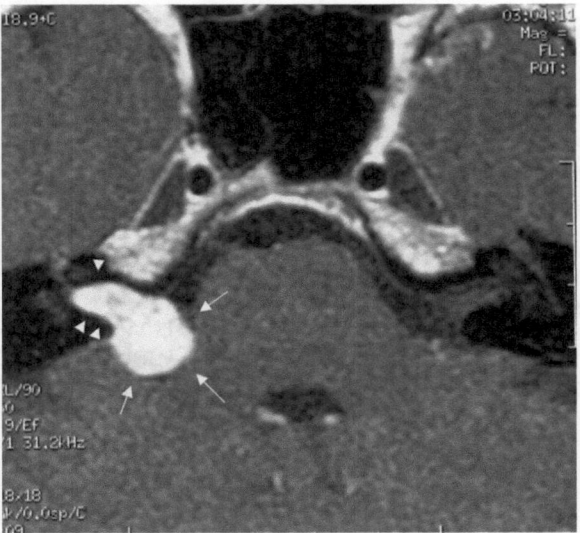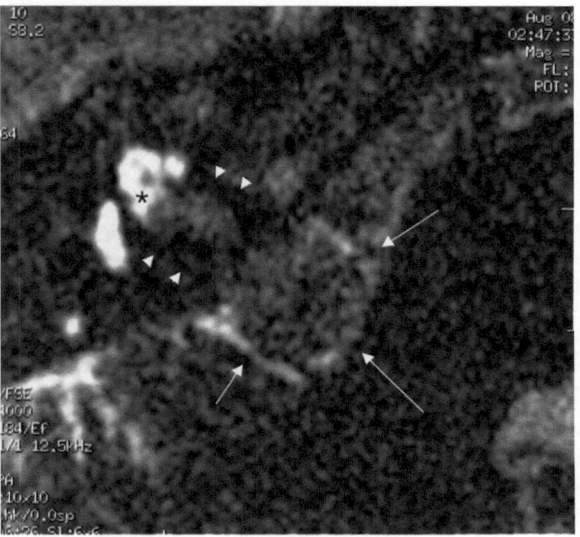

a   b

Fig. 9.2a, b. Typical appearance of cerebellopontine angle–internal auditory canal (CPA–IAC) vestibulocochlear schwannoma. **a** Axial enhanced T1-weighted MR image: strong enhancing mass lesion with canalicular (*arrowheads*) and cisternal (*arrows*) component ("ice cream cone" appearance). **b** Axial high-resolution 3D fast-spin-echo (FSE) T2-weighted MR image: hypointense mass with canalicular (*arrowheads*) and cisternal (*arrows*) component and residual fluid signal in the fundus of the internal auditory canal (*asterisk*)

Three-dimensional spoiled gradient-echo imaging can also be used (NAGANAWA et al. 2001).

On unenhanced T1-weighted images, vestibulocochlear schwannomas are usually isointense to gray matter, with strong enhancement of the lesion after intravenous administration of gadolinium (MULKENS et al. 1993; SMIRNIOTOPOULOS et al. 1993; SWARTZ 1998; Fig. 9.2; Table 9.1). It has been suggested that the intensity and homogeneity of enhancement are produced because their extracellular space is much larger than those of other solid tumors (SMIRNIOTOPOULOS et al. 1993).

On T2-weighted images, the vestibulocochlear schwannoma usually is slightly hyperintense.

High-resolution, thin-slice, strongly T2-weighted MR imaging is also useful for detecting vestibulocochlear schwannomas. Most frequently, 3D FSE/TSE T2-weighted images (or variants of it; CASSELMAN et al. 1993b) and 3D Fourier transformation constructive interference in steady state (3DFT CISS) gradient-echo images are used (CASSELMAN et al. 1993b; NAGANAWA et al. 2001). On these images the mass becomes significantly hypointense to the surrounding CSF. The mass effect of the lesion on the nerves, especially the facial nerve, and vascular structures in the CPA can be clearly evaluated using these sequences (CASSELMAN et al. 1993b; SWARTZ 1998; SARTORETTI-SCHEFER et al. 2000).

The evaluation of the residual fluid signal in the fundus of the internal auditory canal on these sequences is important as it seems that the absence or loss of this signal compromises hearing preservation surgery. Furthermore, the "retro-obstructive" signal loss in the membranous labyrinth, as can be seen on

Table 9.1. Imaging characteristics and suggestive features of the most common lesions of cerebellopontine angle. *IAC* internal auditory canal; *CSF* cerebrospinal fluid

Lesion	T1-weighted	T2-weighted	Enhancement	Suggestive features
Vestibulocochlear schwannoma	Isointense	Hyperintense	Yes	Spherical mass with acute angles, extension in IAC
Meningioma	Isointense	Iso- or hypointense	Yes	Hemispheric mass eccentric to IAC, may cross IAC
Epidermoid cyst	Hypointense	Hyperintense	No	Hyperintense on diffusion-weighted images
Arachnoid cyst	Hypointense	Hyperintense	No	Isointense to CSF, hypointense on diffusion-weighted images

Signal intensities as compared with gray matter

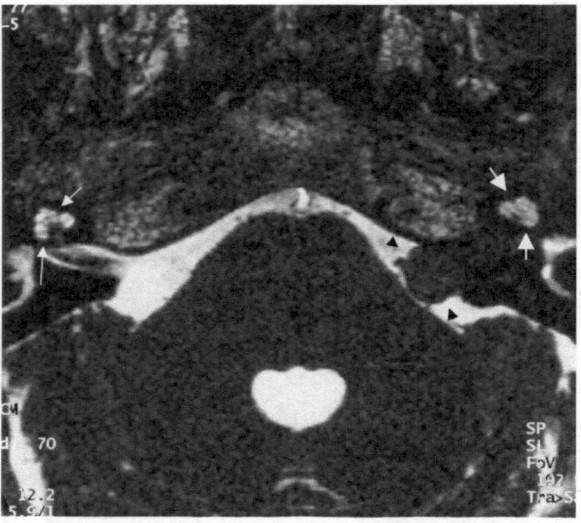

Fig. 9.3. Retro-obstructive signal loss on constructive inter-ference in steady state (CISS) sequence. Axial high-resolu-tion 3D Fourier transformation (FT) CISS MR image: large hypointense mass lesion replacing fluid signal in CPA and IAC compatible with a vestibulocochlear schwannoma (*arrowheads*). The lesion enhanced strongly on T1-weighted MR images (not shown). Note the lack of residual fluid signal in the fundus of the IAC. There is a clear signal drop in the mid and apical turn of the left cochlea (*large arrows*). Compare with the normal signal in the right cochlea (*small arrows*): retro-obstructive signal drop in the left cochlea. (Courtesy of J.W. CASSELMAN)

CISS sequences also seems to compromise hearing preservation surgery. Apparently, this retro-obstruc-tive signal drop is related to the CISS sequence (Fig. 9.3; SOMERS et al. 2001). It is hypothesized that the observed intralabyrinthine fluid signal changes are caused by impairment of the terminal vascular supply by the tumor impacting the IAC (SOMERS et al. 2001).

There are multiple uncommon features of acoustic schwannomas that may be seen during MR evalua-tion including cysts, necrosis, hemorrhage, or adja-cent meningeal reaction (Fig. 9.4; MULKENS et al. 1993; SMIRNIOTOPOULOS et al. 1993; SWARTZ 1998).

Although typically described in meningiomas, a linearly enhancing "dural tail" has occasionally been observed adjacent to vestibulocochlear schwanno-mas (KUTCHER et al. 1991; SWARTZ 1998).

9.2.4
Meningioma

Meningioma is the second most common mass in the CPA. Meningioma of the CPA constitutes up to 10% of all meningiomas and 3–8% of all CPA masses. These arise from the arachnoid villi of the leptomeninges. These villi are most numerous in the large dural sinuses but also occur in smaller veins and along the root sleeves of exiting cranial and spinal nerves. Meningioma has a distinct female predilection with

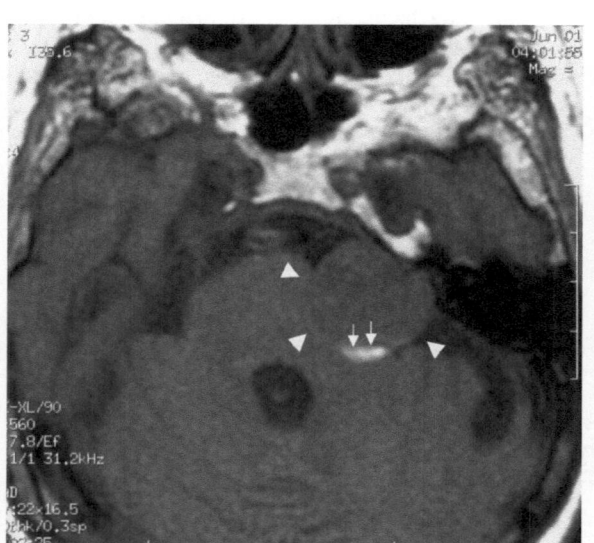

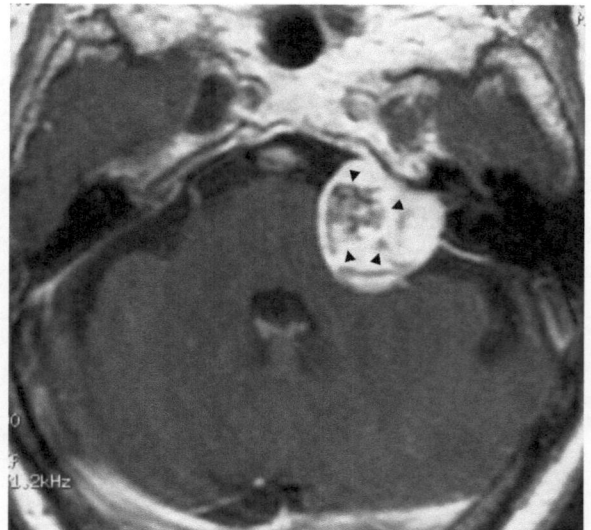

Fig. 9.4a, b. Acoustic schwannoma with intratumoral hemorrhage. **a** Axial non-enhanced T1-weighted MR image: large left CPA–IAC iso-intense mass with characteristic aspect of vestibulocochlear schwannoma (*arrowheads*). Focal area of T1 hyperintensity posteriorly is secondary to hemorrhage (*arrows*). **b** Axial enhanced T1 MR image: strong but inhomogeneous enhancement with scattered areas of non-enhancement (*arrowheads*) consistent with intratumoral cysts or necrosis

a ratio of 2:1. They usually present in the middle-age group (SMIRNIOTOPOULOS et al. 1993; HEIER et al. 1997; SWARTZ 1998).

The clinical presentation of patients with cisternal meningioma varies, depending on the precise location of the tumor. Meningiomas are usually larger at presentation than vestibulocochlear schwannomas. Cranial nerves V, VII, and VIII are usually affected. Meningiomas are usually hemispherical with obtuse angles (Fig. 9.5). They are eccentric to the internal auditory canal and may cross the porus acusticus. Entirely intracanalicular meningiomas have been reported (HAUGHT et al. 1998). Meningiomas often stimulate overgrowth (hyperostosis) of the nearby calvaria, even without histologic infiltration into the bone.

On unenhanced CT scans, meningiomas are usually homogeneously hyperattenuating masses, compared with brain. They enhance strongly after intravenous iodinated contrast material. The CT scans obtained with windows adjusted for bone detail may demonstrate characteristic hyperostosis.

On MR, signal intensity is variable but is usually similar to gray matter on T1-weighted MR images. It can be isointense or hypointense on T2-weighted MR images. Strong enhancement is noted (Table 9.1; SMIRNIOTOPOULOS et al. 1993; HEIER et al. 1997; SWARTZ 1998). A "dural tail" sign is often seen as an area of linear enhancement along the adjacent dura which is continuous with the dural margin of the meningioma (Fig. 9.5). The abnormal enhancement

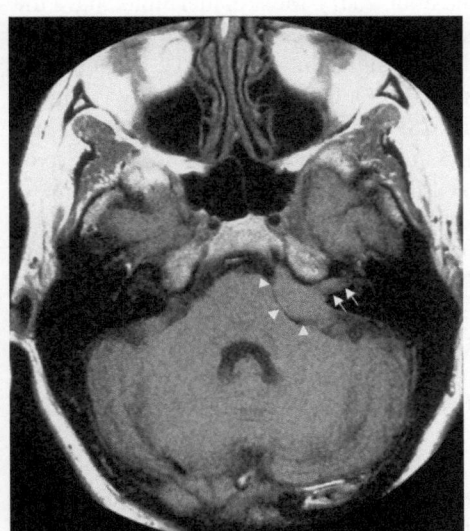

Fig. 9.5a, b. Meningioma with internal auditory canal extension. a Axial unenhanced T1-weighted MR image: isointense hemispherical mass (*arrowheads*) along the posterior side of the left temporal bone extending (*arrows*) into the left internal auditory canal. b Axial and coronal enhanced T1-weighted MR image: strong enhancing hemispherical mass (*arrowheads*) with obtuse angles with the temporal bone. There is a small enhancing component into the left internal auditory canal (*thin arrows*). Note the small dural tail along the posterior side of the temporal bone (*thick arrows*)

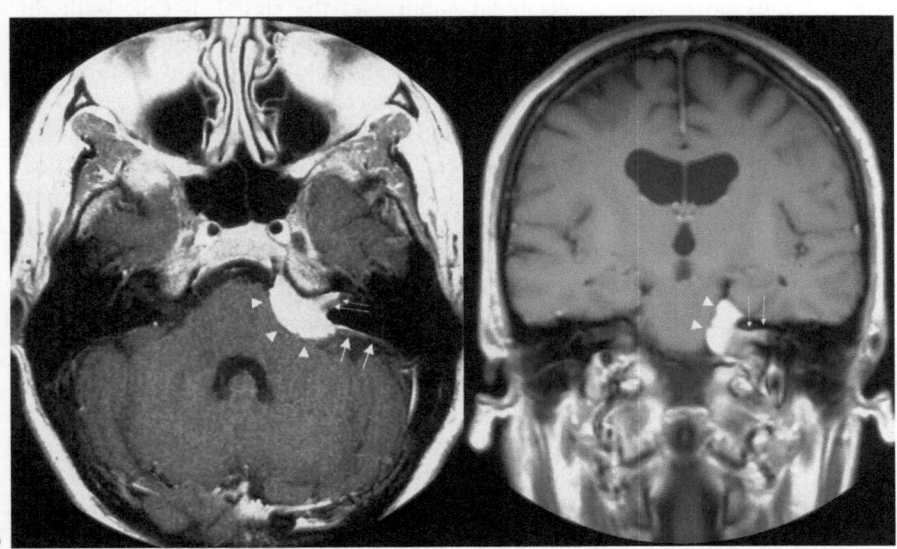

has been ascribed to dural infiltration by tumor, but it may also be caused by non-neoplastic vascular and hyperplastic changes in reaction to the adjacent mass (SMIRNIOTOPOULOS et al. 1993; SWARTZ 1998). The presence of a dural tail is non-specific and has been reported with schwannoma, oligodendroglioma, metastases, and inflammatory processes such as sarcoidosis (KUTCHER et al. 1991; SMIRNIOTOPOULOS et al. 1993; SWARTZ 1998). An IAC extension can be seen in case of larger lesions. Extension of tumor into adjacent intracranial structures, such as Meckel's cave, is also highly suggestive of meningioma (SWARTZ 1998).

9.2.5
Epidermoid Inclusion Cyst

Epidermoid tumors represent approximately 0.2–1.8% of all primary intracranial tumors. The CPA is the most common intracranial location for an epidermoid inclusion cyst (congenital cholesteatoma), but these cysts may also occur in the middle fossa as well as the suprasellar and quadrigeminal plate cisterns. Epidermoid inclusion cysts account for 5% of masses in this region, third only to vestibulocochlear schwannomas and meningiomas. Most intracranial epidermoids and dermoids are not true neoplasms but are considered congenital lesions that arise from inclusion of ectodermal epithelial elements at the time of neural tube closure. These inclusion cysts of skin epithelium are typically unilocular rather than multilocular masses. Lined only by a simple squamous epithelium, epidermoids expand slowly over decades by the continued desquamation of the lining. Epidermoid tumors are thus slow-growing, benign lesions. They have an equal incidence in men and women, typically occurring between 20 and 60 years with a peak incidence in the fourth decade, followed by the third and fifth decades (GAO et al. 1992; SMIRNIOTOPOULOS et al. 1993; HEIER et al. 1997; SWARTZ 1998). An epidermoid readily conforms and molds itself around the surfaces of the adjacent pons, cerebellum, and brain stem. In addition, these tumors can become quite adherent to the surrounding structures and may surround normal vessels and nerves, further limiting resectability.

Signs and symptoms are produced by a slow-growing mass that displaces adjacent neural and vascular structures. Symptoms due to involvement of cranial nerves, brain stem, and cerebellum are most frequent (GAO et al. 1992; SMIRNIOTOPOULOS et al. 1993; SWARTZ 1998).

Intracranial epidermoid tumors generally appear as well-defined lobulated masses. Epidermoids are homogeneous masses of attenuation values near that of water (GAO et al. 1992; SMIRNIOTOPOULOS et al. 1993; SWARTZ 1998; BONNEVILLE et al. 2001). Their relative hypodensity is thought to be due to the high cholesterol and keratin content of the desquamated debris. Calcification can be present. The central portion of the epidermoid cyst is avascular and does not enhance; however, occasionally there may be a thin rim of peripheral enhancement, perhaps caused by displaced normal structures (vessels) rather than the cyst lining itself. Although homogeneous on CT scans, epidermoids often have a lamellated or onion-skin appearance on MR images, reflecting the layer-on-layer accretion of desquamated material (GAO et al. 1992; SMIRNIOTOPOULOS et al. 1993; SWARTZ 1998; BONNEVILLE et al. 2001). Most epidermoids have low to intermediate signal intensity on T1-weighted MR images and a high signal intensity on T2-weighted MR images (Figs. 9.6, 9.7). Usually, the intensity is slightly greater than CSF on all pulse sequences (KALLMES et al. 1997). As on CT, they either do not enhance on postcontrast MR scans or have only a thin rim of peripheral enhancement (GAO et al. 1992; SMIRNIOTOPOULOS et al. 1993; SWARTZ 1998; BONNEVILLE et al. 2001). Hydrocephalus, even in the setting of marked displacement and compression of the brain stem, is usually not seen (KALLMES et al. 1997).

As the signal intensity is close to the signal intensity of CSF, the major differential diagnosis should be made with an arachnoid cyst; therefore, the fluid-attenuated inversion recovery sequence (FLAIR) is more sensitive than conventional sequences in differentiation of epidermoid and arachnoid cysts because it suppresses the signal of CSF. With this sequence, epidermoid cysts have high signal intensity, whereas the signal of arachnoid cysts is suppressed (IKUSHIMA et al. 1997

The 3D CISS sequence also allows a good differentiation between an epidermoid and CSF (Figs. 9.7, 9.8). On the 3D CISS sequence the epidermoid becomes hypointense to CSF and hyperintense compared with brain parenchyma. This is probably caused by the cholesterol crystals and keratin filling the lesion. The 3D CISS sequence has also the advantage of its high spatial resolution due to its very thin sections allowing an exact description of the tumor extension (IKUSHIMA et al. 1997).

Diffusion-weighted imaging is also well known to allow differentiation of epidermoid and arachnoid cysts. On diffusion-weighted images, epidermoid cysts show a clear hyperintensity, whereas arach-

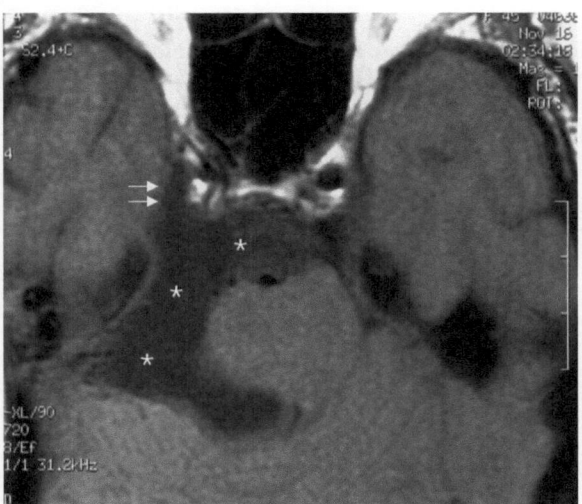
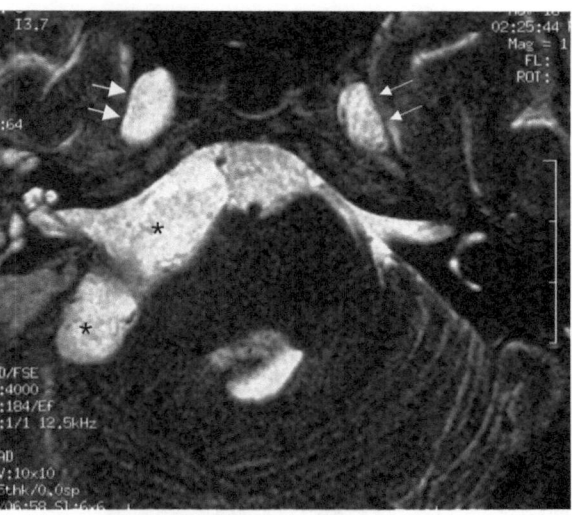

Fig. 9.6a, b. Imaging features of CPA epidermoid on T1/T2-weighted MR images. **a** Axial unenhanced T1-weighted MR image: large hypointense mass in the right CPA (*asterisks*) compressing the brain stem with extension in Meckel's cave on the right side (*arrows*): large epidermoid tumor. **b** Axial high-resolution 3D FSE T2-weighted MR image (imaging plane lower than in **a**): large homogeneous hyperintense mass in the right CPA (*asterisks*) compressing the brain stem as well as the facial and vestibulocochlear nerves. Note the more homogeneous aspect of the right Meckel's cave suggestive of invasion into Meckel's cave (*thick arrows*). Compare with the non-invaded normal left side (*thin arrows*)

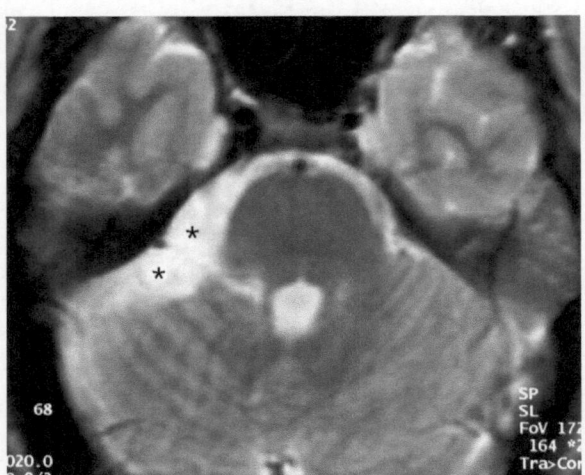

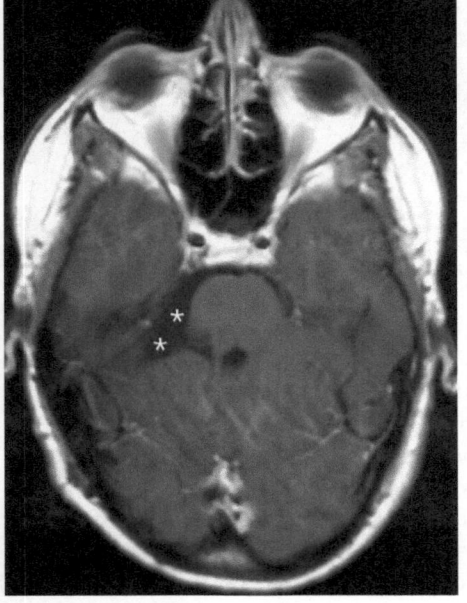

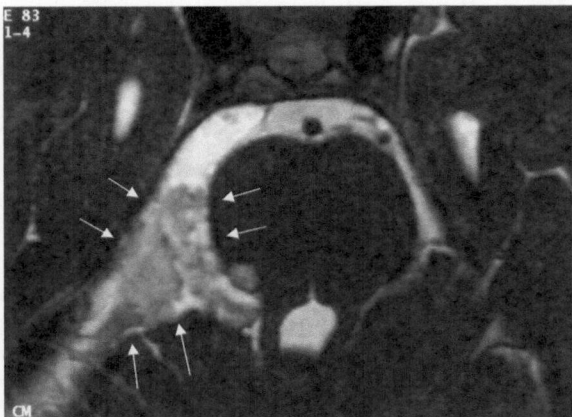

Fig. 9.7a–c. Imaging features of CPA epidermoid on T1/T2-weighted and high-resolution 3DFT CISS images. **a** Axial T2-weighted MR image: homogeneous hyperintense mass (*asterisks*) in the right CPA with compression of brain stem and cerebellum. **b** Axial enhanced T1-weighted MR image: hypointense non-enhancing mass (*asterisks*) in the right CPA with compression of brain stem and cerebellum. **c** Axial high-resolution 3 DFT CISS T2-weighted MR image: inhomogeneous aspect (*arrows*) of the lesion in the right CPA, hypointense to CSF and hyperintense to brain stem: findings characteristic of an epidermoid tumor. (Courtesy of J. CASSELMAN)

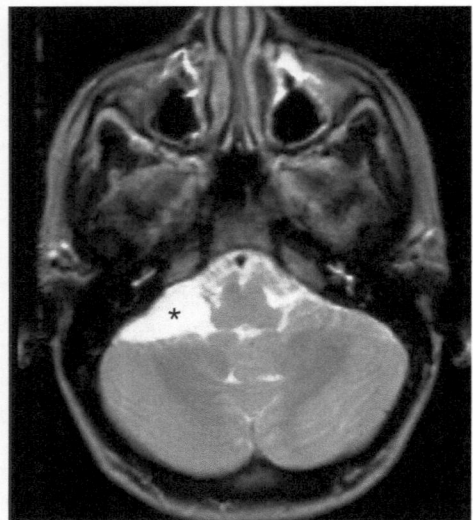

Fig. 9.8a–c. Imaging features of CPA arachnoid cyst on T1/T2-weighted and high-resolution 3DFT CISS images. **a** Axial T2-weighted MR image: homogeneous hyperintense mass (*asterisk*) in the right CPA. On this sequence, the lesion is indistinguishable from an epidermoid tumor. **b** Axial unenhanced T1 MR image: homogeneous hypointense mass in the right CPA (*asterisk*). On this sequence, the lesion is indistinguishable from an epidermoid tumor. **c** Axial high-resolution 3DFT CISS T2-weighted MR image: sharply demarcated lesion with characteristic homogeneous hyperintensity (*asterisk*), equal to CSF hyperintensity: arachnoid cyst. (Courtesy of J. CASSELMAN)

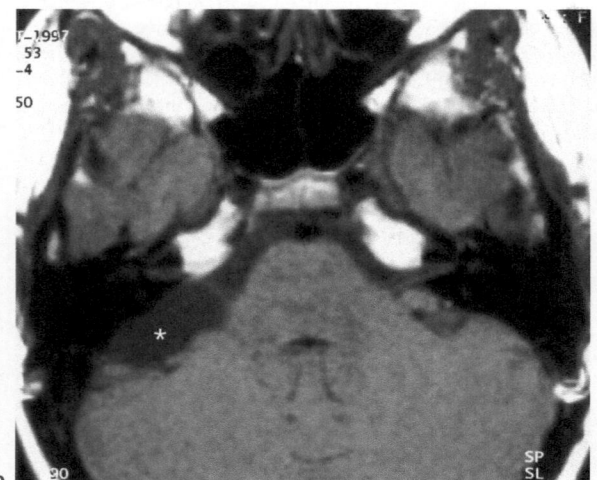

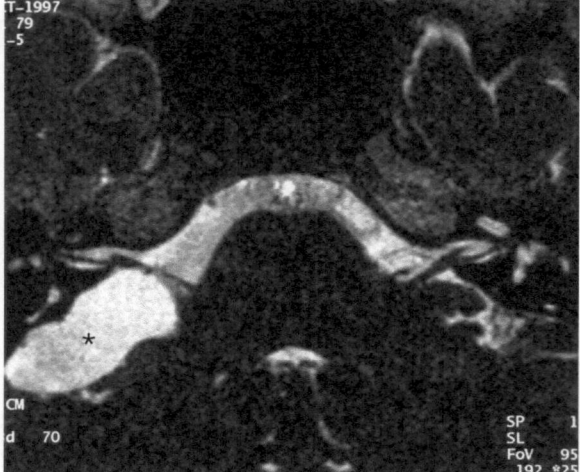

noid cysts show a hypointensity (Fig. 9.9; Table 9.1; BONNEVILLE et al. 2001; CHEN et al. 2001). The hyperintensity of epidermoid tumors on echo-planar diffusion-weighted images is not caused by diffusion restriction in the lesion but instead by the intrinsic T2 shine-through effect on the diffusion-weighted MR sequence (CHEN et al. 2001).

The epidermoid inclusion cyst should be differentiated from the acquired epidermoid (cholesteatoma) and the cholesterol granuloma. The acquired epidermoid is the result of a chronic infection and occurs usually in the middle ear. The lesion is lined with squamous epithelium and arises from herniation of the squamous epithelium of the pars flaccida of the tympanic membrane into the middle ear cavity following repeated episodes of middle ear infection. The cholesterol granuloma is another acquired inflammatory lesion of the petrous bone. On MR images, the

cholesterol granuloma contains high signal intensity areas of T1 shortening, either from lipid or blood products (methemoglobin; (SMIRNIOTOPOULOS et al. 1993).

9.2.6
Other Lesions

A large variety of unusual lesions are encountered in CPA (Table 9.2). The site of origin is the main factor in making a diagnosis for an unusual lesion of the CPA. The CPA masses can primarily arise from the cerebellopontine cistern and other CPA structures, e.g., non-acoustic schwannomas, aneurysm, melanoma (both primary and melanotic), miscellaneous meningeal lesions, or lipoma (Fig. 9.10). Tumors can also invade the CPA by extension from the

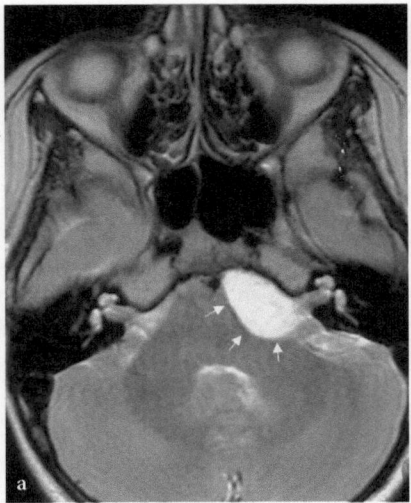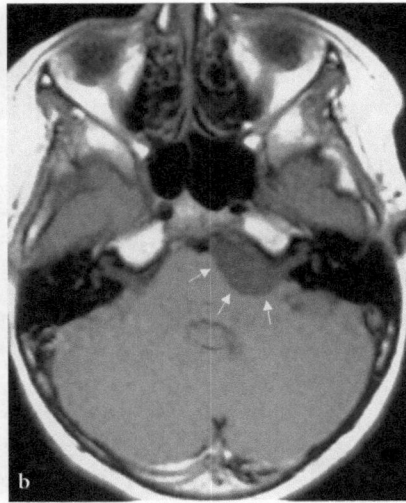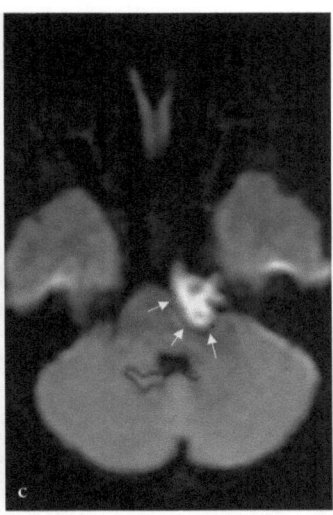

Fig. 9.9a–c. Imaging features of CPA epidermoid on diffusion-weighted images. **a** Axial T2-weighted MR image shows uniform hyperintensity (*arrows*) of the lesion in the left CPA/pre-pontine cistern. **b** Axial T1-weighted unenhanced MR image: low signal intensity cystic mass (*arrows*) in the left CPA/pre-pontine cistern. **c** Axial diffusion-weighted image shows clear hyperintensity in the lesion (*arrows*): findings characteristic of epidermoid tumor. (Courtesy of P. SEYNAEVE)

Table 9.2. Unusual lesions of the cerebellopontine angle

Cisterns	Dermoid cyst
	Lipoma
	Miscellaneous cysts
Nerves	Schwannoma (fifth to twelfth cranial nerve)
Arteries	Aneurysm
	Ectasia
Meninges	Carcinomatous meningitis
	Infectious and inflammatory meningitis
	Primary and metastatic melanoma
Brain stem	Brain stem glioma
	Choroid plexus papilloma
	Lymphoma
	Hemangioblastoma
	Ependymoma
	Medulloblastoma
	Dysembryoplastic neuroepithelial tumor
Skull base	Cholesterol granuloma
	Paraganglioma
	Petrous apicitis
	Chordoma
	Chondroma/chondrosarcoma
	Endolymphatic sac tumor
	Pituitary adenoma

petrous bone or skull base: cholesterol granuloma; paraganglioma; chondromatous tumors; chordoma; endolymphatic sac tumors; pituitary adenoma; and apex petrositis. An exophytic intraaxial lesion can also give rise to a CPA tumor such as a brain stem glioma, choroid plexus papilloma, lymphoma, hemangioblastoma, ependymoma, medulloblastoma, or a dysembryoplastic neuroepithelial tumor (BONN-

EVILLE et al. 2001). A close evaluation of the CT and MRI findings can lead to a preoperative diagnosis. Evaluation of the attenuation at CT, signal intensity at MRI, contrast enhancement, shape and margins of the lesion, mass effect, and adjacent bone reaction is helpful in making the diagnosis (SMIRNIOTOPOULOS et al. 1993; HEIER et al. 1997; SWARTZ 1998; BONNEVILLE et al. 2001).

9.3
Intracanalicular and Intralabyrinthine Schwannomas

9.3.1
Introduction

The majority of tumoral lesions of the internal auditory canal and membranous labyrinth are again schwannomas of the vestibulocochlear nerve; therefore, this paragraph focuses on intracanalicular and intralabyrinthine schwannomas.

However, in the MR evaluation of patients presenting with sensorineural hearing loss, vertigo, and other symptoms of cochlear or vestibular dysfunction, a large scala of other pathologies giving rise to labyrinthine enhancement is also found. Apart from the enhancement of intralabyrinthine schwannomas, inflammatory and infectious labyrinthitis is known

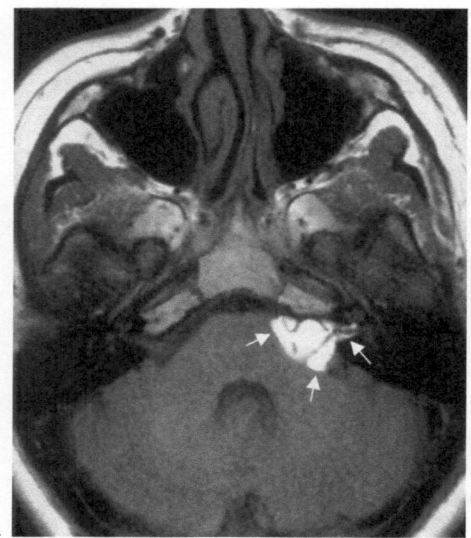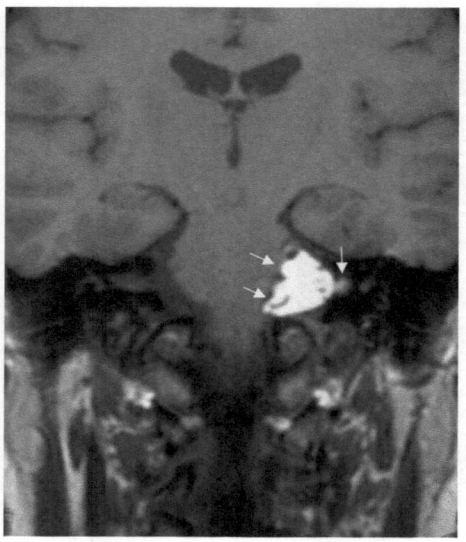

Fig. 9.10a, b. Imaging features of CPA lipoma. **a** Axial T1-weighted unenhanced MR image: high signal mass intensity in the left CPA cistern. The lesion is completely encasing the neural and vascular structures in the CPA. **b** Coronal T1-weighted unenhanced MR image: high signal intensity mass in the left CPA cistern. The signal voids in the lesions are caused by neural and vascular structures traversing the lesion: CPA lipoma. (Courtesy of M. Lemmerling)

to be one of the major causes of gadolinium enhancement of the membranous labyrinth on T1-weighted MR images (Mafee 1995; Swartz 1996).

9.3.2
Intracanalicular and Intralabyrinthine Schwannomas

Intracanalicular vestibulocochlear schwannomas arise from the Schwann cell portion of the vestibulocochlear nerve with a predilection for the branches of the vestibular nerve in the internal acoustic meatus.

Vestibulocochlear schwannomas can be restricted to the internal auditory canal or vestibulocochlear schwannomas can penetrate the cribose area and penetrate in the labyrinth thus giving rise to an intracanalicular schwannoma with intralabyrinthine extension (Doyle and Brackmann 1994; Forton et al. 1994; Swartz 1998).

True or primary intralabyrinthine schwannoma used to be a rare and often incidental finding at autopsy or surgery, but with the widespread use of gadolinium-enhanced MRI they are diagnosed more frequently (Doyle and Brackmann 1994; Forton et al. 1994; Fitzgerald et al. 1999).

Primary intralabyrinthine schwannomas originate from the Schwann cells surrounding the peripheral fibers of the cochlear nerve within the turns of the cochlea or the peripheral vestibular nerve fibers

of the cristae or maculae within the vestibule. Like the more common vestibulocochlear schwannomas of the internal auditory canal and the cerebellopontine angle, intralabyrinthine schwannomas are encapsulated and slow growing. They generally cause symptoms by producing pressure or invasion of adjacent structures (Mafee et al. 1990; Doyle and Brackmann 1994; Forton et al. 1994).

The majority of all described intralabyrinthine neuromas involving the vestibular system present as "Meniere-like" syndromes with incapacitating vertigo and associated sensorineural hearing loss (Doyle and Brackmann 1994; Forton et al. 1994; Fitzgerald et al. 1999). Clinical reports are clearly contradictory in the discussion as to whether clinical symptoms are correlated with the specific location of the tumor within the labyrinth (Doyle and Brackmann 1994; Forton et al. 1994; Fitzgerald et al. 1999).

Surgical intervention is indicated in the presence of disabling vertigo, tumors that demonstrate growth, and tumors that extend beyond the confines of the labyrinth.

9.3.3
Imaging Features

There is no place for CT in the evaluation of patients suspected of having an internal auditory canal or intralabyrinthine schwannoma.

It is well known that enhanced T1-weighted sequences and thin-slice high-resolution T2-weighted sequences form the best sequence combination not only for detection of small intracanalicular and membranous labyrinth lesions (CASSELMAN et al. 1993a,b), but also for assessment of tumor volume (SCHMAL-BROCK et al. 1999) and depiction of nerve involvement (SCHMALBROCK et al. 1999; SARTORETTI-SCHEFER et al. 2000).

Unenhanced T1-weighted sequences are needed to evaluate hyperintense lesions such as subacute hemorrhage and high-level proteinaceous fluid inside the labyrinth. Even a small intracanalicular or intralabyrinthine schwannoma can be suspected on unenhanced T1-weighted images as a small, slightly hyperintense lesion. The enhancement of the schwannoma can be clearly seen on postcontrast T1-weighted images (Figs. 9.11, 9.12). Apart from the fact that enhancement should be focal and nodular in order to distinguish it from labyrinthitis or neuritis, the high-resolution thin-slice T2-weighted sequence aids in the differential diagnosis by showing the absence of any hypointense nodular lesion in the membranous labyrinth or internal auditory canal in case of labyrinthitis or neuritis. Furthermore, enhancement of a schwannoma should persist in time contrary to the temporary enhancement of infectious/inflammatory lesions (MAFEE et al. 1990; CASSELMAN et al. 1993a; DOYLE and BRACKMANN 1994; FORTON et al. 1994; SWARTZ 1996, 1998).

On the thin-slice high-resolution T2-weighted images, in case of a small lesion, one should be able to localize the exact origin of the intracanalicular schwannoma regarding the nerves in the internal auditory canal (CASSELMAN et al. 1993b; SCHMALBROCK et al. 1999). In case of an intracochlear schwannoma, the location of the lesion in the scala tympani or scala vestibuli can be done (Fig. 9.11).

As the tumor growth of these lesions is unpredictable, follow-up imaging with volume measurement becomes very important in the selection of patients who should undergo surgery (SCHMAL-BROCK et al. 1999).

Considerable debate still exists as to whether small intracanalicular and intralabyrinthine schwannomas can be screened by using only high-resolution thin-slice T2-weighted sequences. Several studies have shown high-resolution fast-spin-echo T2-weighted MRI of the internal auditory canal and CPA to have an equal sensitivity to conventional gadolinium-enhanced T1-weighted images. They propose high-resolution fast-spin-echo T2-weighted MRI of the internal auditory canal and CPA as a lower-cost screening examination for causes of sensorineural hearing loss (DANIELS et al. 1998, 2000); however, inflammatory and infectious (viral) lesions involving the labyrinth can be missed using only high-resolution fast-spin-echo T2-weighted images. Diffuse meningeal enhancement can also be overlooked without contrast material. Certain lesions of the otic capsule, such as cochlear otosclerosis and osteogenesis imperfecta, also may appear only after contrast administration (JACKLER 1996). Furthermore, as it seems that volume

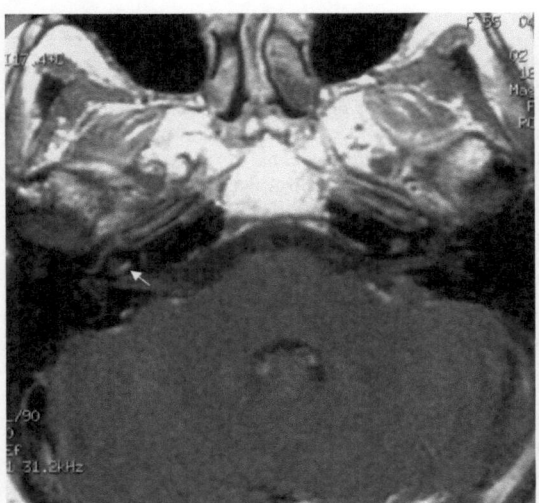 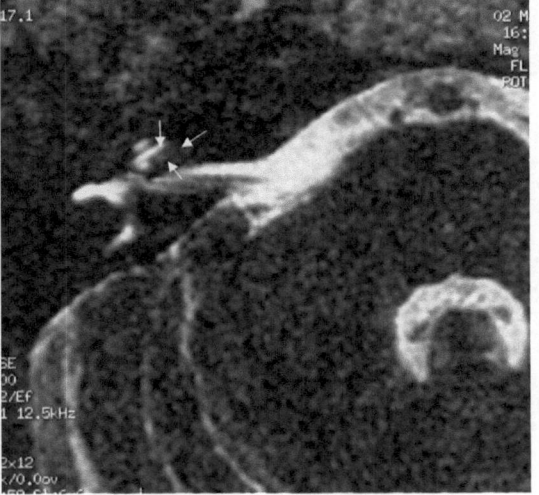

Fig. 9.11a, b. Imaging features of intracochlear schwannoma. **a** Axial T1-weighted enhanced MR image: focal, small enhancing lesion partially filling the mid-cochlear turn (*arrow*). **b** Axial high-resolution 3D FSE T2-weighted image: sharply demarcated, focal zone of signal loss (*arrows*) in the scala tympani of the mid cochlear turn caused by tumor, replacing labyrinthine fluid: small intracochlear schwannoma

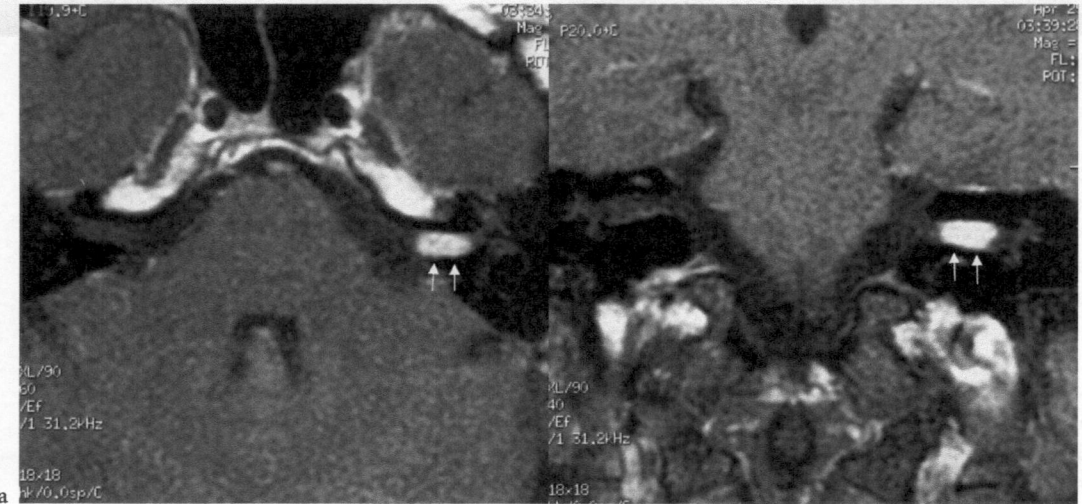

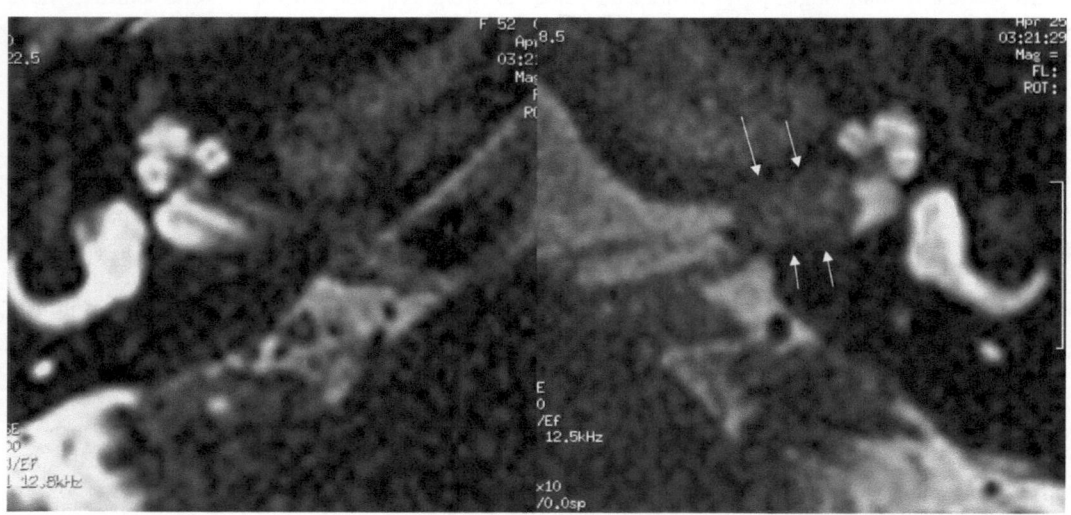

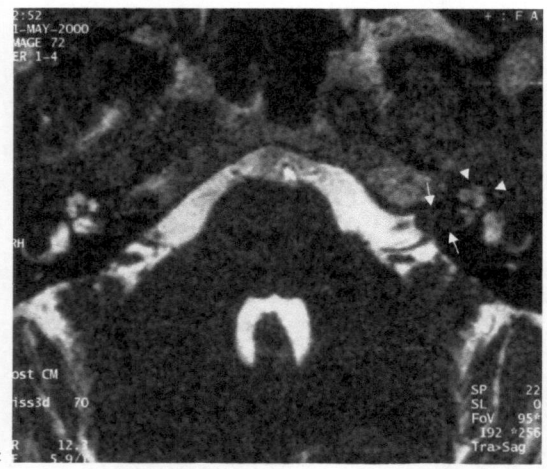

Fig. 9.12a–c. Intracanalicular vestibulocochlear schwannoma with retro-obstructive signal loss on CISS sequence. **a** Axial and coronal enhanced T1-weighted MR image: strong, uniform enhancing mass in the left internal auditory canal (*arrows*) compatible with a vestibulocochlear schwannoma. **b** Axial high-resolution 3D FSE T2-weighted MR image: well-circumscribed oval hypointense mass (*arrows*) in the left internal auditory canal. There is residual fluid signal in the fundus of the internal auditory canal with a normal signal in the membranous labyrinth. **c** Axial high-resolution 3 DFT CISS T2-weighted MR image: same mass in the internal auditory canal (*arrows*) with residual fluid signal in the fundus of the IAC with a clear "retro-obstructive" signal loss in the fundus of the IAC and membranous labyrinth (*arrowheads*). This retro-obstructive signal loss is found only on the 3DFT CISS sequence. Compare with the normal right side. (CISS images courtesy of J. CASSELMAN)

averaging still remains the most important cause of uncertainty in the evaluation of small intracanalicular and intralabyrinthine schwannomas, the thin-slice, small-field-of-view T1-weighted sequence (spin echo or 3D gradient echo) after intravenous administration of gadolinium still remains the gold standard (HERMANS et al. 1997).

Again, in cases of intracanalicular schwannoma, the evaluation of the residual fluid signal intensity in the fundus of the internal auditory canal on thin-slice high-resolution T2-weigthed images and the evaluation of retro-obstructive intralabyrinthine signal loss are important, as these findings are related to hearing preservation surgery (Fig. 9.12; SOMERS et al. 2001).

9.3.4
Other Lesions

A variety of other lesions are found in the membranous labyrinth and internal auditory canal, e.g., meningioma, hemangioma (Fig. 9.13), lipoma, metastasis (Fig. 9.14), traumatic neuroma, arachnoid cysts, etc. (BOHRER and CHOLE 1996; BIGELOW et al. 1998; HAUGHT et al. 1998; KRAINIK et al. 2001); however, as these lesions are extremely rare, reports on their imaging features are limited. Lipomas are easily recognized on MR imaging due to their uniform hyperintensity on unenhanced T1-weighted images with signal loss on a fat-saturation technique. As it is known that CPA or IAC lipomas grow very slowly and have an intimate relation with the adjacent cranial nerves and vessels,

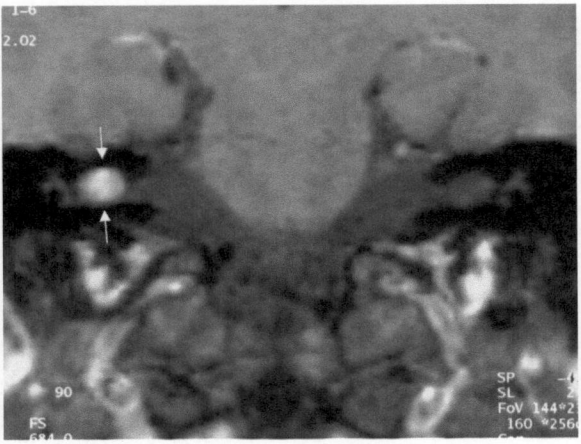
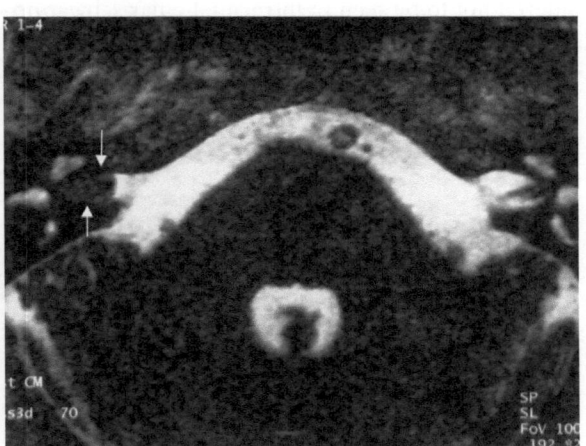

Fig. 9.13a, b. Imaging features of intracanalicular hemangioma. **a** Axial T1-weighted enhanced MR image: focal, sharply demarcated enhancing lesion in the fundus of the internal auditory canal (*arrows*). **b** Axial high-resolution 3D FSE T2-weighted image: oval hypointense lesion in the fundus of the IAC (*arrows*). There is no residual fluid signal in the fundus of the IAC. The lesion is highly suggestive of intracanalicular schwannoma. Pathologic examination revealed intracanalicular hemangioma

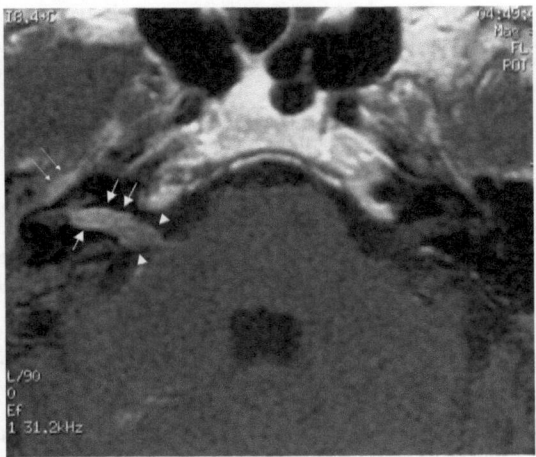
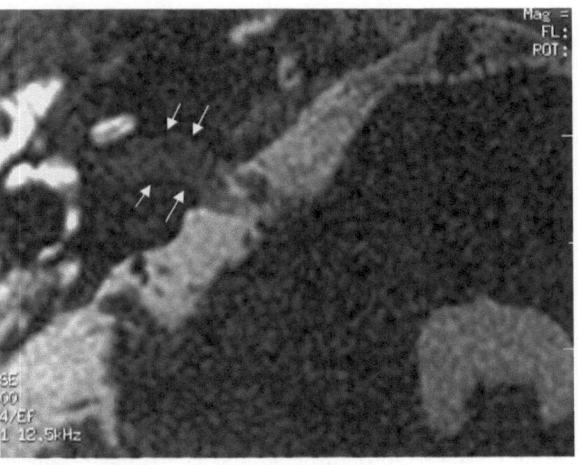

Fig. 9.14a, b. Imaging features of intracanalicular metastasis of a bronchocarcinoma. **a** Axial T1-weighted enhanced MR image: strongly enhancing mass lesion (*thick arrows*) in the right IAC with a small component protruding into the CPA (*arrowheads*). There is also partially enhancing tissue anterior in the middle ear cavity (*thin arrows*). This enhancement is caused by perineural extension of the intracanalicular metastasis along the tympanic segment of the facial nerve. The CT showed enlargement of the tympanic segment of the facial nerve canal (not shown). **b** Axial high-resolution 3D FSE T2-weighted image: mass lesion with fluid replacement in the right IAC (*arrows*) caused by metastatic involvement of the IAC. Note the high signal of the fluid in the middle ear cavity

possibly thus causing a significant postoperative morbidity (BOHRER and CHOLE 1996; BIGELOW et al. 1998), conservative follow-up is regarded the best treatment option. Metastasis in the CPA or IAC can look identical to a schwannoma. The presence of thick linear and extranodular contrast enhancement is reported in cases of metastasis (KRAINIK et al. 2001).

In conclusion, possible imaging features allowing differential diagnosis from schwannoma are high signal on T1-weighted images, heterogeneous contrast enhancement of the lesion, or extranodular contrast enhancement. These three features are considered not to be seen in intracanalicular schwannomas (KRAINIK et al. 2001).

References

Bigelow DC, Eisen MD, Smith PG et al. (1998) Lipomas of the internal auditory canal and cerebellopontine angle. Laryngoscope 108:1459–1469

Bohrer PS, Chole RA (1996) Unusual lesions of the internal auditory canal. Am J Otol 17:143–149

Bonneville F, Sarrazin JL, Marsot-Dupuch K et al. (2001) Unusual lesions of the cerebellopontine angle: a segmental approach. Radiographics 21:419–438

Casselman JW, Kuhweide R, Ampe W et al. (1993a) Pathology of the membranous labyrinth: comparison of T1- and T2-weighted and gadolinium enhanced spin-echo and 3DFT-CISS imaging. Am J Neuroradiol 14:59–69

Casselman JW, Kuhweide R, Deimling M et al. (1993b) Constructive interference in steady state-3DFT MR imaging of the inner ear and cerebellopontine angle. Am J Neuroradiol 14:47–57

Chen S, Ikawa F, Kurisu K et al. (2001) Quantitative MR evaluation of intracranial epidermoid tumors by fast fluid-attenuated inversion recovery imaging and echo-planar diffusion-weighted imaging. Am J Neuroradiol 22:1089–1096

Daniels RL, Shelton C, Harnsberger HR (1998) Ultra high resolution nonenhanced fast spin echo magnetic resonance imaging: cost-effective screening for acoustic neuroma in patients with sudden sensorineural hearing loss Otolaryngol Head Neck Surg 119:364–369

Daniels R, Swalow C, Shelton C et al. (2000) Causes of unilateral sensorineural hearing loss screened by high-resolution fast spin echo magnetic resonance imaging: review of 1070 consecutive cases. Am J Otol 21:173–180

Doyle KJ, Brackmann DE (1994) Intralabyrinthine schwannomas. Otolaryngol Head Neck Surg 110:517–523

Fitzgerald DC, Grundfast KM, Hecht DA et al. (1999) Intralabyrinthine schwannomas. Am J Otol 20:381–385

Forton G, Somers T, Hermans R et al. (1994) Preoperatively diagnosed utricular neuroma treated by selective partial labyrinthectomy. Ann Otol Rhinol Laryngol 103:885–888

Gao P, Osborn AG, Smirniotopoulos JG et al. (1992) Radiologic–pathologic correlation: epidermoid tumor of the cerebellopontine angle. Am J Neuroradiol 13:863–872

Haught K, Hogg JP, Killeffer JA et al. (1998) Entirely intracanalicular meningioma: contrast-enhanced MR findings in a rare entity. Am J Neuroradiol 19:1831–1833

Heier LA, Comunale JP Jr, Lavyne MH (1997) Sensorineural hearing loss and cerebellopontine angle lesions. Clin Imaging 21:213–223

Hermans R, Van der Goten A, De Foer B et al. (1997) MRI screening for acoustic neuroma without gadolinium: value of 3DFT-CISS sequence. Neuroradiology 39:593–598

Ikushima I, Korogi Y, Hirai T et al. (1997) MR of epidermoids with a variety of pulse sequences. Am J Neuroradiol 18:1359–1363

Jackler RK (1996) Cost-effective screening for acoustic neuroma with unenhanced MR: a clinician's perspective. Am J Neuroradiol 17:1226–1227

Kallmes DF, Provenzale JM, Cloft HJ et al. (1997) Typical and atypical MR imaging features of intracranial epidermoid tumors. Am J Roentgenol 169:883–887

Krainik A, Cyna-Gorse F, Bouccare D et al. (2001) MRI of unusual lesions of the internal auditory canal. Neuroradiology 43:52–57

Kutcher TJ, Brown DC, Maurer PK et al. (1991) Dural tail adjacent to acoustic neuroma: MR features. J Comput Assist Tomogr 15:669–670

Mafee MF (1995) MR imaging of intralabyrinthine schwannoma, labyrinthitis, and other labyrinthine pathology. Otolaryngol Clin North Am 28:407–430

Mafee MF, Lachenauer CS, Kumar A et al. (1990) CT and MR imaging of intralabyrinthine schwannoma: report of two cases and review of the literature. Radiology 174:395–400

Mulkens T, Parizel P, Martin JJ et al. (1993) Acoustic schwannoma: MR findings in 84 tumors. Am J Roentgenol 160:395–398

Naganawa S, Koshikawa T, Fukatsu H et al. (2001) MR cisternography of the cerebellopontine angle: comparison of three-dimensional fast asymmetrical spin-echo and three-dimensional constructive interference in the steady-state sequence. Am J Neuroradiol 22:1179–1185

Sartoretti-Schefer S, Kollias S, Valavanis A (2000) Spatial relationship between vestibular schwannoma and facial nerve on three-dimensional T2-weighted fast spin-echo MR images. Am J Neuroradiol 21:810–816

Schmalbrock P, Chakeres DW, Monroe JW et al. (1999) Assessment of internal auditory canal tumors: a comparison of contrast-enhanced T1-weighted and steady-state T2-weighted gradient-echo MR imaging. Am J Neuroradiol 20:1207–1213

Smirniotopoulos JG, Yue NC, Rushing EJ (1993) Cerebellopontine angle masses: radiologic–pathologic correlation. Radiographics 13:1131–1147

Somers T, Casselman J, De Ceulaer G et al. (2001) Prognostic value of magnetic resonance imaging findings in hearing preservation surgery for vestibular schwannoma. Otol Neurootol 22:87–94

Swartz JD (1996) Sensorineural hearing deficit: a systematic approach based on imaging findings. Radiographics 16:561–574

Swartz J (1998) The vestibulocochlear nerve, emphasizing the normal and diseased IAC and CPA. In: Swartz JD, Harnsberger HR (eds) Imaging of the temporal bone, 3rd edn. Thieme, New York

The Clinician's View

I. Dhooge

The most common pathological process in the CPA is the vestibular schwannoma, arising from the eighth cranial nerve, followed distantly by meningiomas; however, a wide variety of lesions can present in the CPA. Although some of these lesions present with a clinical history and physical findings that distinguish them from the more common acoustic neuromas and meningiomas, the majority are differentiated preoperatively only with appropriate radiographic assessment. Preoperative tentative diagnosis allows for more detailed patient counseling, more accurate therapeutic planning, and more predictable surgical outcomes. In some circumstances it may even obviate the need for an unnecessary surgical exploration.

The most frequent tumor found in the CPA is the vestibular schwannoma. Because the most common symptoms of a vestibular schwannoma deal with hearing or equilibrium, the ENT specialist is consulted by the patient. The patient with the „classic" presentation of progressive unilateral sensorineural hearing loss, tinnitus, and disequilibrium is more the exception than the rule. But any unexplained, asymmetrical hearing loss or unilateral tinnitus is, in most cases, followed by MRI. The widespread use of MRI has resulted in the identification of patients with very small, relatively asymptomatic vestibular schwannomas for whom the natural history is still not known.

The question of whether and when to undertake treatment of a vestibular schwannoma is a complex issue. Young patients with progressive neurological deficit or evidence of tumor growth clearly are candidates for surgery; however, there are groups of patients for whom conservative approaches, including long-term observation, may be indicated. Elderly patients without severe neurologic symptoms or evidence of tumor growth are one such group. There is also evidence that some patients with unilateral vestibular schwannoma and a subgroup of patients with NF2 may have tumors that fail to progress rapidly, resulting in stable neurologic function for a long time. Conservative management may be appropriate for these patients. It is extremely important for the clinician to have a correct radiologic estimation of growth (three dimensional) of the tumor.

The choice of therapy (surgery vs stereotactic irradiation vs observation) and the surgical approaches (translabyrinthine vs rectosigmoid vs middle fossa) for the removal of the vestibular schwannoma depends partly on tumor size. Radiographic differentiation between a vestibular schwannoma and meningioma is important, because the relationship of cranial nerves to the tumor is much less predictable than with vestibular schwannoma. Meningiomas represent a more heterogeneous group than vestibular schwannomas. They have a more complex molecular pathogenesis and a more varied histopathology, with a significant proportion exhibiting features of malignancy. Although they make up a small proportion of CPA tumors, meningiomas are of special interest because of the technical problems associated with their removal. This differs somewhat from vestibular schwannomas. Hearing preservation is more likely than in vestibular schwannomas for similar-sized tumors and the rectosigmoid operation is the favored approach for most cases. A preoperative diagnosis is therefore critical for optimal counseling and treatment.

Imaging is also important postoperatively to document complete tumor removal, follow residual tumor, or assess tumor stability after irradiation.

10 Imaging of the Jugular Foramen

H. Tanghe

CONTENTS

10.1
Anatomy

The jugular foramen is an opening in the skull base, located between the temporal and the occipital bone. Asymmetry between the right and left foramen is the rule. The right foramen is the largest in 68% of the cases, equal to the left in 12% and smaller than the left in 20% (Rhoton 2000). This is explained by the asymmetry in the intracranial venous drainage (Fig. 10.1).

Several anatomical structures go through the jugular foramen: the sigmoid sinus; jugular bulb; the inferior petrosal sinus; the meningeal branches of the ascending pharyngeal and the occipital arteries; the glossopharyngeal; vagus; and accessory nerves; the tympanic branch of the glossopharyngeal nerve

(Jacobson's nerve); and the auricular branch of the vagus nerve (Arnold's nerve; Fig. 10.2a; (Rhoton 2000; Sen et al. 2001).

Despite several studies, the exact anatomy of the jugular foramen is uncertain, mostly because of the great variations from person to person (Rubinstein et al. 1995). Hovelaque in 1934 described two compartments: the pars nervosa (anteromedial) and the pars venosa (posterolateral). Rhoton in 1997 and 2000 (Rhoton 2000) proposes a division into three parts at the intracranial orifice: a small petrosal compartment anteromedially, containing the inferior petrosal sinus; a large lateral sigmoid part containing the sigmoid sinus; and an intrajugular part, containing the cranial nerves IX, X, and XI. Within the foramen, there is a bony and fibrous septum between the sigmoid and petrosal part. It is through this area that the cranial nerves pass (Fig. 10.2a–c).

The nerve of Jacobson is the tympanic branch of the glossopharyngeal nerve, originating at the external orifice of the jugular foramen. It traverses the tympanic canaliculus to enter the tympanic cavity

H. Tanghe, MD
Section of Neuroradiology, Department of Radiology, Dijkzigt, Sophia Children's and Daniel Den Hoed Hospitals, Erasmus University Medical Centre, Dr. Molenwaterplein 40, 3015 Rotterdam, The Netherlands

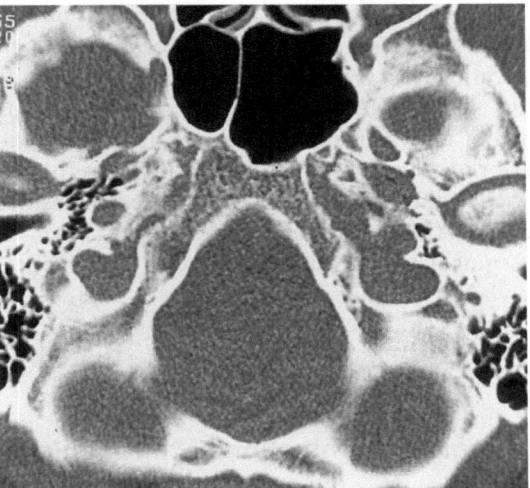

Fig. 10.1. Normal asymmetry of the jugular foramen. The left jugular foramen is larger than the right, due to the asymmetry of the intracranial venous drainage

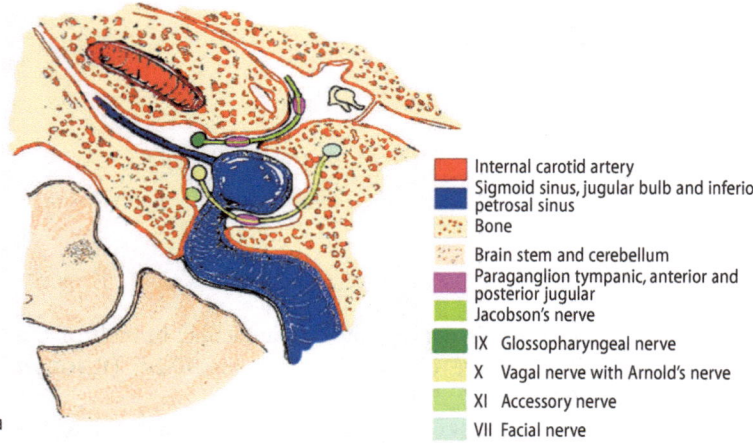

Internal carotid artery
Sigmoid sinus, jugular bulb and inferior petrosal sinus
Bone
Brain stem and cerebellum
Paraganglion tympanic, anterior and posterior jugular
Jacobson's nerve
IX   Glossopharyngeal nerve
X   Vagal nerve with Arnold's nerve
XI   Accessory nerve
VII Facial nerve

Fig. 10.2a–c. Normal anatomy of the jugular foramen. **a** Scheme. **b** Axial CT of the left jugular foramen at the level of the horizontal part of the carotid canal. **c** Axial CT at the level of the vertical part of the carotid canal. The jugular foramen is divided into a medial small pars nervosa and a larger lateral part, the pars vascularis, separated by a bony and fibrous septum. **c** The mastoid canaliculus, containing the Arnold's nerve, is visible running from the lateral wall of the jugular foramen toward the mastoid segment of the facial canal

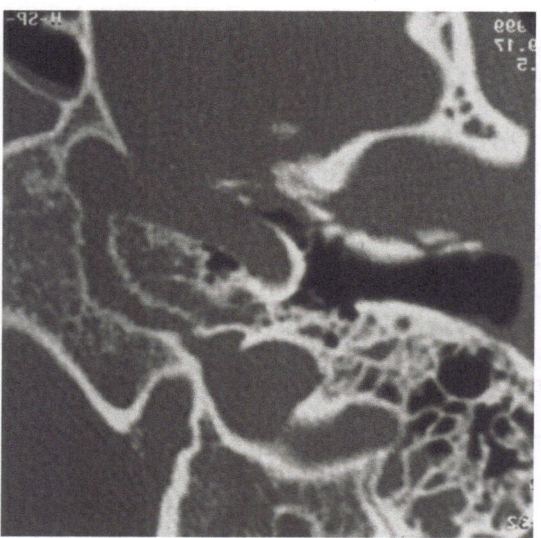

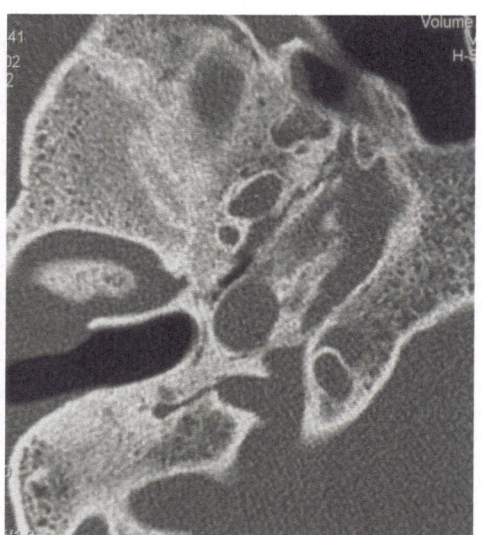

where it gives rise to the tympanic plexus providing the sensory innervation of the middle ear and the parasympathetic innervation via the otic ganglion to the parotid gland (Fig. 10.2a).

The nerve of Arnold, the auricular cutaneous branch of the vagus nerve, arises at the level of the superior vagal ganglion. This branch goes to the lateral wall of the jugular foramen to enter the mastoid canaliculus (Fig. 10.2c), and ascends toward the mastoid segment of the facial canal to exit the temporal bone via the tympanomastoid fissure.

10.2
Radiological Examination of the Jugular Foramen

The evaluation of the jugular foramen and the temporal bone, especially in tumours, requires high-quality cross-sectional imaging with both CT and MR to fully answer all the detailed preoperative questions. For the anatomical variants CT imaging alone is preferable.

The CT examination is best done with a multidetector spiral CT (when available) making ultra-thin sections (0.7 mm) in the axial plane with coronal and sagittal reconstructions. When both CT and MR are used, the task of CT is not to explore the soft tissue extension, but to show the bony anatomy, the condition of the bony margins of the foramen and other structures in the neighbourhood, the extent of the bony destruction of the skull base, and to detect some lesion characteristic features that are not visible on MR, such as the intratumoral calcifications or the hyperostosis of a meningioma.

The primary task of MR is to evaluate the soft tissue extension of the disease, to interpret the signal intensity characteristics and to find additional features not visible on CT such as the presence of intratumoral vessels in a paraganglioma. Our MR imaging protocol for the jugular foramen (on a Philips 1.5-T Integra) consisted of: (a) a non-enhanced axial 3D gradient echo T1-weighted sequence with contiguous slice thickness of 2 mm, starting at C2 level until above the internal auditory canal; (b) this sequence is repeated after the administration of gadolinium in the axial plane; (c) a 2D turbo spin echo (TSE) T2-weighted sequence in the axial plane with slice thickness of 3 mm; and (d) a 2D T1-weighted SE sequence after gadolinium in the coronal plane with slice thickness of 3 mm. In addition, an evaluation of the neck can be necessary in case of a paraganglioma, to find multiplicity. Magnetic resonance venography in the coronal plane can be used to study the patency or invasion of the internal jugular vein, and the sigmoid sinus. In the postoperative situation, after an infratemporal approach with filling up the defect with a fat/muscle graft, the use of a fat-saturated contrast-enhanced T1-weighted image is important to detect recurrent paraganglioma. The diagnosis of recurrent paraganglioma in a previously surgically treated patient can be very difficult.

Angiography is seldom needed for diagnostic purposes, but plays a role in the preoperative embolization (see Chap. 10).

10.3
Overview of the Lesions of the Jugular Foramen

The jugular foramen is a complex region of the skull base with an extensive differential diagnostic list of possible lesions (Table 10.1).

It is important to recognize the "pseudo-lesions" such as the normal asymmetry of the foramen, the anatomical vascular variants (see Chap. 10) and the modality-dependent pitfalls such as the flow-related artefacts on MR (SWARTZ and HARNSBERGER 1998).

The true lesions can be divided into primary lesions located in the foramen and secondary extensions to the jugular foramen (WEBER and MCKENNA 1994).

A practical starting point for the differential diagnosis is to look at the dimension and the bony margin of the jugular foramen on CT. There are four possibilities:
1. The jugular foramen is normal.
2. The foramen is enlarged with an intact cortical outline.
3. The foramen is enlarged with an erosion, destruction of its cortical outlines.
4. The foramen has a normal size but its bony margins are destroyed.

In the first category pseudo-lesions must be regarded as flow-related artefacts on MR, on a dural arteriovenous (AV) fistula and on a thrombosis of the jugular bulb or sigmoid sinus. The possibilities in the second category are: normal asymmetry; schwannoma; meningioma; dural AV fistula; and cholesteatoma. The differential diagnostic list in the third category consists of paraganglioma, metastasis, Ewing's sarcoma and giant cell tumour. The lesions of the fourth category are secondary extensions to the foramen from lesions originating elsewhere such as malignant otitis externa, cholesteatoma, metastasis, chondrosarcoma, chordoma, nasopharyngeal carcinoma and endolymphatic sac tumour (Table 10.1).

10.4
Vascular Lesions

Vascular lesions are discussed in Chap. 10.

10.5
Common Tumours

10.5.1
Paraganglioma

Paragangliomas, also called glomus tumours, are neuroendocrine neoplasm's composed largely of paraganglion chief cells (BURGER and SCHEITHAUER 1994). These tumours arise from glomus bodies also named paraganglia. Normal paraganglia occur in the head and neck region at several places (Table 10.2), frequently located near nerves and vessels (PETRUS and LO 1996; RAO et al. 1999). Within the jugular foramen the paraganglioma can arise from paraganglia located in the adventitia of the jugular bulb or at Jacobson's nerve (nerve IX) or at Arnold's nerve (nerve X). In the middle ear normal paraganglia are found at the cochlear promontory.

Paragangliomas restricted to the middle ear are called glomus tympanicum tumours. Glomus jugulotympanicum and glomus jugulare tumours involve, respectively, the middle ear plus the jugular foramen or the jugular foramen alone. Endocrinological functional activity is rare in head and neck paragangliomas, 93% of the functioning tumours are pheochromocytomas (also a tumour of paraganglionic tissue) and only 7% occur at other sites (MAFFE et al. 2000).

Table 10.1. Differential diagnosis of the jugular foramen lesions, based on the size and the cortical outline on CT: *A* a normal jugular foramen; *B* enlarged foramen with an intact cortical outline; *C* erosion, destruction of the cortical outline in an enlarged foramen; *D* a normal-sized foramen with bony destruction; *AV* arteriovenous

A	B	C	D
MR flow-related artefacts	Normal asymmetry	Paraganglioma	Malignant otitis externa
Thrombosis	Schwannoma	Metastasis	Metastasis
Dural AV fistula	Meningioma	Ewing's sarcoma	Chordoma
	Dural AV fistula	Giant cell tumour	Chondrosarcoma
	Cholesteatoma		Nasopharyngeal carcinoma
			Endolymphatic sac tumour

Table 10.2. Locations of the normal paraganglia in the head and neck region. (From Lo et al. 1993 and Manski et al. 1997)

Name	Relationship
Tympanic	Cochlear promontory in the middle ear
Anterior jugular	Jacobson's nerve (IX) in jugular foramen
Posterior jugular	Arnold's nerve (X) in jugular foramen
Adventitia of the jugular bulb	Jugular bulb in jugular foramen
Intravagale	Ganglion nodosum of the vagal nerve
Extravagale	Along the vagal nerve in the carotid space
Facial	Mastoid segment of the facial canal or ganglion geniculi
Carotid body	Carotid bifurcation
Superior laryngeal	Superior laryngeal nerve
Inferior laryngeal	Recurrent laryngeal nerve
Orbital	Ganglion ciliare in the orbit
Fossa pterygopalatina	Pterygopalatine ganglion
Nasopharynx	
Buccal mucosa	

Paragangliomas may be multiple, either synchronously or metachronously in 3% for sporadic cases to 26% for the familial cases (Fig. 10.3). They can occur in association with pheochromocytoma, thyroid carcinoma, Carney triad (gastric leiomyosarcoma, pulmonary chondroma and paraganglioma) and other endocrine disorders. Familial paragangliomas have a prevalence of 7–9%, with 90% of the cases arising from the carotid body (Rao et al. 1999).

The symptoms depend on the primary site of origin and the extension of the tumour and include a vascular tympanic membrane, conductive hearing loss, pulsatile tinnitus, bruit, vertigo, sensorineural hearing loss and cranial nerve deficit.

Paragangliomas are benign but locally invasive and very vascular tumours. From its origin in the middle ear, the glomus tympanicum first invades the bone between the hypotympanum and the jugular foramen. With further growth they are indistinguishable from a glomus jugulare, hence the term glomus jugulotympanicum. The differentiation between a simple glomus tympanicum and a glomus jugulotympanicum is an important radiological task, because there is a big difference in the operative approach, with the latter requiring extensive skull base surgery. From the jugular foramen the tumour can extend laterally with destruction of the mastoid segment of the facial canal and invasion of the facial nerve. Anteriorly the tumour grows into the total middle ear and further along the petrous bone to the foramen lacerum and the cavernous sinus. Inferior spread produces infiltration of the internal jugular vein and further growth in the carotid loge below the skull base. The intracranial extension is first situated extra-axially in the cerebellopontine angle and in advanced cases not only extra-axially, but also intra-axially in the cerebellum. Glomus vagale tumours, arising from the ganglion nodosum or extravagal, may secondarily extend into the jugular foramen.

The neuroradiological evaluation requires both CT and MRI. Thin-section CT in the axial and coronal planes with bone window gives information about the surrounding bony structures such as the enlargement and erosion of the jugular foramen, the infiltration of the petrous bone, the carotid canal, the facial canal, the hypoglossal canal and the inner ear structures. It also helps in the differential diagnosis with lesions that do not erode the bone such as schwannoma and meningioma (Fig. 10.4). Magnetic resonance shows

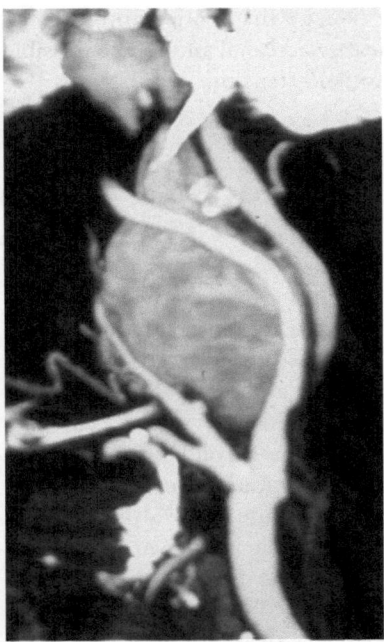

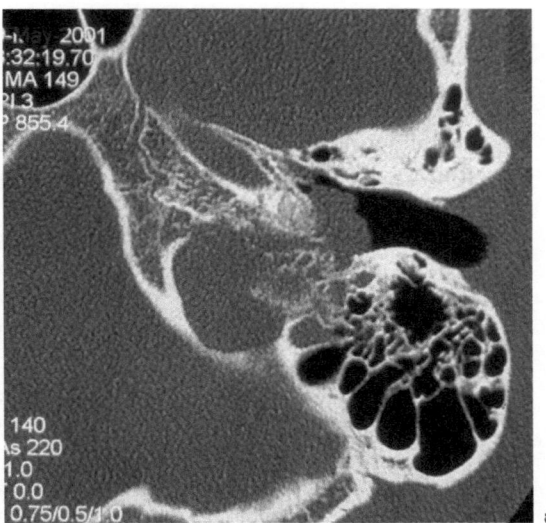

Fig. 10.3. Multiple paragangliomas. Computed tomographic angiography, sagittal maximum intensity projection reconstruction of axial contrast-enhanced thin sections from a multislice spiral CT examination. A large carotid paraganglioma is situated at the bifurcation of the common carotid artery, displacing the internal carotid artery backwards and the external carotid artery anteriorly. In the higher cervical region, a small vagal paraganglioma is typically situated behind the internal carotid artery, which is displaced anteriorly. At the skull base a jugular paraganglioma is visible with its extension in the carotid loge below the skull base

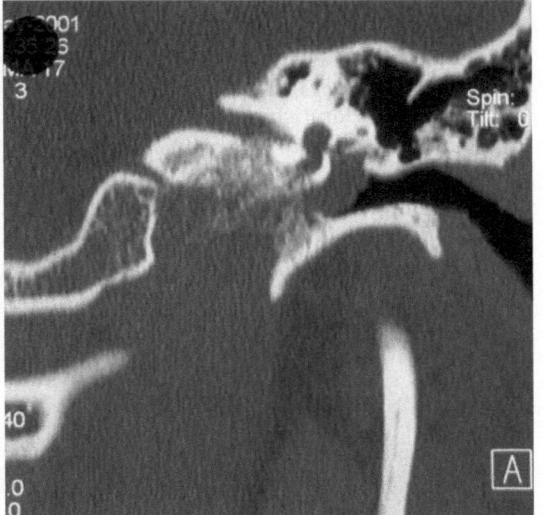

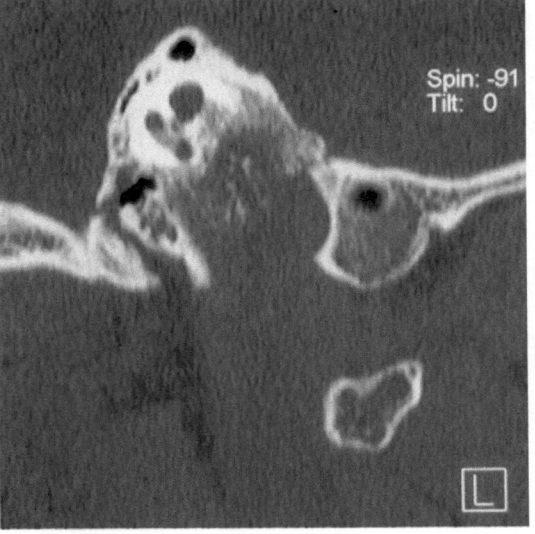

Fig. 10.4a–c. Jugulotympanic paraganglioma type C3. **a** A 0.7-mm axial section from a multislice spiral CT examination. **b** Coronal reconstruction. **c** Sagittal reconstruction, all figures in bone window. The jugular foramen is enlarged. Erosion of the anterior, lateral and superior walls of the foramen with extension of the bony erosion into the medial pars petrosum along the horizontal part of the carotid canal (classification C3). The soft tissue mass invades the bony septum between the jugular foramen and the hypotympanum and extends into the middle ear just to the tympanic membrane. Superiorly the tumour extends into the bone towards the internal auditory canal and the basal turn of the cochlea. The mastoid segment of the facial canal remains intact

the soft tissue extension of the tumour in the ear and below the skull base and intracranially (Fig. 10.5). The MR is equally important in the differential diagnosis by showing the characteristic intratumoral vessels (signal void) and the frequent presence of subacute intratumoral haemorrhage with a high signal on T1- and T2-weighted images. The combination of both features gives a salt-and-pepper appearance on T1-weighted images without contrast. This feature is limited to the larger paragangliomas (>1 cm) and is not pathognomonic, as is also seen in other hypervascular lesions such as metastasis. Use of contrast is necessary to find the smaller tumours such as the glomus tympanicum and for the demonstration of the soft tissue extent in the larger tumours. All paragangliomas have a strong enhancement. Magnetic resonance venography provides information about jugular vein occlusion and collateral venous drainage. Two hallmarks of this tumour are the bony erosion and the rich vascularization (Fig. 10.6); the latter poses special problems of blood loss during operation. Preoperative embolization is needed in the larger tumours (see Chap. 10).

In the previous century, Fisch introduced a classification of glomus temporale tumours useful in the planning of the preoperative embolization and for the selection of the surgical approach (Table 10.3; FISCH and MATTOX 1988). This classification is based on the location of the tumour in the middle ear or in the jugular foramen, on the relationship between the tumour and the carotid canal and on the possible presence of intracranial extension.

10.5.2
Schwannoma

Schwannoma is a benign tumour, composed entirely of Schwann cells. The neurofibroma is a well-differentiated nerve sheath tumour composed predominantly of Schwann cells and, to a lesser extent, fibroblasts and perineural cells (BURGER and SCHEITHAUER 1994). Neurofibromas of cranial nerves are extremely rare. Schwannomas are the second most common extra-axial intracranial tumours, preceded only by meningiomas. They constitute 5–10% of all intracranial neoplasms. The peak incidence is between the third and sixth decades. Degenerative changes are frequent. Tumour-related cysts can occur in the centre or at the periphery of the tumour. Like their intraspinal counterparts, the intracranial schwannomas show a predilection for the sensory nerves, and most often involve the vestibular division of the eight nerve. The fifth cranial nerve is the second most common site of origin. Schwannomas of the cranial nerves three, four and six are rare. Schwannomas of the jugular foramen usually originate from the ninth nerve. The presenting symptoms may be similar to

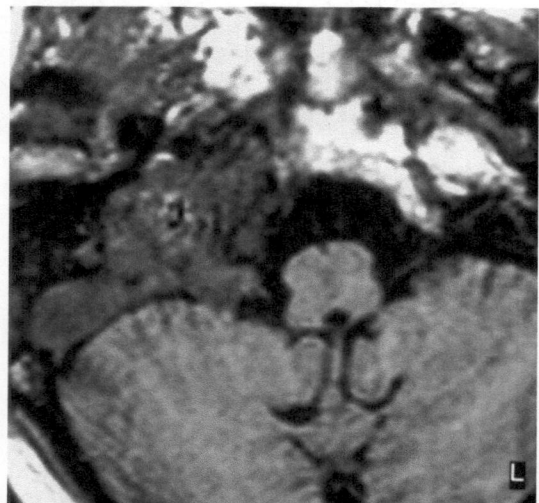 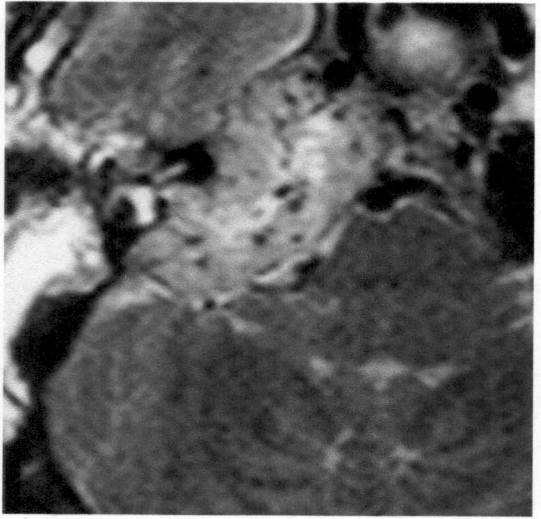

Fig. 10.5a, b. Large jugulotympanic paraganglioma type C4De. **a** A 2-mm axial 3D FT gradient-echo T1-weighted image without contrast. **b** A 3 mm axial TT2-weighted SE image. Magnetic resonance shows better the soft tissue extension. The tumour is located in the jugular foramen, the middle ear, the medial pars petrosum reaching the foramen lacerum and further into Meckel's cave and the cavernous sinus (classification C4). The intracranial extension in the cerebellopontine angle remains extra-axial (classification De). The intratumoral vessels (punctiform zones of signal void) and the salt-and-pepper appearance are clearly visible

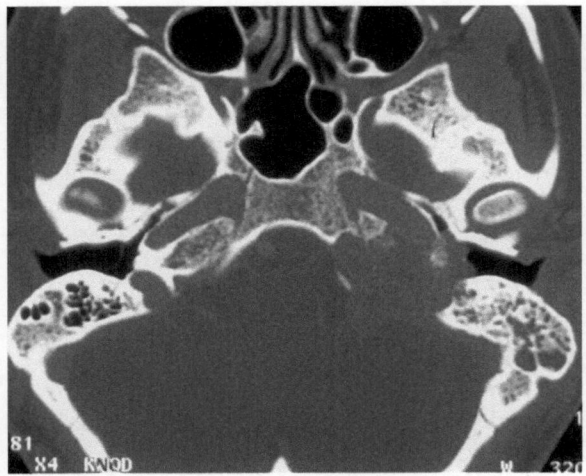

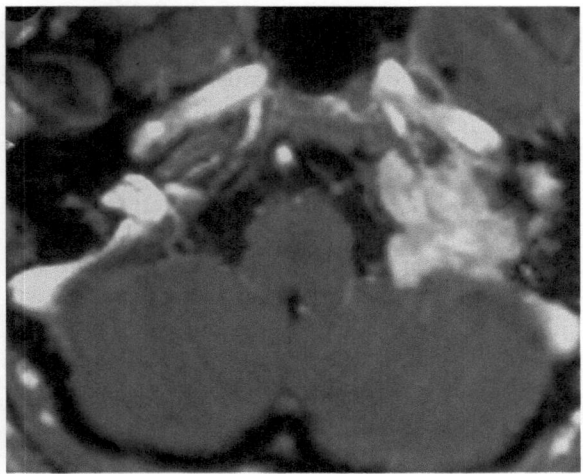

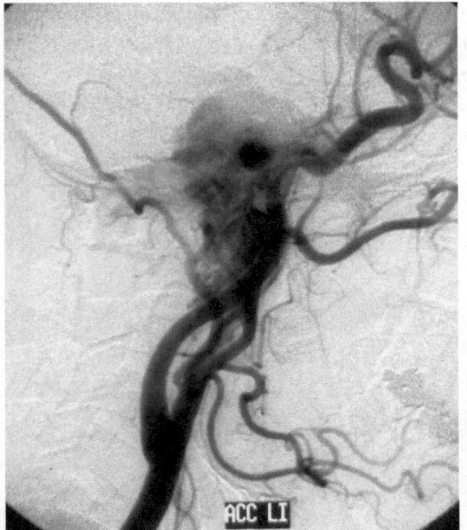

Fig. 10.6a–c. Jugulotympanic paraganglioma type C3De. a A 1-mm axial CT bone window. b A 2-mm axial 3D FT gradient echo T1-weighted image after contrast. c Angiography of the left common carotid artery. The two hallmarks of a paraganglioma of the jugular foramen are the bony erosion (a) and the rich vascularization (c). The tumour erodes the medial wall of the mastoid segment of the facial canal. The intracranial extension remains extra-axial (b). The lesion extends below the skull base in the carotid loge until the C2 level (c)

Table 10.3. Classification of glomus temporale tumours according to Fisch and Mattox (1988)

Type	Description
A	Glomus tympanicum confined to the tympanic cavity
B	Glomus tympanicum extending into the mastoid bone but leaving the cortical outline of the jugular foramen intact
C	Glomus jugulare. The letter C describes the variable extension into the infralabyrinthine portion of the temporal bone and along the carotid canal
C1	Minimal erosion of the vertical segment of the carotid canal
C2	Extensive erosion of the vertical segment of the carotid canal
C3	The erosion extends into the horizontal segment of the carotid canal
C4	The tumour reaches the foramen lacerum and may extend into the cavernous sinus
D	Glomus jugulare with intracranial extension
De1 to De3	Extradural extension, depending on the size
Di1 to Di3	Additional intradural extension, depending on the size

those of a vestibular schwannoma, due to the growth in the posterior fossa (MANZZONI et al. 1997). Unilateral hearing loss was the most common presenting symptom in the series of ELDEVIK et al. (2000). Signs of injury of the vagal or accessory nerves are frequently absent (ELDEVIK et al. 2000).

Schwannoma is the most common lesion that produces a smooth enlargement of the jugular foramen with sharp contours and often a sclerotic rim, well visible on CT scan with bone window (Fig. 10.7a). On CT the tumour is isodense and sometimes hypodense. On MR the signal intensity on the T1-weighted image is low and on the T2-weighted image high. The solid part of the tumour enhances strongly and usually homogeneously. Intratumoral cysts and necrosis are common and favours the diagnosis of schwannoma against meningioma. Intratumoral calcifications are absent. Bony erosions and intratumoral vessels, such as those seen in paraganglioma, are absent. Frequently the tumour has a dumbbell-shaped form with one part in the jugular foramen and the other part in the carotid loge or in the cerebellopontine angle (Fig. 10.7b, c; TAKAHASHI et al. 1997). When the tumour has a large intracranial part, confusion with a vestibular schwannoma is possible, especially because the latter can extend into the jugular foramen. But in a vestibular schwannoma the internal auditory canal is enlarged and in a jugular foramen schwannoma it is normal (ELDEVIK et al. 2000; WEBER and McKENNA 1994).

10.5.3
Meningioma

Meningiomas of the jugular foramen arise from arachnoid villi associated with the jugular bulb or that follow the cranial nerves IX to XI into the jugular foramen. Besides this primary meningioma of the jugular foramen, meningiomas may arise within the temporal bone and extend to the jugular foramen. Also the more common meningioma of the facies posterior of the pars petrosum (cerebellopontine angle menin-

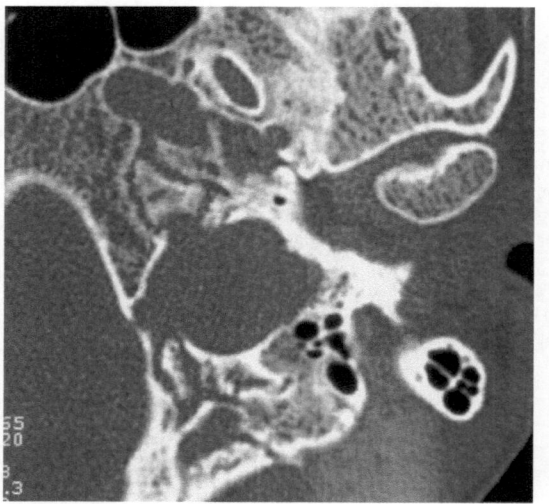

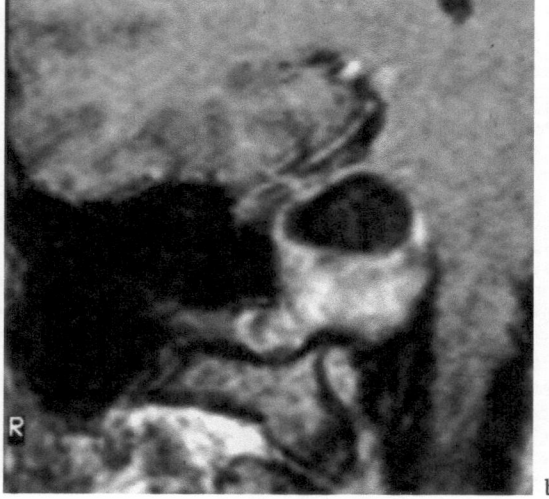

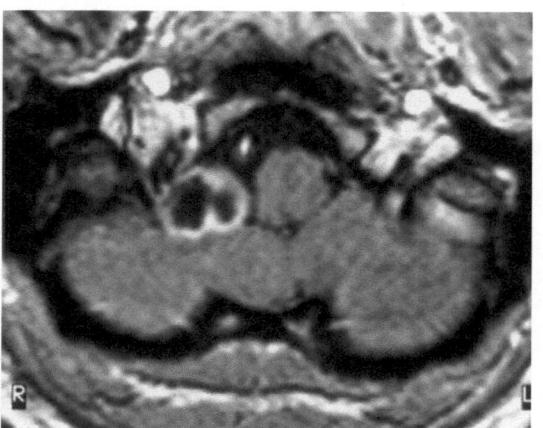

Fig. 10.7a–c. Schwannoma of the lower cranial nerves. **a** Axial CT bone window. **b** A 3-mm coronal T1-weighted SE image after contrast in a different patient. **c** A 2-mm axial 3D FT gradient-echo T1-weighted image after contrast. The CT examination in **a** shows a smooth enlargement of the jugular foramen with intact contours. The tumour in the second patient (**b, c**) has a cystic component and is dumbbell shaped with a large part in the cerebellopontine angle so that it can be confused with a vestibular schwannoma. Note the small component in the jugular foramen (**b**), and the internal auditory canal (not shown) was normal

gioma) can grow into the jugular foramen (RUSSEL and RUBINSTEIN 1989).

On CT a meningioma gives, like a schwannoma, a smooth enlargement of the jugular foramen with an intact cortical outline (Fig. 10.8a). The tumour is isodense or hyperdense in the native CT without contrast. It is the most common tumour in this location that can have intratumoral calcifications (Fig. 10.8a) and practically the only one with bony sclerosis or hyperostosis. When these signs are absent the differential diagnosis with a paraganglioma can be difficult. On MR the signal intensity is low on T1-weighted images and variable on T2-weighted images. After administration of gadolinium, the enhancement is strong and homogeneous (Fig. 10.8b, c). Frequently, there is an enhancement of the adjacent dura with gadolinium. This dural tail sign, although not pathognomonic, is very suggestive for meningioma, but it is among other lesions also described in schwannoma (BOUREKAS et al. 1995). Further features in the differential diagnosis with a paraganglioma are: (a) a meningioma rarely has intratumoral vessels or the same angiographic appearance as a paraganglioma; and (b) bony erosions are absent and the local extension pattern is different. Meningiomas do not have cystic components like a schwannoma.

10.5.4
Other Lesions of the Jugular Foramen (Primary and Secondary)

10.5.4.1
Endolymphatic Sac Tumour

In the late years of the previous century, the endolymphatic sac tumour (ELST) was recognized as a separate entity. The ELST is an adenomatous neoplasm of the papillary pattern originating from the endolymphatic sac's epithelium. Other possible adenomatous tumours of the temporal bone are metastases, direct extensions from extratemporal lesions and the primary middle ear adenomatous tumours of the mixed histological pattern (BATSAKIS and EL-NAGGAR 1993). The endolymphatic sac is the terminal

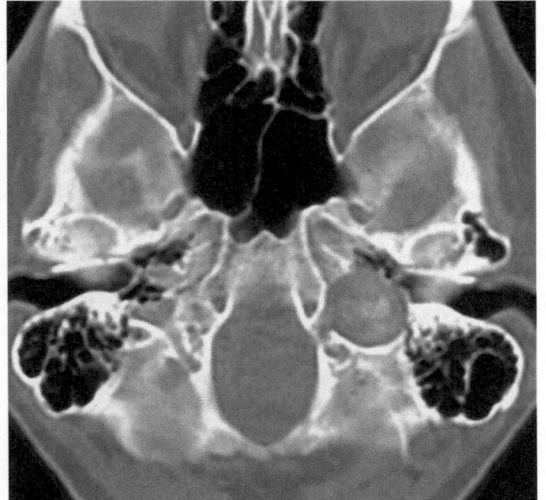
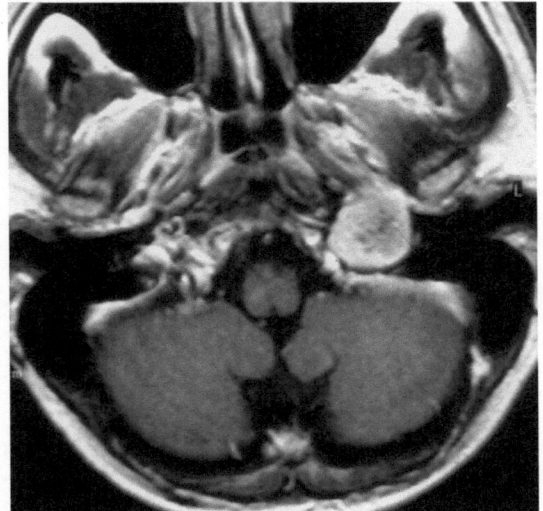
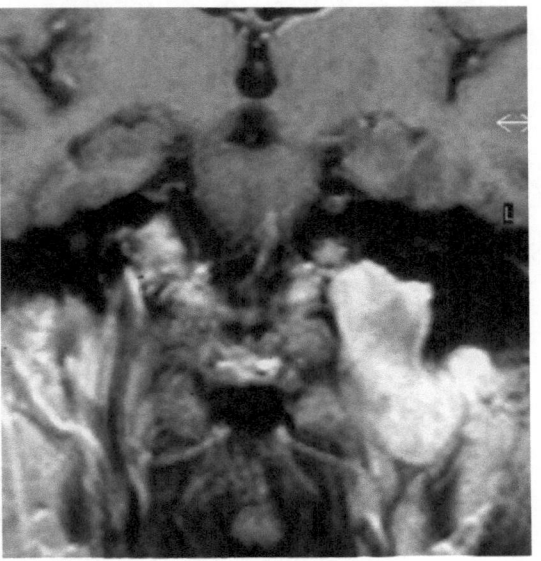

Fig. 10.8a–c. Meningioma. a Axial CT bone window. b, c A 3-mm axial and coronal T1-weighted SE image after contrast. Smooth enlargement of the jugular foramen with intact bony margins. The intratumoral calcifications (a) give an important clue to the diagnosis. The tumour extends below the skull base into the carotid loge. The nonenhancing part in b and c corresponds to the calcifications

saccular enlargement of the endolymphatic duct and lies between the inner and outer layers of the dura and the facies posterior of the pars petrosum. The ELST is centred between the sigmoid sinus and the internal auditory canal (IAC) around the vestibular aqueduct at the facies posterior. There is frequent involvement of the IAC, the jugular foramen and the posterior fossa. When it extends into the middle ear, it is a rare cause of a vascular mass (BATSAKIS and EL-NAGGAR 1993). Several isolated reports have suggested a pos-

sible association of ELST with the von Hippel-Lindau disease, and finally the work of MANSKI et al. in 1997 proved this association (Fig. 10.9a, b). The prevalence of ELST in von Hippel-Lindau disease is 6%, much higher than in the general population (MANSKI et al. 1997). The ELST is a slow-growing, locally aggressive, hypervascular tumour that does not metastasize. The hallmark of the tumour on CT is bony destruction (Fig. 10.9a). The lytic bony margins have a geographic or mixed geographic/moth-eaten pattern. Within

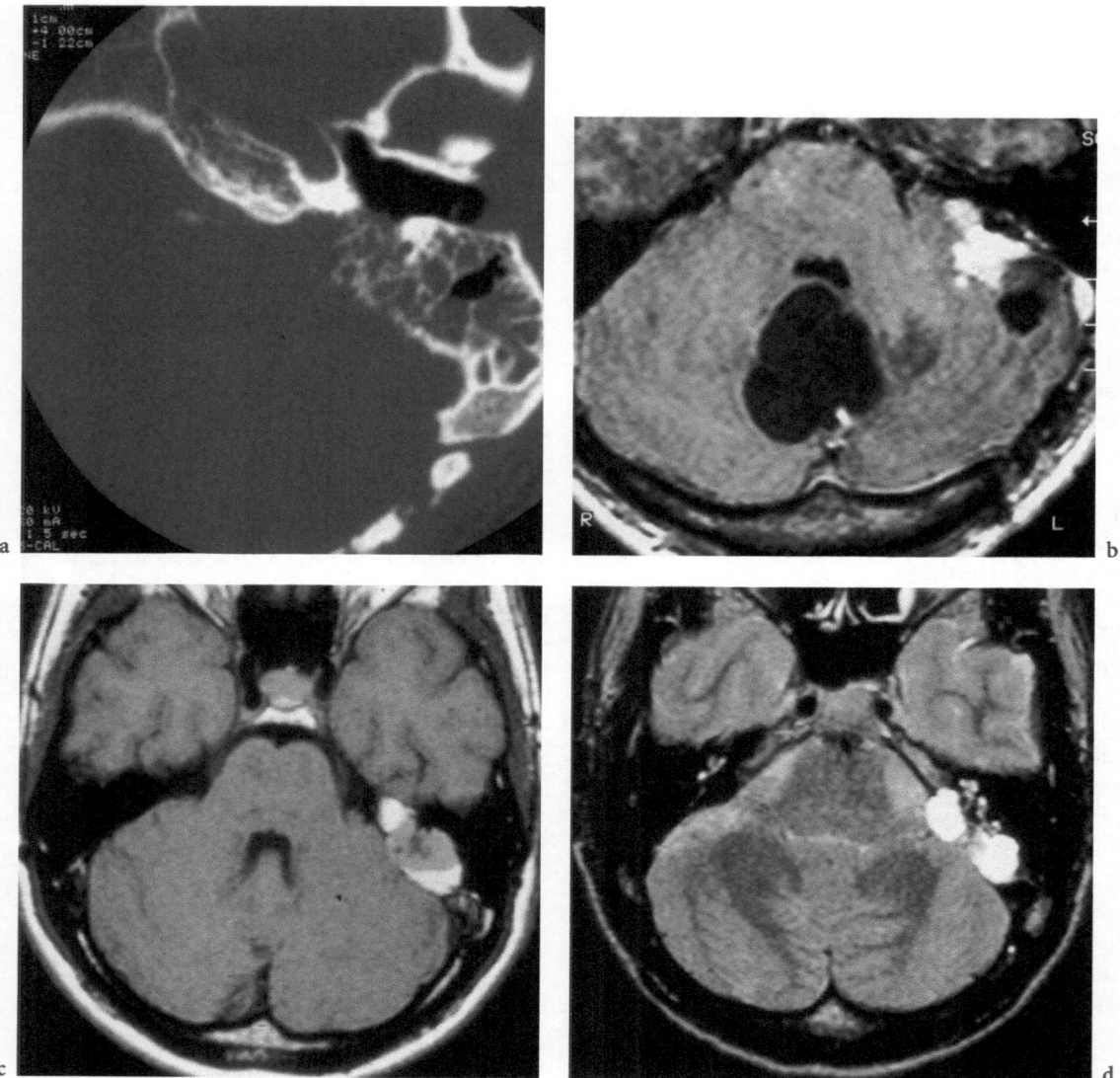

Fig. 10.9a–d. Endolymphatic sac tumour (ELST). **a** A 1-mm axial CT bone window and **b** 3-mm axial T1-weighted SE image after contrast in a patient with von Hippel-Lindau disease. **c** A 3-mm axial non-enhanced T1-weighted SE image and **d** a 3-mm axial T2-weighted SE image in a different patient. The CT in **a** in a patient with von Hippel-Lindau disease shows bony erosions of the jugular foramen and extension along the facies posterior of the pars petrosum. The bony defect in the occipital bone is from a previous operation. The MR in **b** shows the enhancing of the ELST and a haemangioblastoma with a large cystic part and a small mural nodule. The signal intensity of the lesion in the MR of **c** and **d** in a different patient corresponds to blood products

the lesion there are hyperdense areas, corresponding to intratumoral bone with bone trabeculae, as found on histological sections. On MR the ELST is a "blood-product-containing" tumour. On T1- and T2-weighted images the signal intensity (SI) is heterogeneous, with hyperintense areas corresponding to blood-filled cysts, proteinaceous cysts and subacute haemorrhage. In between are smaller foci of marked hypointensity, representing the tumour bone matrix and/or hemosiderin (Fig. 10.9c, d). After administration of gadolinium, the enhancement is strong (Fig. 10.9b). Angiography shows a hypervascular mass which mimics a paraganglioma (Lo et al. 1993). Although both ELST and paraganglioma cause irregular bone destruction, may involve the jugular foramen and are hypervascular, the differential diagnosis is easy when looking at the primary location of the tumour: ELST is located retrolabyrinthine at the facies posterior, and the glomus tumour primarily infralabyrinthine. The typical flow voids on MR of the larger glomus tumours are not seen in the smaller ones and also not in the ELST. The haemangioma, another tumour with prominent intratumoral bone spiculae in this region, has a different location at the IAC, the suprageniculate region or the mastoid genu of the facial canal.

10.5.4.2
Histiocytosis

Langerhans cell histiocytosis occurs predominantly in children (15–60% of children with the disease; Rubinstein et al. 1995). This tumour-like condition is characterized by a lytic bone destruction, which may be extensive. In the temporal bone the disease primary involves the otic capsule, lateral mastoid or the external auditory canal region. The jugular foramen may be secondarily involved. Computed tomography shows a lytic lesion without reactive sclerosis. The soft tissue mass enhances strongly and homogeneously (Fig. 10.10). On MR the lesion can have a heterogeneous SI due to the presence of blood-degradation products (Bonafé et al. 1994).

10.5.4.3
Giant Cell Tumour

Giant cell tumour occurs rarely in the jugular foramen. The radiological features on CT and MR can be indistinguishable from those of a paraganglioma. On angiography this tumour can be as vascular as a paraganglioma (Rosenbloom et al. 1999), although our own case was avascular (Fig. 10.11).

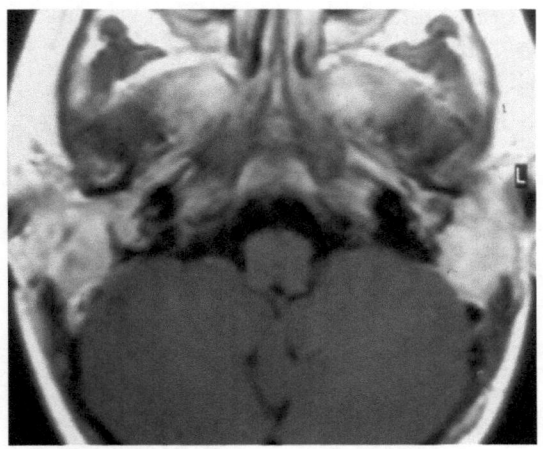

Fig. 10.10. Histiocytosis. A 3-mm axial T1-weighted SE image after contrast in a 2-year-old child. Bilateral homogeneously enhancing lesion of many parts of the temporal bone, including the jugular foramen

10.5.4.4
Metastasis

In an early stage, metastases may be indistinguishable from paraganglioma, but they are more aggressive and destructive, evolve faster and the extension pattern is different. The history is usually key to the diagnosis. A metastasis can be lytic, sclerotic or mixed.

10.5.4.5
Malignant External Otitis

Malignant external otitis (necrotizing external otitis) is a potentially life-threatening infection of the external auditory canal and skull base. The infection occurs mostly in elderly diabetic or immunocompromised patients. The infection begins as a typical external otitis (Fig. 10.12a) and extends from the external auditory canal inferiorly via the fissures of Santorini to involve the soft tissues around the stylomastoid foramen, causing a facial nerve palsy. With further extension the mastoid, middle ear, the parotis, and other soft tissues of the neck become involved, and with posteromedial extension also the jugular foramen. A diffuse skull base osteomyelitis finally results (Fig. 10.12b, c). *Pseudomonas aeruginosa* is the most common pathogen. Infections caused by *Aspergillus* are less frequent and typically begin in the middle ear or mastoid.

Both CT and MR are used for the initial assessment of the extent of the disease. The CT shows the bony erosions and the soft tissue extension, but for the latter MR is better. Neither modality is suited

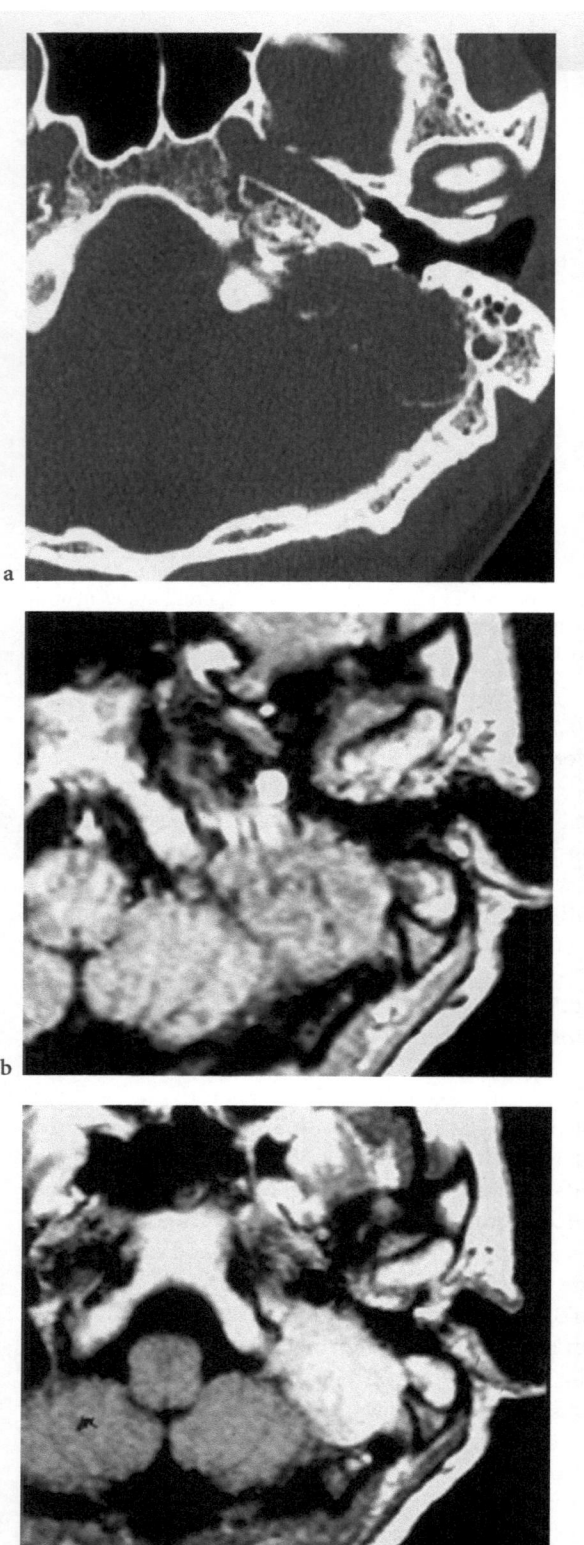

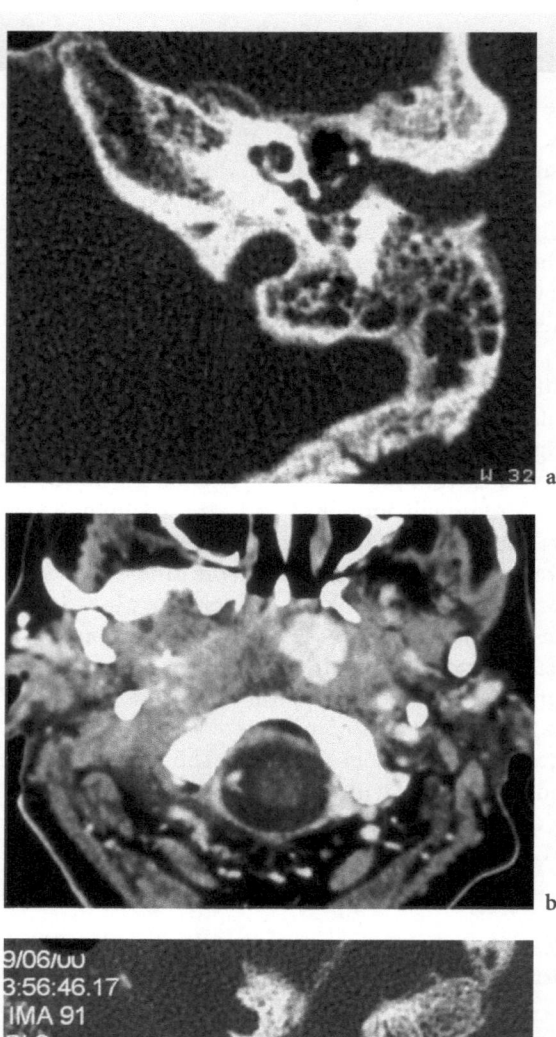

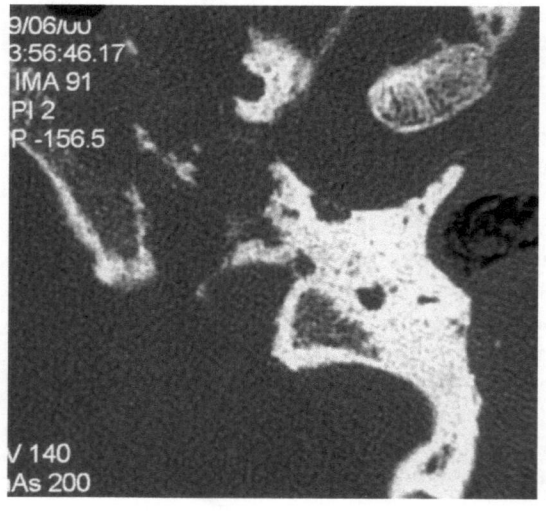

Fig. 10.11a–c. Giant cell tumour. a A 1-mm axial CT bone window. b, c A 2-mm axial 3D FT gradient-echo T1-weighted image without and with contrast. The CT and MR examinations show a destructive lesion in the jugular foramen and pars petrosum, with some intratumoral zones of signal void not due to calcifications but avascular on angiography (not shown). Strong enhancement after contrast (c)

Fig. 10.12a–c. Malignant external otitis. a A 1-mm axial CT bone window in a patient with an early stage of the disease. There is a soft tissue mass in the external and middle ear with minimal erosion of the posterior wall of the external auditory canal. No further extension into the skull base and the jugular foramen is intact. b, c A 1-mm axial CT bone window and 2-mm axial CT after contrast in a different patient shows extensive disease with erosion and destruction of large parts of the temporal bone and skull base, including the jugular foramen. The soft tissue extension below the skull base is bilateral with invasion of both carotid loges and bilateral bacterial arteritis. On the right this leads to a stenosis of the internal carotid artery and on the left to a rupture of the artery with a large pseudo-aneurysm. The patient died from bleeding

for the follow-up of osteomyelitis. Nuclear medicine techniques are a better choice for the treatment follow-up (SLATTERY and HARNSBERGER 1998).

10.5.4.6
Chordoma

Chordoma arises from notochord that forms the embryonal axial skeleton. Remnants of the primitive notochord can occur at any position along the neur-axis, but mostly in the sacrococcygeal region and in the spheno-occipital area. In principle, the chordoma of the skull base is a midline tumours arsing from the clivus, but they can extend to the jugular foramen. On CT the tumour shows a lytic bone destruction without sclerosis. Bony sequestration within the tumour mass occurs. On MR the lesion frequently has a heterogeneous signal intensity, because of old intratumoral haemorrhage, high-protein mucinous collections and bony sequestrations. The enhance-ment after contrast is moderate to marked (WEBER and MCKENNA 1994).

References

Batsakis GJ, El-Naggar AK (1993) Papillary neoplasm (Heff-ner's tumors) of the endolymphatic sac. Ann Otol Rhinol Laryngol 102:648–651

Bonafé A, Joomye H, Jaeger P, Fraysse B, Manelfe C (1994) Histiocytosis X of the petrous bone in the adult: MRI. Neuroradiology 36:330–334

Bourekas EC, Wildenhain P, Lewin JS, Tarr RW, Dastur KJ, Raji MR, Lanzieri CF (1995) The dural tail sign revisited. AJNR 16:1514–1516

Burger PC, Scheithauer BW (1994) Atlas of tumor pathology: tumors of the central nervous system. AFIP, Washington

Eldevik OP, Gabrielsen TO, Jacobsen EA (2000) Imaging find-ings in schwannomas of the jugular foramen. AJNR 21: 1139–1144

Fisch U, Mattox D (1988) Microsurgery of the skull base. Thieme, New York

Hovelaque A (1934) Osteologie, vol 2. Doin, Paris, pp 155–156

Lo WWM, Applegate LJ, Carberry JN, Solti-Bohman LG, House JW, Brackmann DE, Waluch V, Li JC (1993) Endolymphatic sac tumors: radiologic appearance. Radiology 189:199–204

Maffe MF, Raofi B, Kumar A, Muscato C (2000) Glomus faciale, glomus jugulare, glomus tympanicum, glomus vagale, carotid body tumors and simulating lesions. Radiol Clin North Am 38:1059–1076

Manski TJ, Hefner DK, Glenn GM, Patronas NJ, Pikus AT, Katz D, Lebovics R, Sledjeski K, Choyke PL, Zbar B, Linehan M, Oldfield EH (1997) Endolymphatic sac tumors: a source of morbid hearing loss in von Hippel-Lindau Disease. J Am Med Assoc 277:1461–1466

Manzzoni A, Sanna, M, Saleh E, Achilli V (1997) Lower cranial nerve schwannoma involving the jugular foramen. Ann Otol Rhinol Laryngol 106:370–379

Petrus LV, Lo WMM (1996) Primary paraganglioma of the facial nerve canal. AJNR 17:171–174

Rao AB, Koeller KK, Adair CF (1999) Parangliomas of the head and the neck: radiologic–pathologic correlation. Radiographics 19:1605–1632

Rhoton AL (2000) Jugular foramen. Neurosurgery 47: S276–S285

Rosenbloom JS, Storper IS, Aviv JE, Hacein-Bey L, Bruce JN (1999) Giant cell tumors of the jugular foramen. Am J Otolaryngol 20:176–179

Rubinstein D, Burton BS, Walker AL (1995) The anatomy of the inferior petrosal sinus, glossopharyngeal nerve, vagus nerve, and accessory nerve in the jugular foramen. AJNR 16:185–194

Russel DS, Rubinstein LJ (1989) Pathology of tumours of the nervous system, 5th edn. Arnold, London

Sen C, Hague K, Kacchara R, Jenkins A, Das S, Catalano P (2001) Jugular foramen: microscopic anatomic features and implications for neural preservation with reference to glomus tumors involving the temporal bone. Neurosurgery 48:838–848

Slattery WH, Brackmann DE (1996) Skull base osteomyelitis, malignant otitis externa. Otolaryngol Clin North Am 29: 795–806

Swartz JD, Harnsberger HR (1998) Imaging of the temporal bone. Thieme, New York

Takahashi M, Adachi T, Sako K (1997) Dumbbell-shaped jugular foramen schwannoma. Eur Arch Otorhinolaryngol 254:474–477

Weber AL, McKenna MJ (1994) Radiologic evaluation of the jugular foramen; anatomy, vascular variants, anomalies and tumors. Neuroimaging Clin North Am 4:579–598

The Clinician's View

I. DHOOGE

please see 'The Clinician's View' at the end of chapter 11.

11 Vascular Temporal Bone Lesions

H. Tanghe

CONTENTS

11.1
Imaging Strategies in Pulsatile Tinnitus

Tinnitus is a "sound in one ear or both ears, such as buzzing, ringing, or whistling, occurring without an external stimulus" (AMERICAN HERITAGE DICTIONARY 2000). Tinnitus can be classified as pulsatile (coinciding with the heartbeat) or continuous, and subjective (perceived only by the patient) or objective (perceptible to another person).

Pulsatile tinnitus (PT) can be caused by (a) vascular anatomical variants, (b) vascular tumours, (c) vascular malformations, (d) acquired vascular lesions, (e) vascularized chronic inflammatory tissue of the middle ear, or (f) other diseases such as otosclerosis, Paget's disease and benign intracranial hypertension (Table 11.1; SWARTZ and HARNSBERGER 1998; WEISSMAN and HIRSCH 2000; WALDVOGEL et al. 1998).

H. TANGHE, MD
Section of Neuroradiology, Department of Radiology, Dijkzigt, Sophia Children's and Daniel Den Hoed Hospitals, Erasmus University Medical Centre, Dr. Molenwaterplein 40, 3015 Rotterdam, The Netherlands

Table 11.1. Overview of vascular temporal bone lesions

Pseudo-lesions
Vascular anatomical variants
Tumours with rich vascularity
Acquired vascular lesions
Vascularized chronic inflammation tissue
Vascular malformations

The pre-imaging evaluation of a patient consists of a detailed history, looking for hearing loss, vertigo, headaches and a medical examination including a neuro-otological and audiological evaluation.

In general, the diagnostic yield of the radiological evaluation in PT is low. The imaging analysis starts with a CT – thin sections with bone algorithm in the axial and coronal plane – of the temporal bone and adjacent structures of the skull base. The anatomy of the carotid canal and the jugular foramen is carefully studied. For the anatomical vascular variants and small soft tissue masses, such as a small glomus tympanicum, no further study is needed. For larger masses an MRI examination is complementary and the CT study can be done without intravenous contrast. For acquired vascular lesions and vascular malformations the initial CT can be complemented with a CT angiography or CT venography (dural sinus occlusive disease) when a modern multiple-row-detector CT machine is available; otherwise, an MR angiography/venography can be done. In case of an objective PT, you can start with a CT angiography or MR angiography. A conventional digital subtraction angiography (DSA) is necessary for vascular malformations to demonstrate the angio-architecture and in case of endovascular treatment.

11.2
Vascular Anatomical Variants

Vascular anatomical variants of the temporal bone are a frequent cause of PT or a vascular retrotympanic mass that often clinically cannot be differentiated from a paraganglioma (Table 11.2). This differentiation is important prior to biopsy or therapy. Often these variants are an incidental asymptomatic finding on a CT done for other reasons. The radiological diagnosis is possible with MRI, MR angiography and with CT. For some variants, such as the dehiscent jugular bulb, the bone detail available with CT is important. On MR spin-echo sequences, the signal void of the abnormally located artery or vein may be identical to the signal void of the cortical bone and the air in the ear and the anomaly can be missed. A gradient-echo sequence gives a high signal from the vessel with better differentiation from the cortical bone.

11.2.1
Arterial Variants

11.2.1.1
Aberrant Internal Carotid Artery

The aberrant internal carotid artery (ICA), also called the aberrant flow of the internal carotid artery in the tympanic cavity (LASJAUNIAS et al. 2001), enters the skull base through an enlarged inferior tympanic canaliculus with a characteristic narrowing of the vessel. The fundamental cause is a segmental agenesis, absence of the cervical part of the internal carotid artery with the subsequent absence of the vertical part of the bony carotid canal. The ascending pharyngeal artery, with its tympanic branch (going through its own enlarged inferior tympanic canaliculus), serves as a collateral pathway to the normal horizontal part of the ICA. At the end of the inferior tympanic canaliculus, the artery enters the middle ear cavity and is located behind the tympanic membrane at the promontorium tympani as a "vascular mass", not covered by bone, before entering the horizontal part of the carotid canal through a bony dehiscence. An aberrant ICA can be associated with a persistent stapedial artery (vide infra; TANGHE 1994; WEISSMAN and HIRSCH 2000).

This anomaly can present with objective or subjective pulsatile tinnitus and conductive hearing loss. On otoscopy the ENT surgeon finds a vascular-appearing retrotympanic mass that mimics a paraganglioma. A misdiagnosis as a glomus tympanicum must be avoided: the operation can result in a debacle (SWARTZ and HARNSBERGER 1998; TANGHE 1994).

The CT features are characterized as follows (Table 11.3):

Table 11.2. Vascular anatomical variants. *ICA* internal carotid artery

Arterial	Venous
The aberrant ICA	High jugular bulb
Hyostapedial artery variants	Dehiscent jugular bulb
Laterally displaced ICA	Jugular bulb diverticulum
Isolated agenesis of the ICA	
Pharyngo-tympano-stapedial artery	
Splitting of the petrous ICA	

Table 11.3. The CT appearance of the "aberrant ICA"

Absence of the vertical part of the carotid canal
Enlarged inferior tympanic canaliculus
The vertical segment of the ICA enters the temporal bone through enlarged inferior tympanic canaliculus, running more posteriorly and laterally than normal
Absence of the normal bony posterior margin of the horizontal part of the carotid canal
Soft tissue density in the middle ear at the level of the promontory, joining the horizontal carotid canal through the bony defect mentioned above and simulating a paraganglioma
"Stenosis" at the entry point in the horizontal carotid canal

1. Absence of a normal-appearing vertical segment of the carotid canal.
2. Absence of the bony wall in the posterolateral portion of the horizontal segment of the carotid canal.
3. A round soft tissue mass in the middle ear at the promontorium. Especially in a coronal section this mass can look similar to a glomus tympanicum.
4. On axial CT this mass is in continuity with the horizontal segment of the carotid canal.
5. The aberrant ICA enters the tympanic cavity through an enlarged inferior tympanic canaliculus, located more laterally and posteriorly compared with a normal vertical ICA segment (Fig. 11.1; TANGHE 1994). On conventional MRI the diagnosis of an aberrant ICA is difficult because of the lack of contrast between the low signal of bone, the signal void of the ICA and the air in the middle ear and mastoid portion. Flow-sensitive MR images or MR angiography (MRA) allow the diagnosis. Conventional angiography is not necessary for the diagnosis (WEISSMAN and HIRSCH 2000).

11.2.1.2
Partial Persistence of the Stapedial Artery

The so-called persistent stapedial artery is in fact a partial persistence of the stapedial artery, different from the full persistent variant which is very rare (LASJAUNIAS et al. 2001). The partial persistent variant

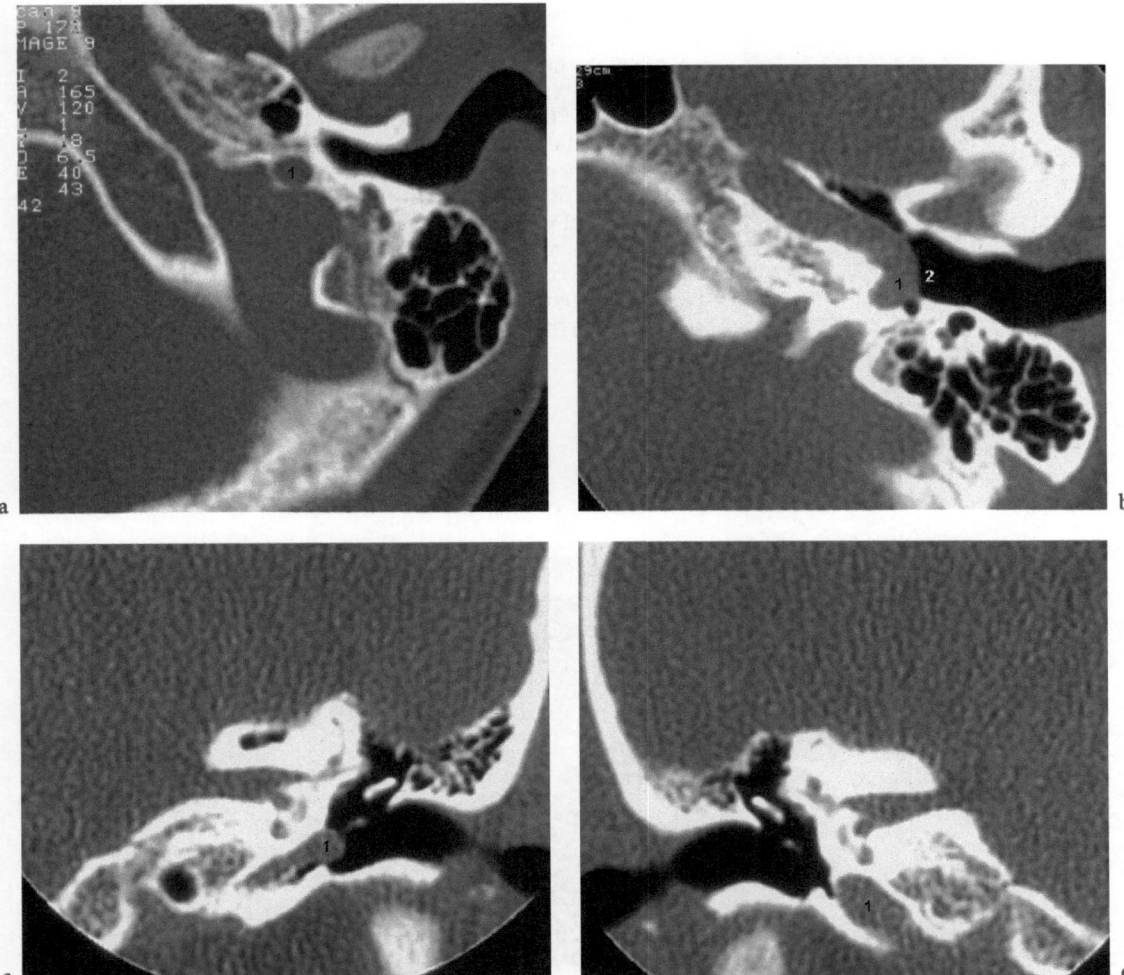

Fig. 11.1a–d. Aberrant internal carotid artery. **a** Axial CT at the level of the enlarged inferior tympanic canaliculus (*1*). This canal is located more laterally and is smaller than the normal vertical part of the carotid canal. **b** Axial CT at the level of the horizontal part of the carotid canal. Part of the lateral bony wall is absent (1) and the carotid artery comes close to the tympanic membrane (2). **c** Coronal CT at the level of the genu in a different patient. The carotid artery reaches the tympanic membrane (3). The inferior tympanic canaliculus is smaller than the normal vertical part of the carotid canal at the opposite site in **d** (*1*)

is an intratympanic origin of the middle meningeal artery. The artery originates from the ICA between the vertical and the horizontal portions of the carotid canal. It enters the middle ear cavity anteroinferiorly, runs along the promontory, passes between the crura of the stapes and enters the tympanic segment of the facial canal causing an enlargement of this canal. At the level of the first genu it leaves the facial canal through its own foramen and enters the extradural space of the middle cranial fossa, becoming the middle meningeal artery (MMA; TANGHE 1994). It can be associated with an aberrant ICA (Fig. 11.2) and with an aneurysmal enlarged ICA (Fig. 11.3).

This vascular variant is most often an incidental finding at operation or on a CT examination (easily overlooked) and rarely symptomatic with pulsatile tinnitus.

A persistent stapedial artery cannot be diagnosed with MR or even MRA. The CT features are pathognomonic (Table 11.4; TANGHE 1994): (a) absence of the foramen spinosum, because there is no MMA to go through; (b) erosion of the promontory; (c) widening of the proximal tympanic segment of the facial canal to accommodate the artery; and (d) absence of the MMA from the internal maxillary artery on angiography.

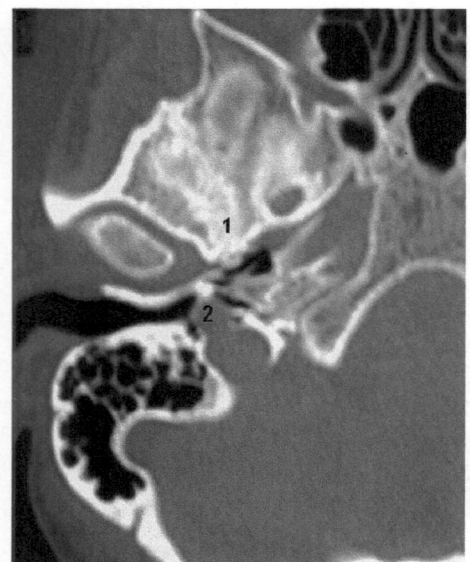

Fig. 11.2a–e. Persistent stapedial artery, associated with an aberrant internal carotid artery. **a** Axial CT. The foramen spinosum is absent (*1*), compared with the normal left side. The carotid artery is in contact with the tympanic membrane through a bony defect at the end of inferior tympanic canaliculus (*2*). There is no bony margin between the inferior tympanic canaliculus and the jugular foramen. **b** Axial CT. The carotid artery lies in the middle ear with a large bony defect in the horizontal part of the carotid canal. Note the origin of the persistent stapedial artery. **c** Coronal CT at the level of the oval window (*1*). **d, e** Coronal and axial CT at the level of the proximal tympanic segment of the facial canal (*1*, in **d** and **e**). The facial canal at the level of the oval window is still normal in size, but it is enlarged at his proximal tympanic segment, to accommodate the persistent stapedial artery. The labyrinthine segment of the facial canal is normal (*2* in **e**)

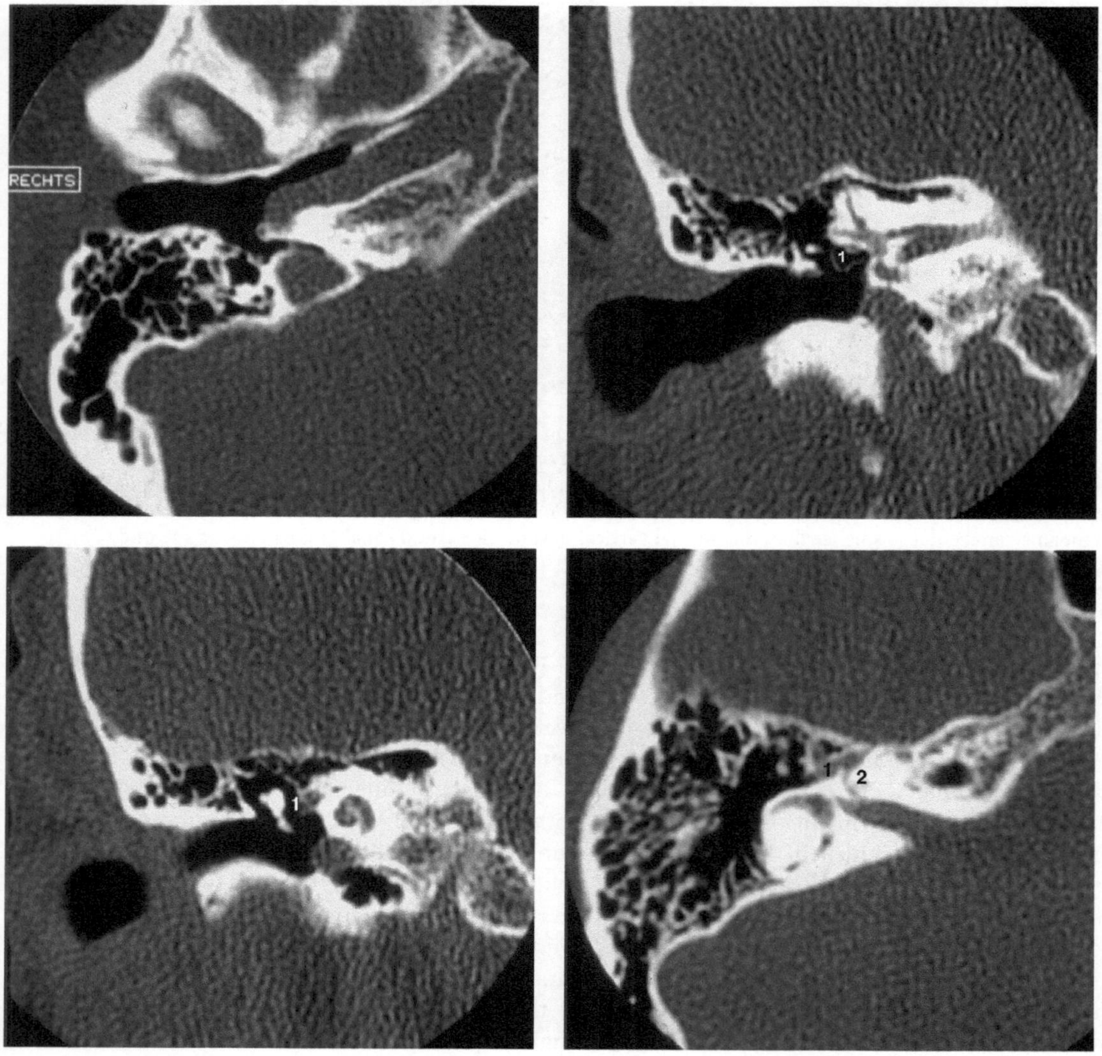

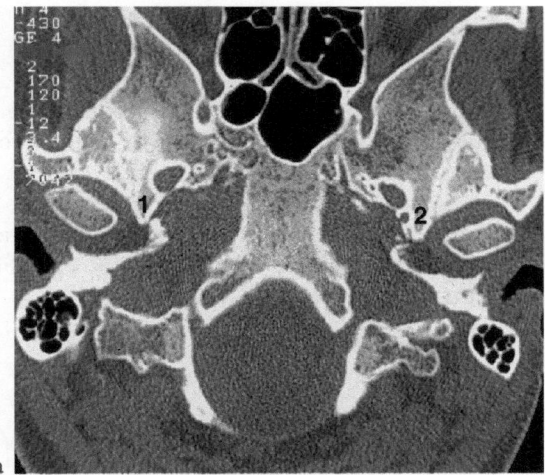
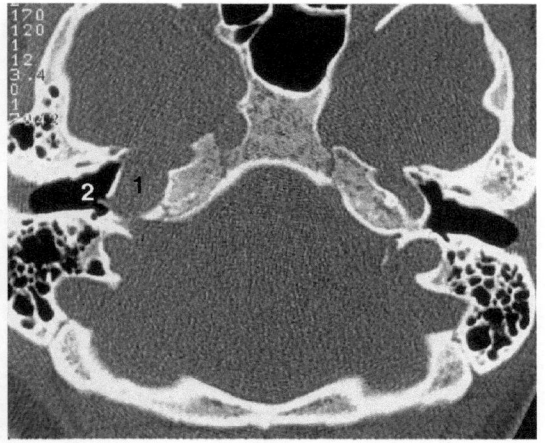
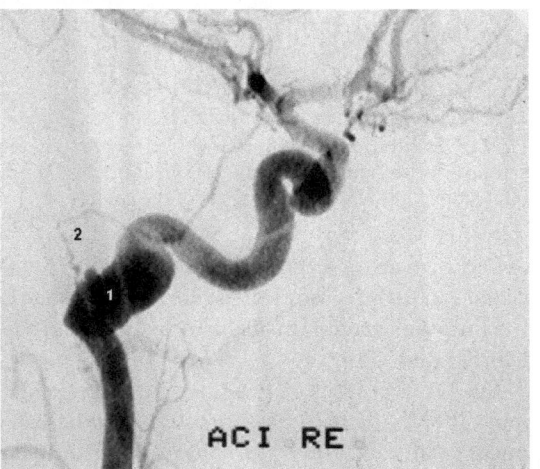

Fig. 11.3a–c. Persistent stapedial artery, associated with aneurysmal enlargement of the carotid artery. **a** Axial CT of the skull base. The foramen spinosum is absent on the right side (*1*) and normal on the left side (*2*). **b** Axial CT at the level of the horizontal part of the carotid canal. The canal is enlarged (*1*). Also note the origin of the persistent stapedial artery (*2*). **c** The angiogram in the same patient shows the fusiform aneurysmal enlargement of the carotid artery (*1*) and the persistent stapedial artery (*2*)

11.2.1.3
Splitting of the Petrous ICA

In this case two channels carry the flow into the petrous portion. Both channels belong to the ascending pharyngeal artery system and the internal carotid artery can still be considered segmentally agenetic (Fig. 11.4; LASJAUNIAS et al. 2001).

11.2.2
Venous Variants

11.2.2.1
The High or High-Riding Jugular Bulb

The jugular bulb is considered high when it extends above the level of the floor of the internal auditory canal. On a T1-weighted MR sequences after gadolinium this variant can simulate an enhancing tumour in the medial temporal bone. But the bony margins of

Table 11.4. The CT appearance of the partial persistent stapedial artery

Absence of the foramen spinosum
Erosion of the promontory
Widening of the proximal tympanic segment of the facial canal

the jugular foramen are intact and well corticated. In case of doubt a CT with bone algorithm can be done (TANGHE 1994; WEISSMAN and HIRSCH 2000).

11.2.2.2
Dehiscent Jugular Bulb

A dehiscent jugular bulb lacks a complete cortical covering and lies in part in the hypotympanum of the middle ear. It usually presents as a vascular retrotympanic mass behind the posteroinferior quadrant of the tympanic membrane (SWARTZ and HARNSBERGER 1998; TANGHE 1994; WEISSMAN and HIRSCH 2000).

On MR the diagnosis is difficult because MR cannot demonstrate the presence or absence of the

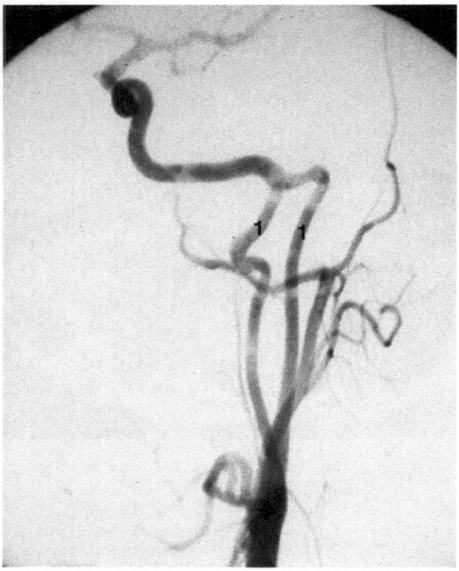

Fig. 11.4. Splitting of the internal carotid artery. Angiogram. The carotid artery is split in two parts (*1*) from its origin at the carotid bifurcation, until the horizontal part of the carotid canal

cortical covering of the jugular foramen. The dehiscence can be inferred from a more lateral position of the bulb on coronal images and by the presence of a lateral lobulation.

On CT the dehiscent jugular bulb is visible as a mass low in the medial part of the middle ear. This mass is in continuity with the jugular bulb in the foramen trough a bony defect (Fig. 11.5).

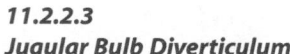

11.2.2.3
Jugular Bulb Diverticulum

A jugular diverticulum is a protrusion of the jugular bulb superior and medial to the jugular foramen. It does not extend into the middle ear, but can be associated with PT, because of turbulence of the venous flow. The tympanic membrane is normal and the anomaly cannot be seen at otoscopy (Fig. 11.6; WEISSMAN and HIRSCH 2000).

11.3
Acquired Vascular Lesions

Numerous acquired vascular lesions can cause PT (Table 11.5) A detailed description is beyond the scope of this chapter (SWARTZ and HARNSBERGER 1998; WEISSMAN and HIRSCH 2000; LO and SOLTI-BOHMAN 1996).

Aneurysm of the petrous portion of the carotid artery can cause PT, but at this location they are rare (Fig. 11.3). Intracranial aneurysms are far more frequent.

Atherosclerotic stenotic disease at the carotid bifurcation in the neck may produce turbulence of flow but gives only occasionally PT. Despite its high prevalence as a cause of asymptomatic carotid bruit, atherosclerosis is not a common cause of symptomatic pulsatile tinnitus (SANDOK et al. 1982).

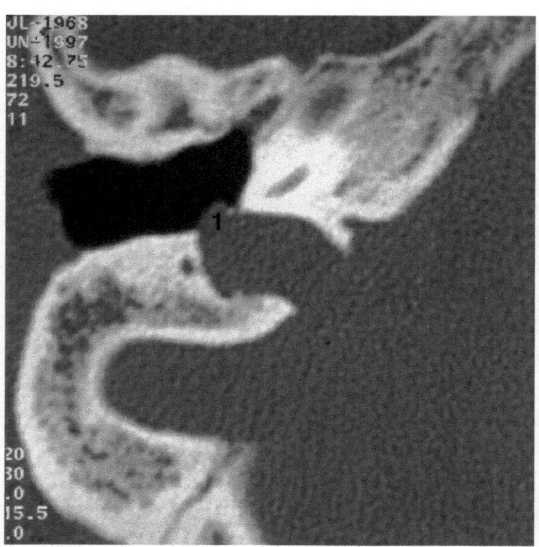

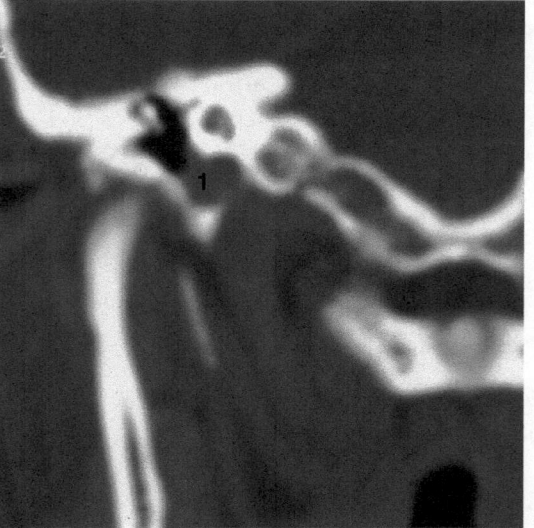

Fig. 11.5a, b. Dehiscent jugular bulb. **a** Axial CT. The jugular bulb protrudes in the middle ear through a bony defect in the jugular foramen (*1*). **b** Coronal CT in a different patient. There is a mass low in the medial part of the middle ear. This mass is in continuity with the jugular bulb in the foramen through a bony defect (*1*)

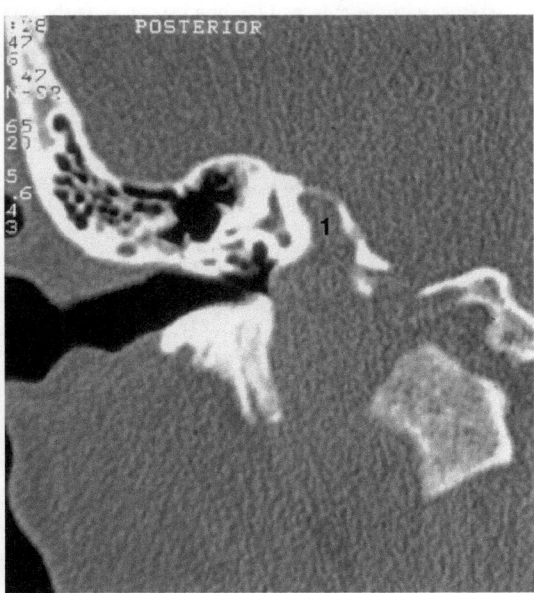

Fig. 11.6. Jugular bulb diverticulum. Coronal CT. There is a protrusion of the jugular bulb superior and medial to the jugular foramen. Such a protrusion is called a diverticulum (*1*). It does not extend into the middle ear

Table 11.5. Acquired vascular lesions

Petrous carotid aneurysm
Atherosclerotic carotid artery disease
Fibromuscular dysplasia
Spontaneous carotid dissection
Thrombosis of dural sinus with intracranial hypertension

Fibromuscular dysplasia of the internal carotid artery most frequently gives intracranial ischemia, but PT is the second most frequent manifestation (SISMANIS et al. 1994).

Other acquired vascular lesions that can give tinnitus are: spontaneous dissection of the internal carotid artery; idiopathic intracranial hypertension with sinus thrombosis; and a vascular compression of the eighth nerve in the cerebellopontine angle

11.4
Endovascular Therapy of Vascular Tumours

Paraganglioma is the most common tumour causing PT or a vascular tympanic membrane (LASJAUNIAS et al. 2001). Other less common vascular tumours are meningioma, haemangioma of the facial nerve, endolymphatic sac tumour (see Chap. 10), cavernous hae-

mangioma of the middle ear and vascular metastasis such as Grawitz tumour (Table 11.6; WEISSMAN and HIRSCH 2000). A meningioma located in the temporal bone can clinically mimic a paraganglioma. When it protrudes in the middle ear, the ENT surgeon sees on otoscopy a vascular retrotympanic mass, indistinguishable from a paraganglioma. Meningiomas and metastasis can be as vascular as paraganglioma. For a detailed discussion of the imaging features of these tumours see Chap. 10.

Paragangliomas have a characteristic angiographic appearance with enlarged feeding arteries, an early and intense tumour blush and early draining veins (Fig. 11.7a). The intratumoral arterioles in the periphery of the tumour are smaller than those in the centre. There are multiple intratumoral direct communications between arterioles and venules with arteriovenous shunting. Large paragangliomas (type C2 or more, according to the classification of FISCH and MATTOX 1988) have a lot of feeding vessels and large intratumoral arteriovenous shunts, making them almost impossible to resect without a preoperative embolization (Fig. 11.7b, c; CONNORS and WOJAK 1999).

In 75–85% of the cases the angioarchitecture of a paraganglioma is multicompartmental (Table 11.7). The tumour may be divided into several parts completely separated from each other. A complete compartment may be overlooked if the corresponding arteries are not injected. There are four important compartments, each with its own set of feeding vessels: (a) an inferior and medial compartment; (b) a posterolateral compartment; (c) an anterior compartment; and (d) a superior compartment (Table 11.7z; MORET et al. 1982).

The pre-embolization angiographic protocol consists of a study of the ICA, and the vertebral, internal maxillary, occipital and ascending pharyngeal arteries. It is further important to look at the relationship of the tumour to the internal vein, the inferior petrosal sinus and other dural sinus. Especially the detection of extraluminal compression or intraluminal tumour extension is important for the surgeon. This information can be obtained from the venous phase of the vertebral and carotid angiography and from the CT and MRI.

Table 11.6. Tumours of the temporal bone that may present with pulsatile tinnitus or a vascular retrotympanic mass

Paraganglioma
Haemangioma
Meningioma
Endolymphatic sac tumour
Vascular metastasis

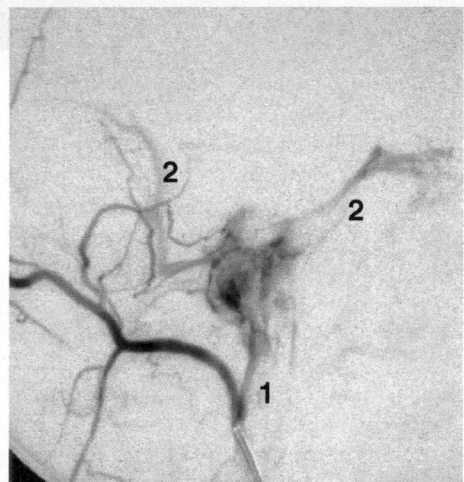

Fig. 11.7a–c. Glomus jugulotympanicum. **a** Occipital artery. The posterior part of the tumour is fed by the stylomastoid artery (*1*). The angiographic appearance is characteristic, with an enlarged feeding artery, an early and intense tumour blush and early draining veins (*2*). **b, c** Angiogram of the common carotid artery before and after embolization. The tumour is very vascular with an intense tumour blush (*1* in **b**). The small tumour blush left, after embolization, comes from feeding from the internal carotid artery via the caroticotympanic ramus (1 in **c**). This vessel usually cannot be catheterized selectively.

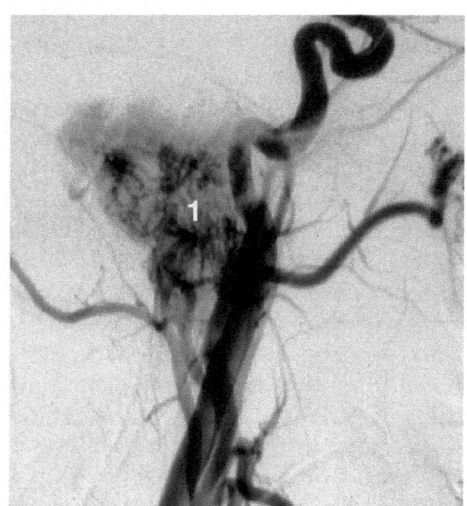

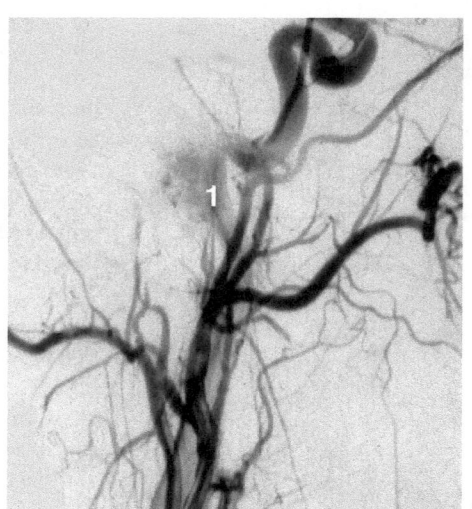

Table 11.7. Angioarchitecture of paraganglioma: compartment and feeding vessels. For each compartment the feeding vessels are arranged starting from the principal vessel to additional feeding vessels with increasing volume of that tumour compartment. (From MORET et al. 1982)

Compartment	Feeding vessels
Inferomedial	Inferior tympanic branch (ascending pharyngeal artery)
	Neuromeningeal trunk (ascending pharyngeal artery)
	Lateral clival branch of the ICA
	Meningeal branches of the vertebral artery
Posterolateral	Stylomastoid artery (occipital artery or posterior auricular artery)
	Meningeal branches of the occipital artery
	Meningeal branches of the vertebral artery
Anterior	Anterior tympanic artery (internal maxillary artery)
	Caroticotympanic artery (ICA)
	Cavernous branches of the ICA
Superior	Middle meningeal artery
	Accessory meningeal artery

The goal of the embolization is the diminution of the peroperative blood loss and the drying of the operative field, making the operation technically possible and shorter in duration. These goals are reached by an intratumoral devascularization of the tumour parenchyma and not by a proximal occlusion of the feeding vessel!

The embolization is carried out with a microcatheter with superselective catheterization of the different feeding vessels. As embolization material we use particles polyvinyl alcohol (PVA), with a size of 150–250 µm. In case of a good intratumoral catheter position smaller particles, <90 µm, can be used to reach the centre of the tumour through the small-sized peripheral intratumoral arterioles. The problem of large intratumoral arteriovenous shunts can be dealt with by the use of liquid embolization material or by selective occlusion of the shunt with an intratumoral coil (Fig. 12).

To prevent complications the dangerous anastomoses between the vertebral, internal carotid and external carotid arteries must be known (Fig. 11.8; Lasjaunias et al. 2001; Connors and Wojak 1999; Moret et al. 1982). Furthermore, it is important to remember that several cranial nerves receive their blood supply by the vessels we intend to embolize: the ninth, tenth, eleventh and twelfth cranial nerves by the ascending pharyngeal artery, the facial nerve by the middle meningeal and accessory meningeal artery, and the third, fourth, fifth and sixth cranial nerves by the accessory meningeal artery. Use of particles which are too small or of glue in conjunction with an improper catheter position can result in definitive cranial nerve palsy.

11.5
Vascular Malformations

Vascular malformations may cause PT, usually objective and sometimes subjective. Often the patient has in addition an audible bruit or a pulsatile thrill. When these signs are present, the angiography can be the initial imaging study. It is important to know that not only intracranial or skull base vascular malformations, but also cervical vascular lesions, such as vertebral arteriovenous fistulas, can cause PT. Every high-flow vascular lesion of which the venous drainage comes through or near the jugular bulb can cause PT (Table 11.8); therefore, the angiographic protocol

should not only include the internal and the external carotid arteries but also the vertebral artery. In some cases the vascular lesion can be located contralateral to the side of the PT. For example, a left-sided dural carotid–cavernous fistula can drain through the right cavernous sinus into the right inferior petrosal sinus to the jugular bulb. Both cavernous sinus plexuses exist anteriorly and posteriorly (Lasjaunias and Berenstein 1987).

11.5.1
Dural Arteriovenous Fistulas

Dural arteriovenous fistulas (DAVF) are the most common cause of objective PT in the patient with a normal otoscopic examination (Weissman and Hirsch 2000). The DAVF are abnormal shunts located in the dura. They can occur at any site in the dura, but most frequently they are located near a venous sinus. They are classified according to their

Table 11.8. Vascular malformations that can cause pulsatile tinnitus

Dural arteriovenous fistula
Carotid–cavernous fistula: direct or dural
Vertebral arteriovenous fistula
External carotid fistula
Brain arteriovenous malformations

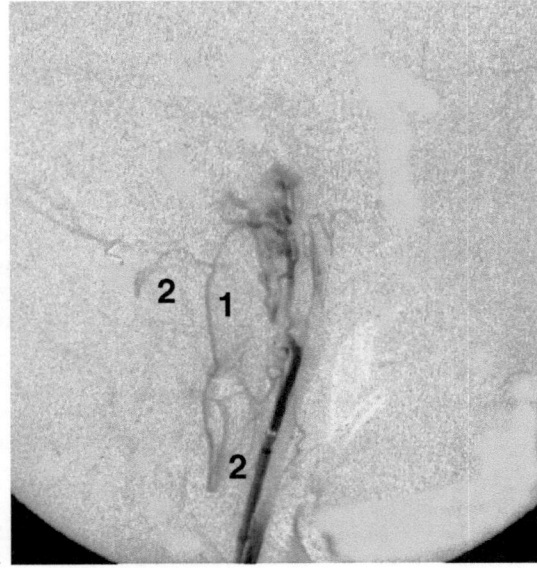
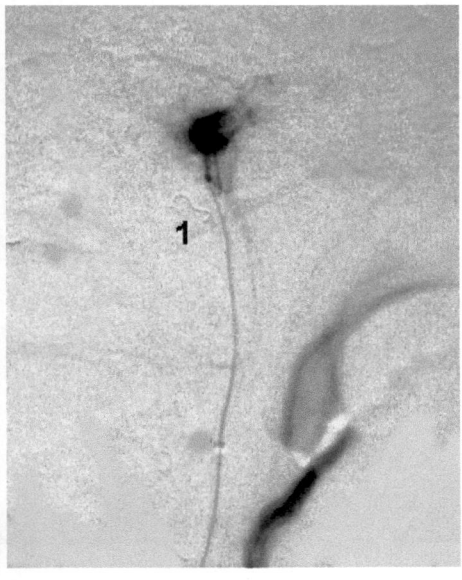

Fig. 11.8a, b. Dangerous anastomosis. **a** Selective injection of the inferior tympanic artery with the microcatheter shows the tumour blush in the middle ear. There is also a visualization of the vertebral artery (2) at the C2–C3 level via the dens arcade (1). **b** After closure of the dens arcade with a microcoil (1), the feeding artery can safely be embolized

location, or to the type of venous drainage. This last classification is important for determining the natural history, the prognosis and the indication for treatment (Table 11.9; COGNARD et al. 1995). Type-I lesions have a benign natural history and these lesions are only treated when the pulsatile tinnitus cannot be tolerated by the patient. Type-IIa lesions are less benign with intracranial hypertension occurring in 20% of the cases. In type IIb the risk for an intracranial bleeding is 10%, in type III the risk is 40% and in type IV 65%. Patients with a DAVF type V developed progressive myelopathy in 50% of the cases. The DAVF are frequently invisible on conventional CT or MR examinations, and the examination must be complemented by MR angiography and venography techniques.

Table 11.9. Classification of dural arteriovenous fistula (DAVF) according to the type of venous drainage. (From COGNARD et al. 1995)

Type I	Antegrade into the venous sinus
Type IIa	Into the venous sinus with reflux in the sinus
Type IIb	Into the venous sinus with reflux in cortical veins
Type III	Direct cortical venous drainage
Type IV	Type III with venous ectasia
Type V	Spinal venous drainage

The treatment of choice is endovascular, via the arterial or venous route (Fig. 11.9). Arterial embolization of the feeding vessels with particles (polyvinyl alcohol foam, PVA) leads to revascularization in most cases. It is beyond the scope of this chapter to go further in detail into the endovascular treatment. Surgery is an option in case of failure of the endovascular treatment. When the nidus of the DAVF is small, than stereotactic radiosurgery is an option.

11.5.2
Vertebral Arteriovenous Fistula

Vertebral arteriovenous fistulas (VAF) are less common lesions. The most frequent cause is trauma, but they may also occur spontaneously, sometimes associated with fibromuscular dysplasia and neurofibromatosis type I. The clinical manifestations can vary: spinal cord or vertebrobasilar ischemia, spinal cord compression, nerve root compression, intraspinal bleeding and pulsatile tinnitus. A bruit is present in nearly 100% of cases. The lesion consists of an abnormal arteriovenous communication between the cervical part of the vertebral artery and the internal jugular vein usually high in the neck. Secondary venous drainage can occur via the occipital veins and the intraspinal epidural venous plexus with spinal cord compression. The treatment of choice is endovascular.

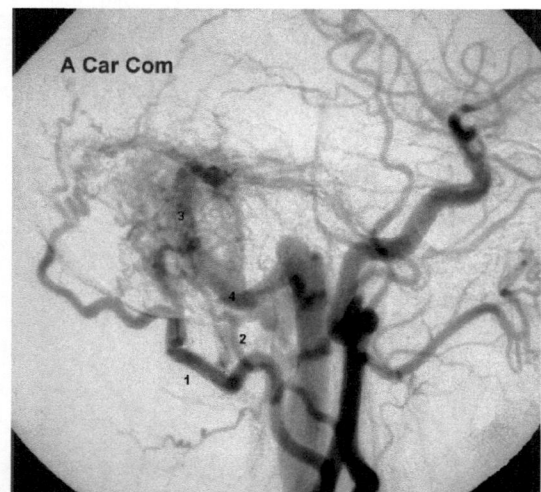
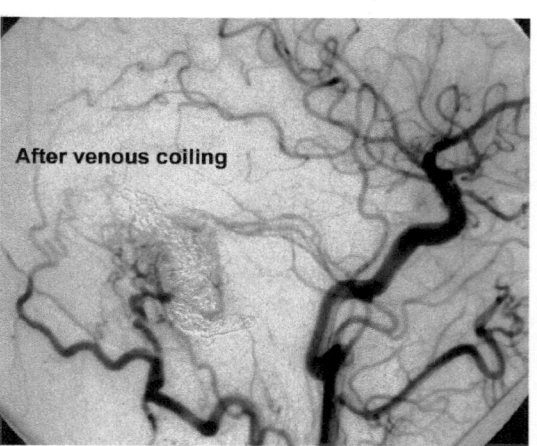

Fig. 11.9a, b. Dural arteriovenous fistula of the transverse sinus, type I. **a** Angiogram of the common carotid artery before embolization. There are multiple feeding arteries from the external (*1, 2*) and internal carotid artery. The nidus is located in the dural wall of the transverse sinus (*3*).The early venous drainage is antegrade through the homolateral transverse sinus (type I; *4*). **b** After venous embolization with coils in the "sick" part of the transverse sinus, the fistula is closed

References

American Heritage Dictionary of the English Language, 4th edn (2000) American Heritage Dictionaries, Boston

Cognard C, Gobin YP, Pierot L, Bailly AL, Houdart E, Casasco A, Chiras J, Merland JJ (1995) Cerebral dural arteriovenous fistulas: clinical and angiographic correlation with a revised classification of venous drainage. Radiology 194:671–680

Connors JJ III, Wojak JC (1999) Paragangliomas. In: Connors JJ III, Wojak JC (eds) Interventional neuroradiology, strategies and practical techniques. Saunders, Philadelphia

Fisch U, Mattox D (1988) Microsurgery of the skull base. Thieme, New York

Lasjaunias P, Berenstein A (1987) Surgical neuroangiography, 1st edn, vol 2. Endovascular treatment of craniofacial lesions. Springer, Berlin Heidelberg New York

Lasjaunias P, Berenstein A, Ter Brugge KG (2001) Surgical neuroangiography, 2nd edn, vol 1. Springer, Berlin Heidelberg New York

Lo WWM, Solti-Bohman LG (1996) Vascular tinnitus. In: Som PM, Curtin HD (eds) Head and neck imaging, 3rd edn. Mosby Year-Book, St. Louis

Moret J, Delvert JC, Bretonneau CH, Lasjaunias P, de Bicetre CH (1982) Vascularization of the ear: normal–variations–glomus tumors. J Neuroradiol 3:209–260

Sandok BA, Whisnant JP, Furlan AJ (1982) Carotid artery bruits: prevalence survey and differential diagnosis. Mayo Clin Proc 57:227–230

Sismanis A, Stamm MA, Sobel M (1994) Objective tinnitus in patients with atherosclerotic carotid artery disease. Am J Otol 15:404–407

Swartz JD, Harnsberger HR (1998) Imaging of the temporal bone. Thieme, New York

Tanghe H (1994) Congenital malformations and anatomic variations of the ear. Riv Neuroradiol 7:417–422

Waldvogel W, Mattle HP, Sturzenegger M, Schroth G (1998) Pulsatile tinnitus; a review of 84 patients. J. Neurol 245:137–142

Weissman JL, Hirsch BE (2000) Imaging of tinnitus: a review. Radiology 216:342–349

The Clinician's View

I. DHOOGE

Glomus tumors are more common than almost any other middle ear neoplasm, and second only to acoustic tumors in the temporal bone overall.

In 1941, Guild first described „glomic tissue" in the temporal bone. The correlation between this tissue and what we now call glomus tumors was not made until 1945, by Rosenwasser, who reported a „carotid body tumor" of the middle ear and mastoid. There are typically three glomus bodies in each ear. The glomus bodies are usually found accompanying Jacobsen's (CN IX) or Arnold's (CN X) nerve or in the adventitia of the jugular bulb; however, the physical location is usually the mucosa of the promontory (glomus tympanicum), or the jugular bulb (glomus jugulare). Although usually histologically benign, glomus tumors are locally destructive, spreading along paths of least resistance. Spread is multidirectional and simultaneous. Because of the location and the vascular nature of the tumors, it is not surprising that the most common complaint of symptomatic patients is pulsatile tinnitus. On physical examination, the hallmark of a jugulotympanic glomus tumor is a red or reddish-blue mass seen behind the tympanic membrane. In the 1940s and 1950s surgical approaches to the temporal bone were limited and recurrence after resection of glomus tumors was common, as were injuries to the facial nerve. Radiation therapy for glomus tumors became popular largely for these reasons. Since the 1970s, the advances in skull-base neurotologic surgery have allowed a resurgence in the surgical management of temporal bone glomus tumors.

Because the clinical characteristics and growth rates of these tumors are variable, management has been recommended from observation alone through radiation therapy and surgical management. The classification proposed by A. De La Cruz is particularly useful in planning the management of patients with glomus tumors.

Imaging studies are indispensable for three-dimensional imaging of bone invasion and delimitation of the inner ear structures and the carotid artery. Magnetic resonance imaging can more clearly delineate the tumor–brain interface and the relationship of the lesion to the intradural structures. Angiographic studies are indicated for assessment of the individual blood supply pattern and for interventional embolization of the tumor. Additionally, this technique ensures preoperative identification of additional glomus lesions, if present.

It is important to make the distinction between tumors confined to the middle ear and mastoid from tumors that involve the jugular bulb. Surgery of limited tumors is feasible without major risk. Patients with jugular bulb, carotid artery, or transdural tumors should be aware of the additional risk inherent in complete removal of their tumors. Specifically, facial nerve transposition is generally necessary and carries the attendant risk of facial paresis. Furthermore, these patients should be aware of the risk of lower cranial nerve injury and possible vascular complications as well. Modern imaging studies should therefore accurately delineate the extent of glomus tumors of the temporal bone for planning therapeutic strategies and accurate counseling of the patient.

12 Petrous Apex Lesions

M. Lemmerling

CONTENTS

12.1
The Normal Petrous Apex

The petrous apex is the most anterior and medial portion of the temporal bone, and articulates with the clivus at the petroclival junction. The petrous apex is pneumatized to a variable degree, and this degree of pneumatization or aeration correlates with the amount of pneumatized air cells in other parts of the temporal bone (Yetiser et al. 2002). Pneumatization of the petrous apex is present in 33% of all temporal bones, and of these, all parts of the apex are pneumatized in only approximately 40% of the cases (Hentona et al. 1994). The non-pneumatized portions of the temporal bone apex show a high signal on both, T1- and T2-weighted MR images (Fig. 12.1). This is due to their fatty bone marrow content. The pneumatized portions in the normal petrous apex show no signal in normal conditions.

12.2
Lesions of the Petrous Apex

Petrous apex lesions are rare, and they are often noted incidentally, unrelated to the presenting clini-

M. Lemmerling, MD, PhD
Medische Beeldvorming, A.Z. St. Lucas, Groenebriel 1,
9000 Ghent, Belgium

cal manifestation (Leonetti et al. 2001); however, in the presence of petrous apex lesions, a variety of clinical symptoms is noted, such as hearing loss, dizziness, headaches, and tinnitus (Muckle et al. 1998). Usually these lesions can be precisely defined using imaging techniques such as CT and MR. Although MR-guided biopsies through a transsphenoidal access have been attempted in the petrous apex region (Bootz et al. 2001), such procedures are usually unnecessary if an experienced radiologist studies the lesion. Magnetic resonance specifically plays an important role in the differentiation of petrous apex lesions, which can often be easily detected with CT, but where CT does not always permit correct differentiation of the imaging finding (Pisanischi and Langer 2000). The importance of MR in this matter has been emphasized since the late 1980s and early 1990s (Griffin et al. 1987; Greenberg et al. 1988; Jackler and Parker 1992; Arriaga and Brackmann 1991). The study of the spontaneous signal intensities of these lesions on T1- and T2-weighted images, and of the enhancement pattern of the internal matrix of the lesions, often allows to provide a correct diagnosis with a very high degree of confidence (Curtin and Som 1995). Consequently, the radiologist plays an important role in the process of decision making with regard to whether the area in question needs surgical therapy, and influences the process of deciding on the exact type of surgery that should be performed (Chang et al. 1998; Profant and Steno 2000; Brackmann and Toh 2002). Magnetic resonance scanning is helpful in evaluating complete removal, complication, recurrence, or formation of complicating granulation tissue (Pisanischi and Langer 2000).

12.2.1
"Don't Touch" Lesions

On the basis of MR, two "don't touch" entities in the petrous apex can be confused with pathologic lesions that need surgery: asymmetric presence of fatty marrow and trapped fluid in petrous air cells

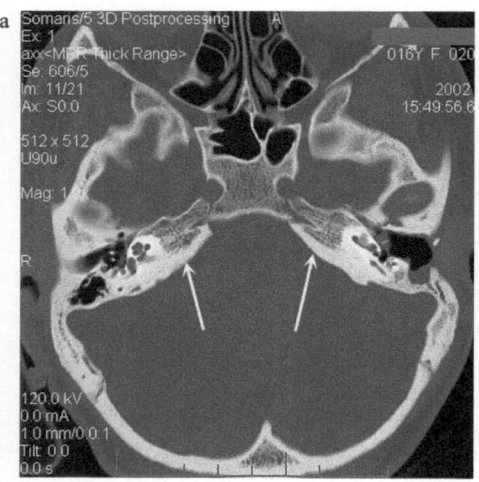

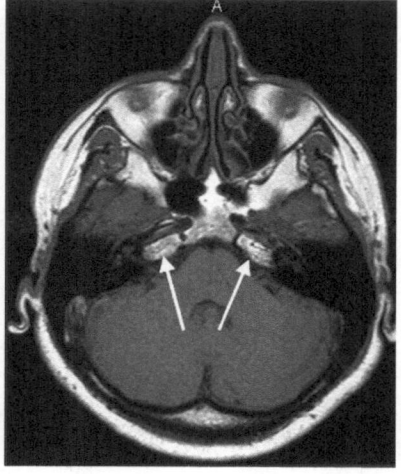

Fig. 12.1a, b. The normal petrous apex as it is seen in most patients. On CT image (**a**) the bone marrow in the petrous apex is seen bilaterally (*arrows*). On axial T1-weighted MR image (**b**) a hyperintense signal is noted bilaterally, lateral to the hyperintense clivus, indicating the presence of fatty bone marrow in the non-pneumatized apex (*arrows*)

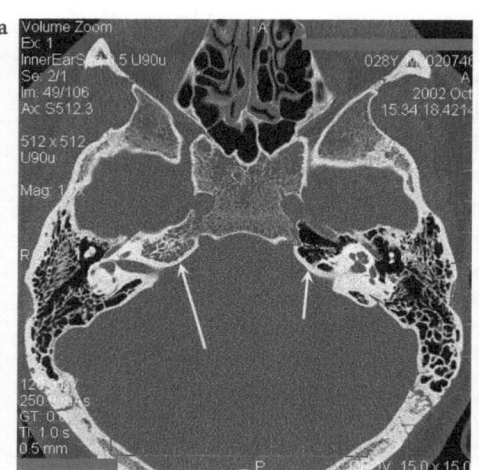

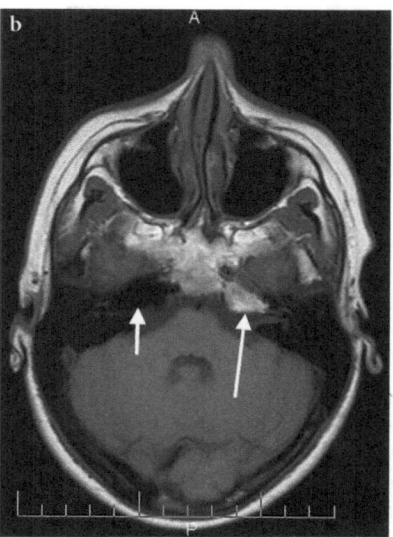

Fig. 12.2. Asymmetrical pneumatization of the petrous apex on CT (**a**), with pneumatization on the left side (*small arrow*) and non-pneumatization on the right side (*large arrow*). Note that on T1-weighted MR image (**b**) a high signal is seen in the apex on the left side (*large arrow*), which should not be mistaken for tumor. The signal is identical to that of fat in other locations (e.g., clivus, mandibular head, pterygopalatine fossa): normal fatty bone marrow in the non-pneumatized apex. The right petrous apex is pneumatized and shows no signal (*small arrow*)

(PALACIOS 2001). Although both have specific imaging characteristics, radiologists do not always confidently define these two non-surgical petrous apex lesions (MOORE et al. 1998).

12.2.1.1
Asymmetric Presence of Fatty Marrow

In case of asymmetric presence of fatty marrow the radiologist should notice that the area with high signal in the petrous apex region has the same signal intensity as fat on all sequences (ROLAND et al. 1990; MOORE et al. 1998) (Fig. 12.2). If there is still any doubt, CT of the region can be performed and will show a less pneumatized petrous apex on the side that was considered suspicious on the MR examination. Fat-suppressed MR techniques can also give the solution.

12.2.1.2
Fluid-filled Petrous Apex Air Cells

The petrous apex is aerated to a variable degree. It is believed that the degree of aeration as such is not responsible for the eventual presence of clinical symptoms (YETISER et al. 2002). In some cases pneumatized petrous apex cells can be fluid filled. Such cells have an intermediate or high signal on the T1-weighted images and a high signal on the T2-weighted images. Trapped fluid is mostly confused with cholesterol granuloma, but the latter does not enhance except for a thin rim, whereas trapped fluid often enhances moderately. The presence of trapped fluid in other mastoid cells often accompanies the fluid trapping in the apex (Fig. 12.3). Computed tomography is also able to assure the radiologist

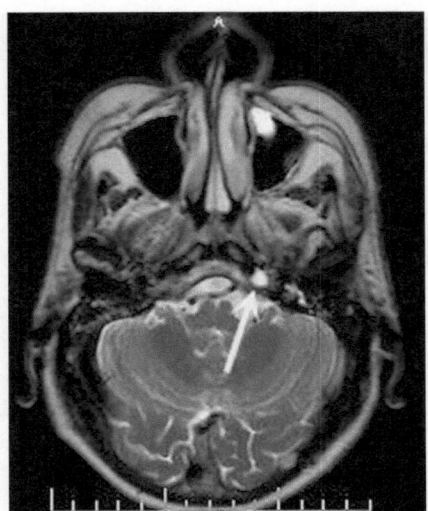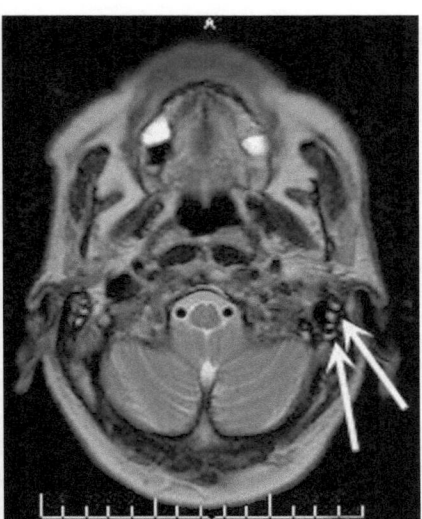

Fig. 12.3. Fluid trapping in pneumatized petrous apex cells shows a high signal on T2-weighted image (*arrow*, **a**) and is often accompanied by other mastoid cells (*arrows*) that also contain trapped fluid (**b**)

that the petrous apex is opacified in a non-expansile way in case of fluid trapping.

12.2.2
True Petrous Apex Lesions

Petrous apex lesions have been classified in different ways by different authors. Whereas some divide the lesions into cystic and solid lesions, others distinguish destructive and non-destructive lesions. The two most frequent lesions in the petrous apex that need surgery are the cholesterol granuloma and cholesteatoma (CHANG et al. 1998). Both are cystic and destructive/expansile lesions and account for, respectively, 60 and 9% of all petrous apex lesions (MUCKLE et al. 1998). The differentiation between both lesions is very important because of their completely different therapeutic management. Cholesterol granuloma can be drained internally into the mastoid or middle ear, whereas cholesteatoma needs a more aggressive removal, which often mandates the sacrifice of hearing (CHANG et al. 1998; PROFANT and STENO 2000; BRACKMANN and TOH 2002). The experience of the surgeon is another important factor in the choice of the surgical approach (HABERKAMP 1997).

12.2.2.1
Cholesterol Granuloma or Cyst

Cholesterol granuloma, also called cholesterol cyst or giant cholesterol cyst, is the most common primary lesion of the petrous apex, and accounts for 60% of all lesions in that region (MUCKLE et al. 1998). They

rarely occur bilaterally (JARAMILLO and WINLE-TAYLOR 2001). Cholesterol cysts contain a brownish liquid glistening with cholesterol crystals (LO et al. 1984; GRAHAM et al. 1985). Repetitive cycles of hemorrhage and granulomatous reaction – the reason why such cysts are also referred to as granulomas – initiated by an obstruction of the ventilation outlet of the apex are believed to cause cholesterol cysts (NAGER and VANDERVEEN 1976).

Cholesterol cysts are most often seen in young adults and are treated surgically, by drainage of the petrous apex. The petrous apex can be achieved through different approaches, such as the transcanal infracochlear, transmastoid infralabyrinthine, middle fossa, translabyrinthine, and transotic approaches. Determination of the best approach depends on the hearing status of the affected ear, on one hand, and the relationship between the petrous apex lesion and the surrounding neurovascular structures, on the other hand. The translabyrinthine approach is useful in non-hearing ears, whereas the transcanal infracochlear approach with stenting is preferred in hearing individuals, if anatomy permits (BRACKMANN and TOH 2002).

On MR cholesterol cysts are hyperintense on both T1- and T2 weighted images (Fig. 12.4; MAFEE et al. 1994). Some have a hypointense rim on both T1- and T2-weighting (GREENBERG et al. 1988). The contralateral apex is often pneumatized.

12.2.2.2
Primary Cholesteatoma or Epidermoid Cyst

Primary cholesteatoma of the petrous apex is also referred to as epidermoid cyst. The term 'cyst' is

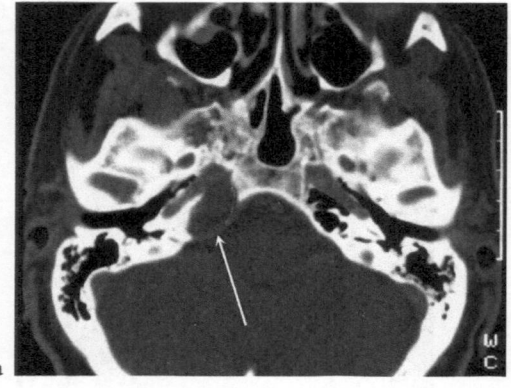
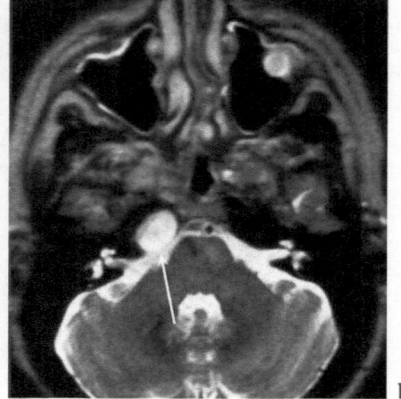
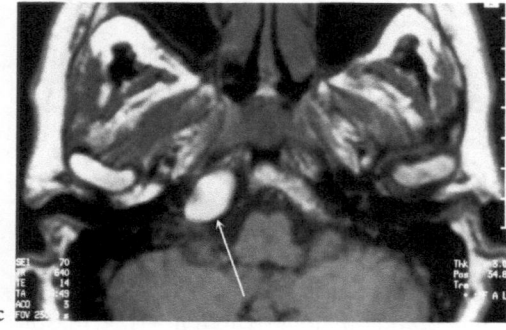

Fig. 12.4a–c. Cholesterol cyst or cholesterol granuloma (*arrow*)? Computed tomography (**a**) shows a round cystic lesion in the petrous apex on the right side. The finding is, however, non-specific. On MR the well-defined mass is hyperintense on both the T2 (**b**)- and T1 (**c**)- weighted images. Note that the contralateral apex is partially pneumatized

confusing since they contain desquamated keratin, which is a solid material. As already mentioned epidermoid cysts are much rarer than the cholesterol cyst (MUCKLE et al. 1998).

Petrous apex cholesteatoma require surgical management and the removal is again done through different approaches, according to different parameters, such as the size of the cholesteatoma, the degree of hearing loss, and the remaining facial nerve function (PROFANT and STENO 2000).

On MR epidermoid cysts are hyperintense on T2-weighted images and hypointense on T1-weighted images (MAFEE et al. 1994). After injection of gadolinium, epidermoid cysts do not enhance or only their capsule enhances (Fig. 12.5).

12.2.2.3
Other Petrous Apex Lesions

Petrous apicitis was a frequent occurrence in the past but has become rare with the appropriate use of antibiotics in the treatment of middle ear disease. Inflammatory/infectious disease of the petrous apex is especially seen in the well-pneumatized apex and is treated by means of surgical drainage. The petrous apex is heterogeneously hyperintense on T2-weighted images, shows a heterogeneous and mixed

signal on T1-weighted images, and enhances heterogeneously after intravenous injection of gadolinium (Fig. 12.6). This enhancement pattern allows differentiation from cholesterol granuloma, which is a non-enhancing lesion. This inflammatory/infectious condition can become aggressive, leading to bone erosion and asymmetric clouding of the petrous tip. This latter condition is best studied with CT (CHOLE and DONALD 1983). In rare cases petrous apicitis can become extremely aggressive and develop to nasopharyngeal abscess formation or cause facial nerve paralysis (FITZGERALD 2001). Extension into the neck has been reported in a child (SOMERS et al. 2001).

Primary mucoceles of the petrous apex are rare, and their MR appearance varies depending on the degree of hydration or inspissation of the contents. They are best treated by an infralabyrinthine approach (LARSON and WONG 1992). Their signal on T1-weighted images increases with the increasing protein concentration. In some cases it can be difficult to distinguish them from primary cholesteatoma.

Petrous apex arachnoid cysts are uncommon. They are rarely symptomatic and are amenable to simple surgical drainage (CHANG et al. 1998). Petrous apex cephaloceles are other uncommon lesions that are usually

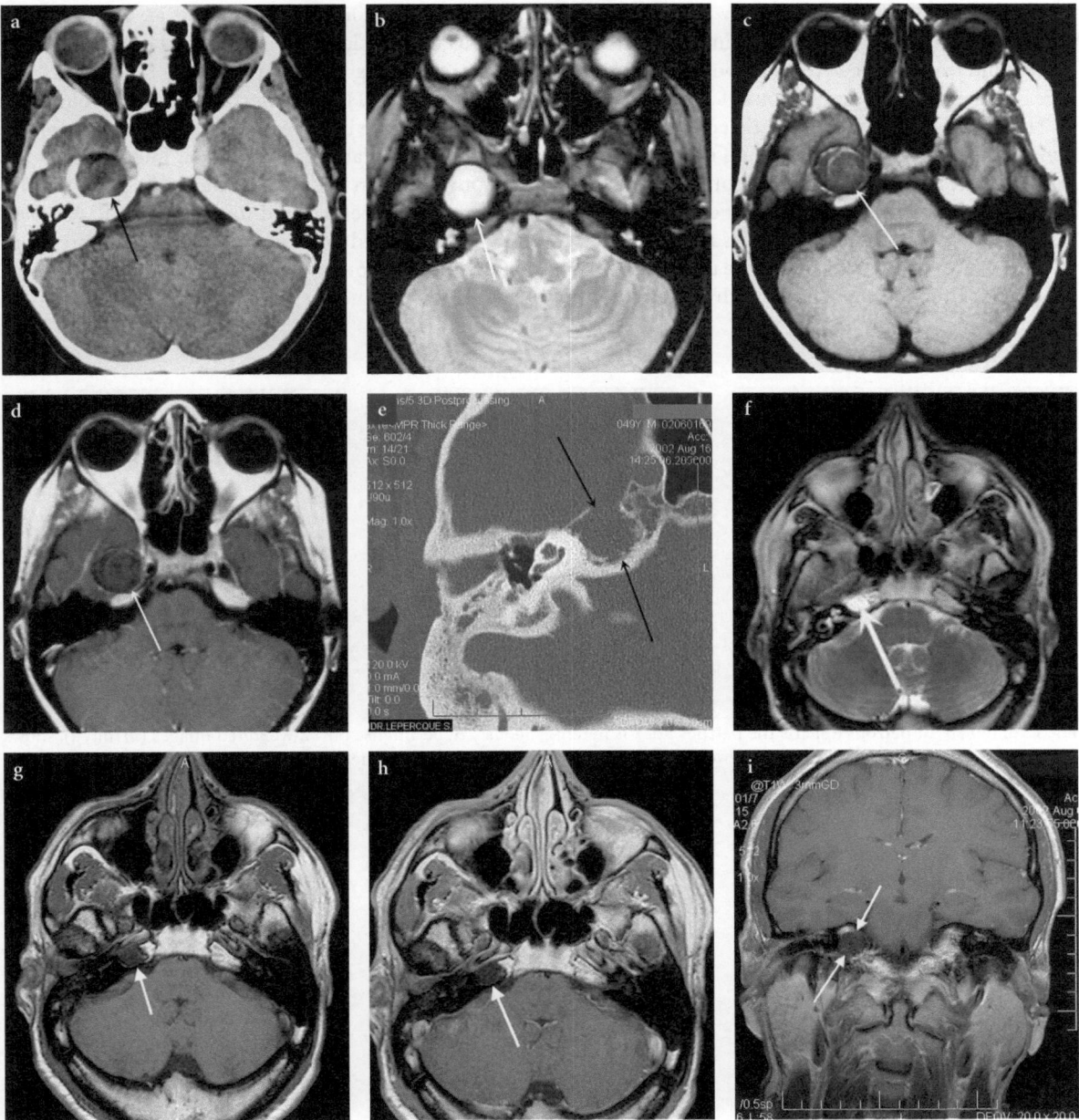

Fig. 12.5a–i. Epidermoid cyst or congenital cholesteatoma. Computed tomography (**a**) shows an ovoid and destructive mass in the petrous apex on the right side (*arrow*) in a child. The CT is unable to differentiate. On MR typical signs of an epidermoid cyst are noted: hyperintense signal on T2-weighted image (*arrow*, **b**), hypointense signal on T1-weighted image (*arrow*, **c**), and only capsular enhancement after intravenous injection of gadolinium (*arrow*, **d**). Computed tomography is also shown in a 49-year-old patient with a destructive lesion in the right petrous apex (*arrows*, **e**). Again, CT is aspecific, but MR proves that the lesion is an epidermoid: the mass is hyperintense on T2-weighted image (*arrow*, **f**), hypointense on T1-weighting (*arrow*, **g**), and shows no enhancement at all on axial (*arrow*, **h**) and coronal (*arrows*, **i**) T1-weighted images after intravenous injection of gadolinium

incidental, but they can occasionally be symptomatic. They represent a protrusion of meninges and cerebrospinal fluid from the posterolateral portion of Meckel's cave into the petrous apex (MOORE et al. 2001).

The petrous apex can be directly invaded by benign or malignant lesions arising from the meninges (Fig. 12.7), nasopharynx, temporal bone, or even parotid region (Fig. 12.8). Primary neoplasms arising from the bony or cartilaginous tissues of the petroclival junction are also found in the apex region, and are discussed in another chapter (chap. 5).

Osseous sarcoidosis presenting as a destructive petrous bone lesion (NG and NIPARKO 2002), as well as petrous apex blastomycosis (BLACKLEDGE and NEWLANDS 2001), are other very rare petrous apex lesions that have been reported.

The interpretation of the signal intensities of the petrous apex can become confusing in patients who have recently been treated for hematologic diseases. The activated red bone marrow causes a decrease in signal intensity on both T1- and T2-weighted images (Fig. 12.9).

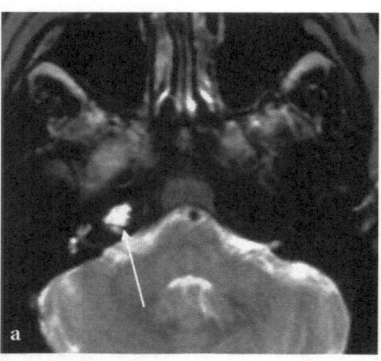 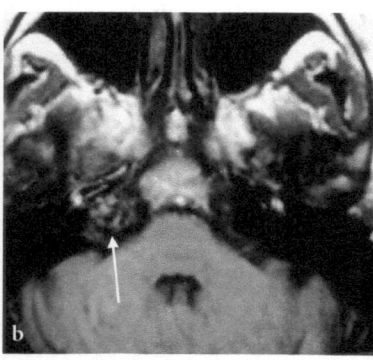 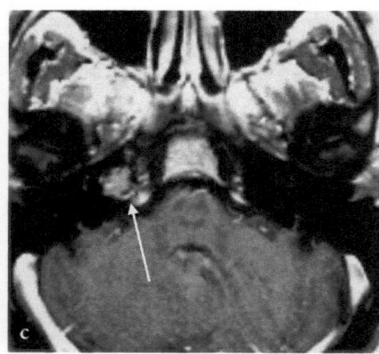

Fig. 12.6. In case of petrous apicitis the petrous apex is heterogeneously hyperintense on T2-weighted images (*arrow*, **a**), shows a heterogeneous and mixed signal on T1-weighted images (*arrow*, **b**), and enhances heterogeneously after intravenous injection of gadolinium (*arrow*, **c**)

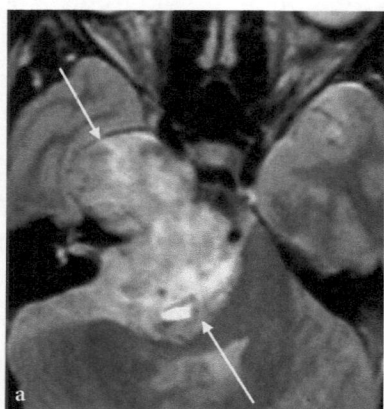 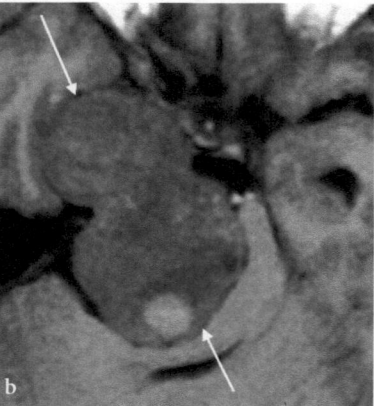 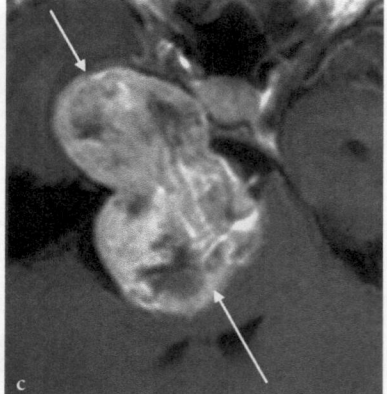

Fig. 12.7a, b. Meningioma. A dumbbell-shaped tumor with heterogeneous high signal intensity on T2-weighted image is growing around the petrous apex (*arrows*, **a**). The mass shows a heterogeneous low signal on T1-weighted image (*arrows*, **b**) and enhances strongly and heterogeneously after intravenous injection of gadolinium (*arrows*, **c**)

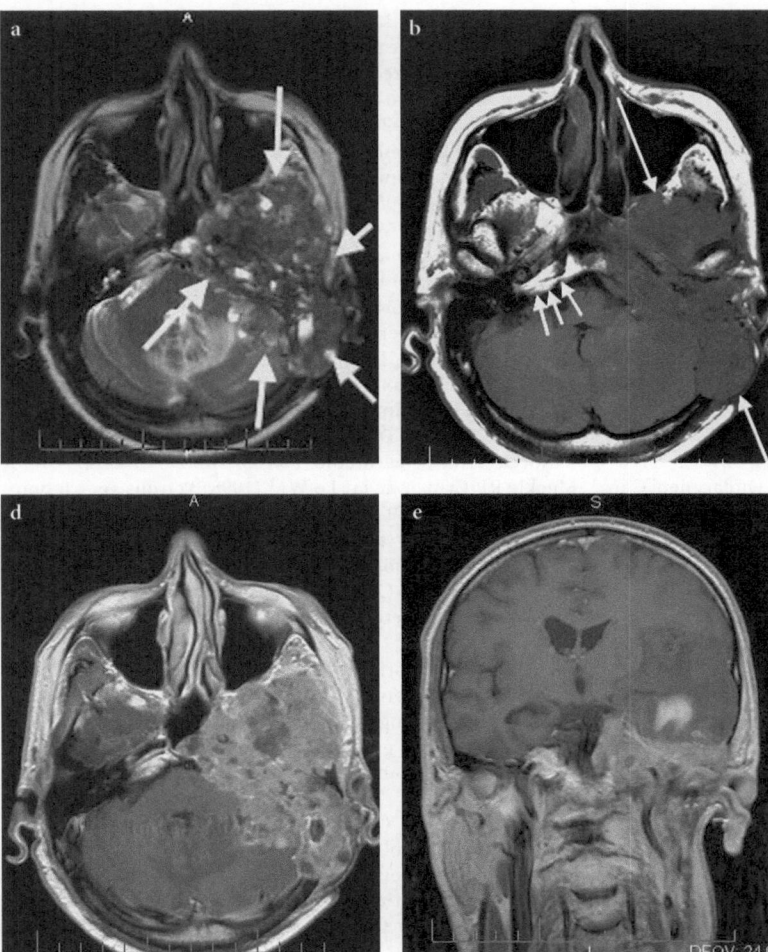

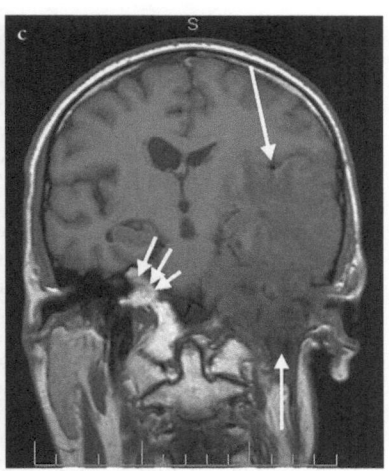

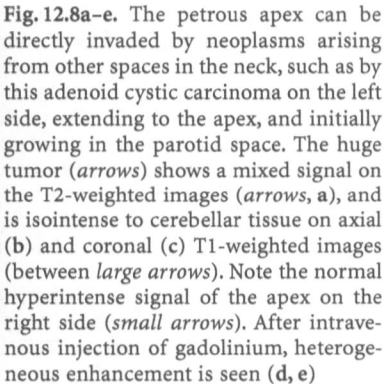

Fig. 12.8a–e. The petrous apex can be directly invaded by neoplasms arising from other spaces in the neck, such as by this adenoid cystic carcinoma on the left side, extending to the apex, and initially growing in the parotid space. The huge tumor (*arrows*) shows a mixed signal on the T2-weighted images (*arrows*, **a**), and is isointense to cerebellar tissue on axial (**b**) and coronal (**c**) T1-weighted images (between *large arrows*). Note the normal hyperintense signal of the apex on the right side (*small arrows*). After intravenous injection of gadolinium, heterogeneous enhancement is seen (**d, e**)

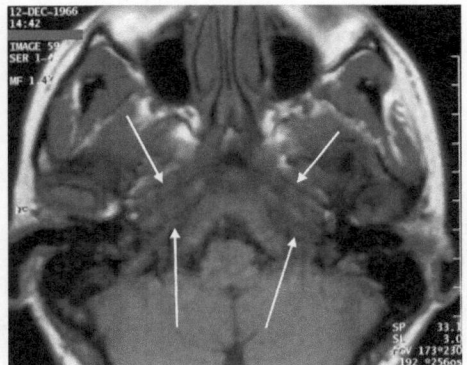

Fig. 12.9. The hyperintense signal intensity on T1-weighted image that is normally seen in the non-pneumatized petrous apex, and that is caused by its fatty bone marrow content, is not present in this hematology patient. The normal soft tissue fat planes, such as those in the cheek and in the pterygopalatine fossa, still show their high signal. Note, however, that the high signal that is normally present in the bony structures in the clivus and the mandibular heads has also disappeared: the red bone marrow is activated due to therapy and has replaced the normal fatty bone marrow. *Arrows* point to the whole gray midline structure that is bilaterally present

References

Arriaga MA, Brackmann DE (1991) Differential diagnosis of primary petrous apex lesions. Am J Otol 12:470–474; 13: 297

Blackledge FA, Newlands SD (2001) Blastomyocosis of the petrous apex. Am J Neuroradiol 9:1205–1214

Bootz F, Keiner S, Schulz T, Scheffler B, Seifert V (2001) Magnetic resonance imaging-guided biopsies of the petrous apex and petroclival region. Otol Neurotol 22:383–388

Brackmann DE, Toh EH (2002) Surgical management of petrous apex cholesterol granulomas. Otol Neurotol 23: 529–533

Chang P., Fagan PA, Atlas MD, Roche J (1998) Imaging destructive lesions of the petrous apex. Laryngoscope 108: 599–604

Chole RA, Donald PJ (1983) Petrous apicitis. Clinical considerations. Ann Otol Rhinol Laryngol 92:544–551

Curtin HD, Som PM (1995) The petrous apex. Otolaryngol Clin North Am 28:473–496

Fitzgerald DC (2001) Nasopharyngeal abscess and facial paralysis as complications of petrous apicitis: a case report. Ear Nose Throat J 80:305–312

Graham MD, Kemink JL, Latack JT, Kartush JM (1985) The giant cholesterol cyst of the petrous apex: a distinct clinical entity. Laryngoscope 95:1401–1406

Greenberg JJ, Oot RF, Wismer GL, Davis KR, Goodman ML, Weber AE, Montgomery WW (1988) Cholesterol granuloma of the petrous apex: MR and CT evaluation. Am J Neuroradiol 9:1205–1214

Griffin C, DeLaPaz R, Enzmann D (1987) MR and CT correlation of cholesterol cysts of the petrous bone. Am J Neuroradiol 8:825–829

Haberkamp TJ (1997) Surgical anatomy of the transtemporal approaches to the petrous apex. Am J Otol 18:501–506

Hentona H, Ohkudbo J, Tsutsumi T, Tanaka H, Komatsuzaki A (1994) Pneumatization of the petrous apex. Nippon Jibiinkoka Gakkai Kaiho 97:450–456

Jackler RK, Parker DA (1992) Radiographic differential diagnosis of petrous apex lesions. Am J Otol 13:561–574

Jaramillo M, Windle-Taylor PC (2001) Large cholesterol granuloma of the petrous apex treated via subcochlear drainage. J Laryngol Otol 115:1005–1009

Larson TL, Wong ML (1992) Primary mucocele of the petrous apex: MR appereance. Am J Neuroradiol 13:203–204

Leonetti JP, Shownkeen H, Marzo SJ (2001) Incidental petrous apex findings on magnetic resonance imaging. Ear Nose Throat J 80:200–202, 205–206

Lo WWM, Solti-Bohman LG, Brackmann DE, Gruskin P (1984) Cholesterol granuloma of the petrous apex: CT diagnosis. Radiology 153:705–711

Mafee MF, Kumar A, Heffner DK (1994) Epidermoid cyst (cholesteatoma) and cholesterol granuloma of the temporal bone and epidermoid cysts affecting the brain. Neuroimaging Clin North Am 4:561–578

Moore KR, Harnsberger HR, Shelton C, Davidson HC (1998) 'Leave me alone' lesions of the petrous apex. Am J Neuroradiol 19:733–738

Moore KR, Fischbein JN, Harnsberger HR, Shelton C, Glastonbury CM, White DK, Dillon WP (2001) Petrous apex cephaloceles. Am J Neuroradiol 22:1867–1871

Muckle RP, Cruz A de la , Lo WM (1998) Petrous apex lesions. Am J Otol 19:219–225

Nager CT, Vanderveen TS (1976) Cholesterol granuloma involving the temporal bone. Laryngoscope 85:204–209

Ng M, Niparko JK (2002) Osseous sarcoidosis presenting as a destructive petrous apex lesion. Am J Otolaryngol 23: 241–245

Palacios E, Valvassori G, D'Antonio M (2001) 'Don't touch me' lesions of the petrous apex. Ear Nose Throat J 80:140

Pisaneschi MJ, Langer B (2000) Congenital cholesteatoma and cholesterol granuloma of the temporal bone: role of magnetic resonance imaging. Top Magn Reson Imaging 11:87–97

Profant M, Steno J (2000) Petrous apex cholesteatoma. Acta Otorhinolaryngol 120:164–167

Roland PS, Meyerhoff WL, Judge LO, Mickey BE (1990) Asymmetric pneumatization of the petrous apex. Otolaryngol Head Neck Surg 103:80–88

Somers TJ, De Foer B, Govaerts P, Pouillon M, Offeciers E (2001) Chronic petrous apicitis with pericarotid extension into the neck in a child. Ann Otol Rhinol Laryngol 110: 988–991

Yetiser S, Kertmen M, Taser M (2002) Abnormal petrous apex aeration. Review of 12 cases. Acta Otorhinolaryngol Belg 56:65–71

The Clinician's View

I. DHOOGE

The petrous apex lies between the inner ear and the clivus. It can be the site of very different lesions: cholesteatomas; granulomas; infection; cysts; neuromas; and chondromas. Patients with petrous apex lesions present with various symptoms and physical findings. Cranial nerve deficits often occur early in the course of disease. The sphenoid and ethmoid sinuses can become involved with growth anteriorly, eventually leading to a nasopharyngeal mass and eustachian tube dysfunction. Lateral growth causes hearing loss, vertigo, and facial paralysis secondary to inner ear and IAC involvement.

In most cases, surgical excision is the mainstay of therapy. Unfortunately, lesions at the petrous apex have traditionally been areas of difficult exposure. Advances in radiologic imaging during the past decade have made it possible to differentiate reliably among benign cystic lesions, normal anatomic variants, and neoplastic lesions of the petrous apex. In the differential diagnosis, it is important to characterize the substance of the lesion, to distinguish between mucus, fat, cholesterol granuloma, and cholesteatoma. It is also important to characterize the border of the lesion as expansile or invasive, which may differentiate between benign lesions and malignant neoplasms. When surgery is considered it is important for the surgeon to have information concerning the size of the lesion and its relationship to vital structures, including the internal auditory canal, cochlea, vestibular labyrinth, carotid artery, and jugular bulb. The use of either conventional angiography or magnetic resonance angiography can be helpful in defining the relationship with surrounding vascular structures, and in ascertaining collateral flow.

Solid tumors and cholesteatoma may require destructive procedures, with cranial nerve and major vessel sacrifice for complete removal. Cystic lesions may be approached conservatively. Complete tumor removal is difficult and often impossible due to the proximity of vital structures and difficult access; however, it offers the best long-term survival with the lowest recurrence rate.

13 Imaging of Facial Nerve Pathology

N. Martin-Duverneuil, A. Behin, J. Chiras

CONTENTS

Introduction

Facial nerve involvement represents a relatively rare occurrence in which the anatomical complexity of the facial nerve anatomy appears closely intricate with a large etiological diversity. Contrary to the frequency of Bell's palsy, the most common inflammatory disease involving the facial nerve, tumoral pathology accounts for only 5% of peripheral facial palsies. Misleading clinical presentation is not uncommon, facial palsy being variously associated with other sometimes predominant clinical findings and an often long delayed diagnosis resulting in a compromised facial nerve function (May and Schaitkin 2000; Zimmerman et al. 2000).

Neuroimaging of the facial nerve thus appears as the best current method to study accurately the entire course of the facial nerve from its origin in the nuclei of the brain stem to its parotid ends, through its cisternal, canalicular, and petrous canals (Martin et al. 1992a). The most important goal of such a study is the detection of often small lesions, requiring the most adequate association of high-resolution thin-section CT and MR, allowing diagnostic suspicion and a precise assessment of tumoral extension in a preoperative grafting evaluation.

N. Martin-Duverneuil, MD; A. Behin, MD; J. Chiras, MD
Department of Neuroradiology Charcot, GH Pitié-La Salpêtrière, 47, Bd de l'Hôpital, 75013 Paris, France

13.2 Tumoral Pathology

Benign schwannomas are the most common tumors involving the facial nerve (Mafee et al. 1988; Martin et al. 1992b). They may occur in any portion of the nerve, with a predilection for the geniculate ganglion and the mastoid segment: the involvement of intracranial and parotid segments is rarer, just as the involvement of facial nerve branches, such as the petrous nerve, the nerve of the stapedius muscle, or the chorda tympani (Figs. 13.1–13.3; Martin et al. 1992b; Lidov et al. 1991; Sterkers and Corlieur 1986; Sullivan et al. 1987).

Magnetic resonance imaging accurately depicts schwannomas as well-delineated, nodular, often small expansive masses restricted to a portion of the nerve and variously extending along its course. They most often appear as T1 isointense and T2 iso- or hyperintense lesions with a strong homogeneous enhancement after gadolinium administration. Assessment of the tumor extension along the facial nerve is best obtained with MRI, allowing essential preoperative evaluation of the surgical grafting procedure after tumor removal (Figs. 13.1, 13.2; Martin et al. 1992b; Inoue et al. 1987; Lidov et al. 1991).

Their CT appearance (Inoue et al. 1987; Iwanaga et al. 1984; Kienzle et al. 1986; Lidov et al. 1991; Mafee et al. 1988; Millen et al. 1990) is an evocative, sharp, well-delineated enlargement of the facial canal. A large extension involving the tympanic segment may cause conductive hearing loss by interfering with ossicular function. On the other hand, facial schwannomas closely located in the internal auditory canal (IAC) more likely cause sensorineural hearing loss than facial paralysis, and may display a regular enlargement of the porus of the IAC with an enhancing soft tissue mass variously extending to the pontocerebellar angle similar to the much more frequent acoustic schwannomas (Fig. 13.1). An evocative focal antero-superior erosion of the porus or a limited enlargement of the initial portion of the labyrinthine segment will thus be accurately requested. Lastly, an

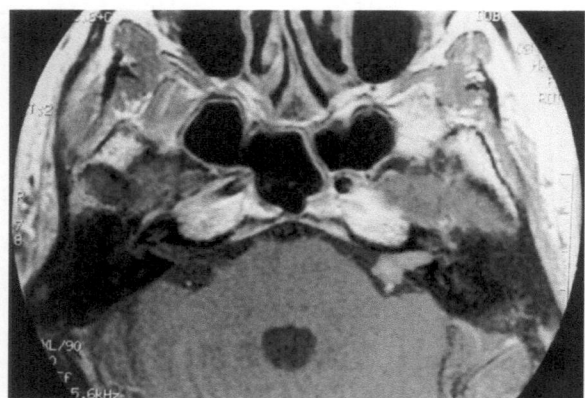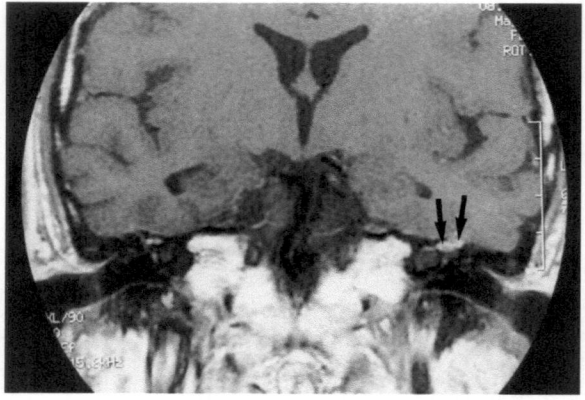

a   b

Fig. 13.1a, b. Facial nerve schwannoma. Contrast-enhanced axial (**a**) and coronal (**b**) T1-weighted MR images. Homogeneously enhancing mass of the cerebello-pontine and canalicular portions of the facial nerve (**a**). The coronal image demonstrates the nodular enlargement and enhancement of the adjacent labyrinthine and tympanic portions of the geniculate ganglion (*arrows*, **b**)

extension to the parotid segment with enlargement of the stylomastoid foramen can be in close contact with the adjacent jugular foramen. The permeability of the homo- and contralateral jugular veins must be precisely evaluated preoperatively.

Owing to the frequently small size of such lesions, congenital anatomical variations, such as frequent dehiscences of the facial canal, must be kept in mind as they may easily simulate small localized facial schwannomas or, on the contrary, display in early tumoral processes a misleading normal CT without any significant enlargement of the facial canal (IWANAGA et al. 1984; LATACK et al. 1983).

Large schwannomas can also develop along the whole course of the facial nerve or appear as a large heterogeneously enhancing mass which protrudes into the overlying intracranial temporal fossa as in their most frequent location in the geniculate ganglion (Fig. 13.2; KIENZLE et al. 1986).

Calcifications are extremely uncommon; their detection should lead to the diagnosis of other rarer lesions such as hemangiomas or meningiomas (Fig. 13.3). Computed tomography remains essential to preoperatively evaluate the petrous bone pneumatization even in cases of characteristic MR appearance of facial schwannomas.

Association with other expansive lesions, such as acoustic schwannomas or meningiomas, must orientate to the more complex neurofibromatosis type 2.

Other rarer benign tumors can involve the facial nerve or the adjacent facial canal with a resulting similar clinical presentation. Most of these tumors, as observed with facial schwannomas, are small sized and can thus be easily overlooked on routine head imaging. Careful attention should be drawn to

technique, with no more than 3-mm-thick routine T1 slices before and after gadolinium administration. Whenever any doubt persists, complementary coronal and/or sagittal slices should be performed. Contrast-enhanced 3DFT MRI of the intrapetrous facial nerve has also been proposed, allowing millimetric or infra-millimetric T1 thick slices that confer the ability to examine the facial nerve, a posteriori, in any desired plane, from a single acquisition (GIRARD et al. 1994).

Ossifying hemangiomas are the second most frequent benign tumors involving the facial canal (CURTIN et al. 1987; LO et al. 1989a; MARTIN et al. 1992c). These benign though rare extraneural lesions are histopathologically classified as capillary, cavernous, venous, arteriovenous, or mixed forms, cavernous patterns being the most frequently observed. These usually small-sized lesions (<1 cm) predominate in the fundus of the IAC, the labyrinthine segment, and the geniculate ganglion area, probably due the complex temporal embryogenesis and the important anastomotic network surrounding the Scarpa ganglion and the geniculate ganglion area.

Initially developed extraneurally, these lesions primarily exert an extrinsic compression of the facial nerve before invading it, thus requiring an accurate technique to obtain an early detection of this small-size lesion allowing surgical removal before neural invasion.

The CT appearance of hemangiomas (CURTIN et al. 1987; LO et al. 1986, 1989b) is that of an expansive mass involving the fundus of the IAC or the geniculate ganglion with unsharp margins. Intratumoral bone spicules or "honeycomb" bone are more characteristic but inconstant. The vascular component

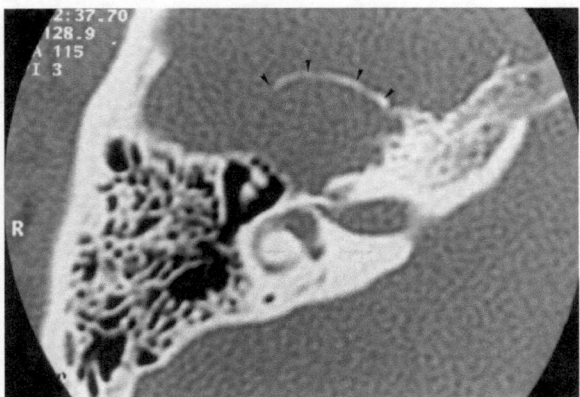

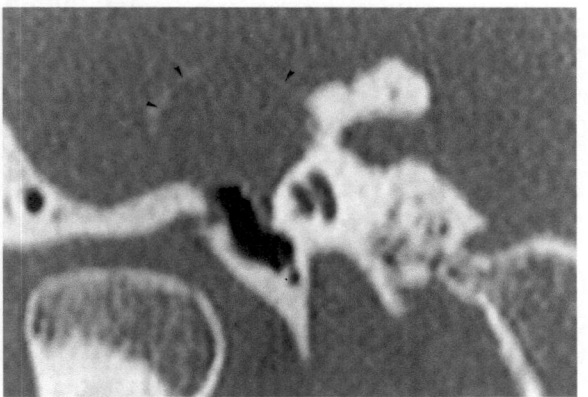

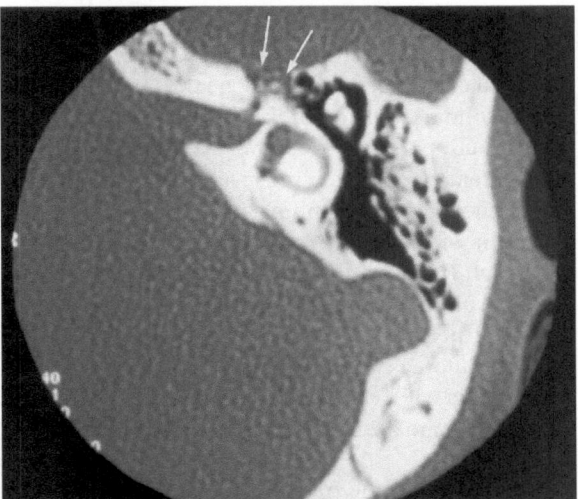

Fig. 13.2a–c. Facial nerve schwannoma. Axial (**a**) and coronal (**b**) CT scans. Contrast-enhanced axial T1-weighted MR image (**c**). Marked expansion of the geniculate area extending into the temporal fossa. Note the well-delineated linear osseous margins circumscribing the mass (*arrows*, **a, b**). The homogeneous enhancing mass of the geniculate ganglion (*arrowheads*) extends to involve the distal intracanalicular segment of the facial nerve (*arrow*)

explains the strong enhancement observed after contrast administration, better detected on MR which precisely assesses the extension along the facial nerve in an accurate preoperative evaluation (MARTIN et al. 1992c; LO et al. 1989b). Contrary to facial schwannomas, and even if hemangiomas can be well-delineated tumors, tumoral enhancing boundaries are often irregular.

Such patterns are difficult to differentiate from the much rarer intratemporal meningiomas (LARSON et al. 1995). Predominantly occurring in the geniculate ganglion area, probably arising from arachnoid lining cells issued from the overlying dura, they display a similar appearance, with unsharp enlarged bone margins, inconstant calcifications, and strong enhancement after contrast administration; both clinically cause facial palsy, sometimes progressive or frequently recurrent when small.

Intratemporal differential diagnosis must also include epidermoid cysts (Fig. 13.4; GAO et al. 1992; TAMPIERI et al. 1989). These usually slowly growing lesions also predominate as well-delineated erosive lesions in the geniculate ganglion area. They develop along the peri-labyrinthine cells with a T1 hypo- and T2 hyperintense cystic appearance. Contrary to the

Fig. 13.3. Facial nerve schwannoma. This axial CT scan shows a slight expansion of the tympanic segment of the geniculate ganglion (*arrows*). Note the unusual appearance of fine bone formation suggesting the hypothesis of ossifying hemangioma

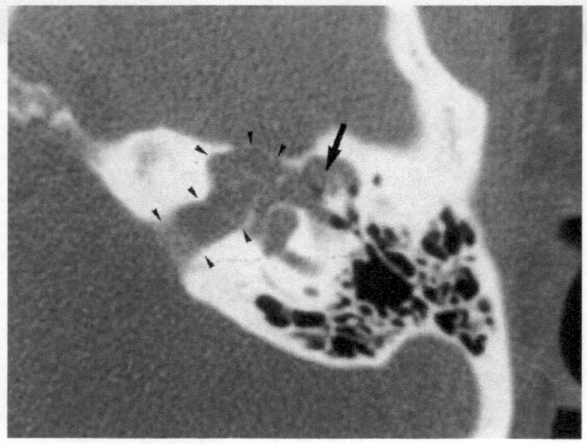

Fig. 13.4. Epidermoid cyst. Axial CT scan showing a marked soft enlargement of the intracanicular segment extending to the labyrinthine segment and the geniculate ganglion area (*arrowheads*). A soft tissue mass is seen filling the attical cavity (*arrow*)

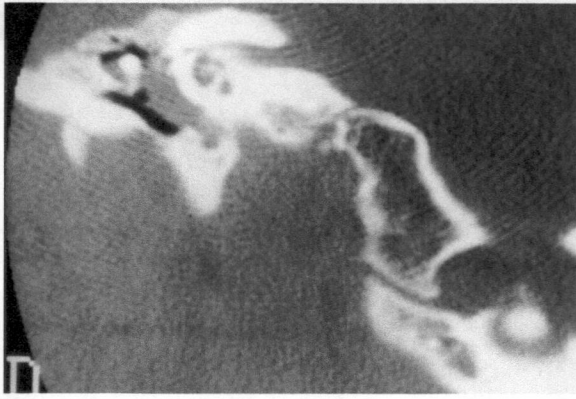

Fig. 13.5. Chemodectoma. Coronal CT scan showing the well-delineated small lesion developed in the tympanic cavity. The initial normal-sized tympanic segment of the facial canal is seen at the upper part of the lesion

other intratemporal masses, no enhancement is seen after contrast administration.

In tympanic locations, chemodectomas (Fig. 13.5) can also appear as small, well-delineated strongly enhancing masses (MARTIN et al. 1989, 1990; VEILLON 1991; BARTELS 1991; ISHII et al. 1991), but they preferentially develop in the tympanic cavity along the cochlear promontory. Secondary erosions of the ossicular chain, the cochlea, and more rarely the tympanic facial canal may occur and, if pulsatile tinnitus is the most frequent clinical finding with an evocative blue eardrum, conductive or perceptive hearing loss are possible; on the contrary, facial palsy is rarely predominant. Angiography will confirm the diagnosis.

Tympanic cholesteatomas can also mimic a small facial schwannoma when they are located close to the facial canal, predominantly near the oval window with secondary erosion of the facial canal (Fig. 13.6). If any doubt persists, MR shows a T1 iso- and T2 iso/hyperintense nonenhancing lesion which eliminates the diagnosis of schwannoma. In chronic otitis media, inflammatory tissue surrounding cholesteatoma may also result (through the osseous erosion of the facial canal) in an inflammatory enhancing involvement of the facial nerve (Fig. 13.7). The less erosive cholesterol granulomas also frequently depicted in chronic otitis media will be easily differentiated on MR based on their T1 and T2 spontaneous hyperintense signal (Fig. 13.8).

Lastly, besides the frequent acoustic schwannoma already seen with facial schwannoma, meningiomas, lipomas, and/or epidermoid cysts are discussed in the IAC and pontocerebellar angle (Fig. 13.9). Clinical findings are often more complex and intricate, associating various brain stem compression symp-

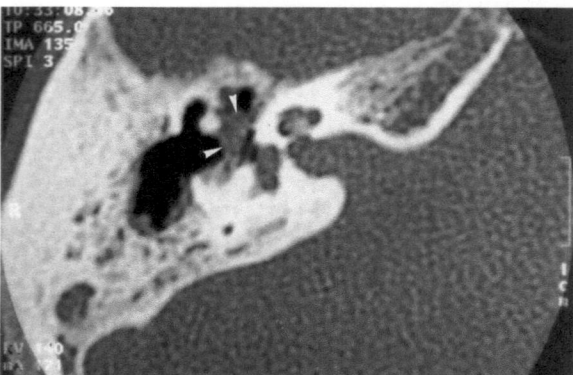

Fig. 13.6. Tympanic cholesteatoma. Axial CT scan showing a small cholesteatoma eroding the lateral part of the tympanic segment of the facial canal, simulating a small facial nerve schwannoma (*arrows*)

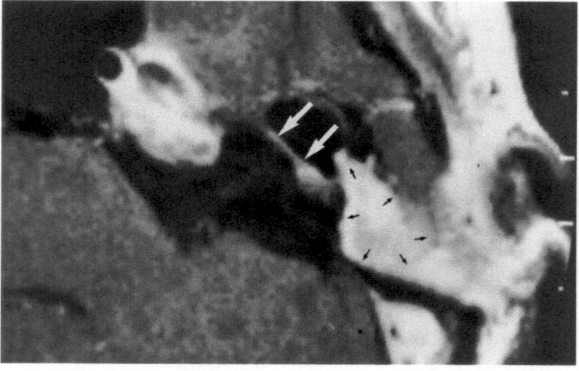

Fig. 13.7. Chronic otitis media with cholesteatoma and inflammatory granuloma. Patient presenting with facial paralysis. Axial enhanced T1-weighted MR image showing the intense enhancement of the inflammatory tissue surrounding the large antral cholesteatoma (*black arrows*). An adjacent linear marked enhancement involves the tympanic segment of the facial nerve (*white arrows*)

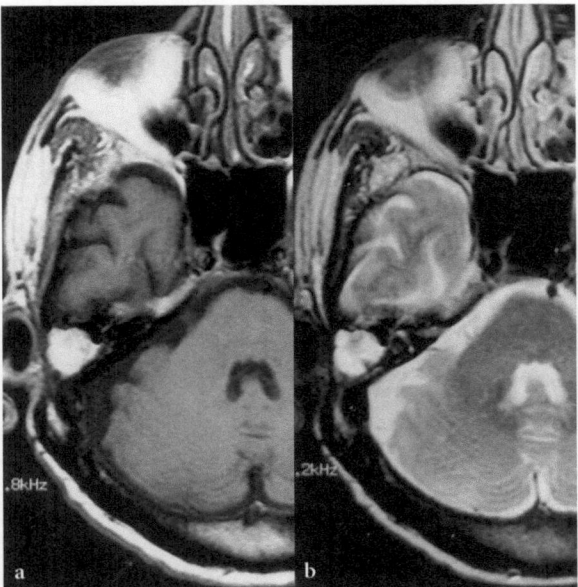

Fig. 13.8a, b. Cholesterol granuloma. Axial nonenhanced T1 (a)- and T2 (b)-weighted MR images showing a spontaneous well-delineated attico-antral mass

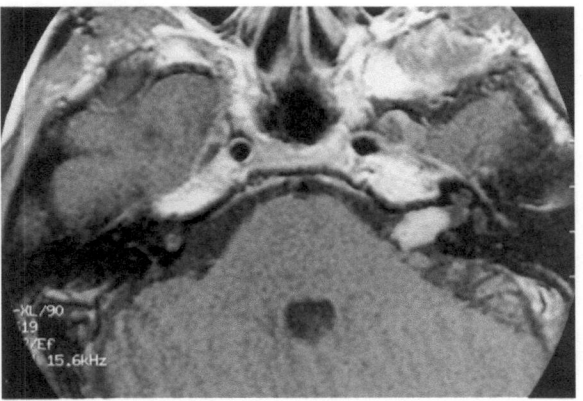

Fig. 13.9. Acoustic schwannoma. Axial enhanced T1-weighted MR image showing a well-delineated enhanced intracanicular mass respecting the distal fundus

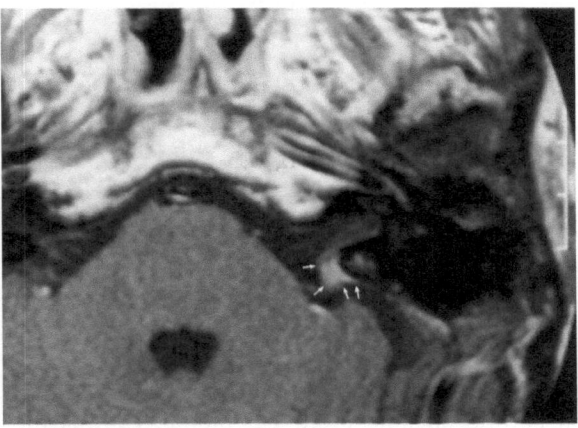

Fig. 13.10. Meningioma. Axial enhanced T1-weighted MR image showing a small enhancing mass posteriorly adjacent to the porus. A small dural tail is seen (*arrows*)

toms, hearing loss, vertigo, and facial paralysis. But meningiomas (Fig. 13.10) are rarely centered on the IAC, appearing as dural-based strongly enhancing masses with a frequently evocative enhancing thickening of the adjacent dura. Extension to the IAC is rare and often large and limited. Calcifications as reactive adjacent hyperostosis are not uncommon. Rarer lipomas display a characteristic nonenhancing CT hypodensity with a T1 hyper- and T2 hypointense pattern, whereas epidermoid cysts do not differ from intratemporal location as often large nonenhancing T1 hypo- and T2 iso/hyperintense masses compressing the adjacent neural structures (GAO et al. 1992; TAMPIERI et al. 1989).

Neuroimaging of the facial nerve, often superimposable to imaging for facial paralysis, should in all cases include a T2 axial sequence displaying the brain stem and the cerebral hemispheres. Involvement of the intraaxial facial fibers located beyond the facial nuclei during their pathway to the cisternal segment must be evaluated on MR. Pathologies can be quite varied including tumoral, vascular, inflammatory, or demyelinating diseases, which can be easily overlooked in an imaging assessment strictly focalized on the temporal bone.

Except benign lesions, malignant tumors can also involve the facial nerve. Malignant schwannomas are extremely rare, appearing in most cases as enhancing heterogeneous lobulated lesions enlarging the facial canal (MUHLBAUER et al. 1987). Prognosis is poor, still worse when associated with neurofibromatosis. Pulmonary, subarachnoid, or spinal metastases are rare but possible.

Isolated metastases involving the facial nerve without any simultaneous involvement of the temporal bone are quite rare, most often secondary to adenocarcinomas (CONLEY et al. 1991). Owing to a similar clinical presentation, preoperative diagnosis can be difficult with benign lesions (Fig. 13.11).

On the other hand, facial nerve can be secondarily involved in tumoral pathology of the petrous bone. Contiguous petrous lesions, such as, for example, squamous carcinomas, pharyngo-laryngeal carcinomas, can extend to petrous bone, as well as hema-

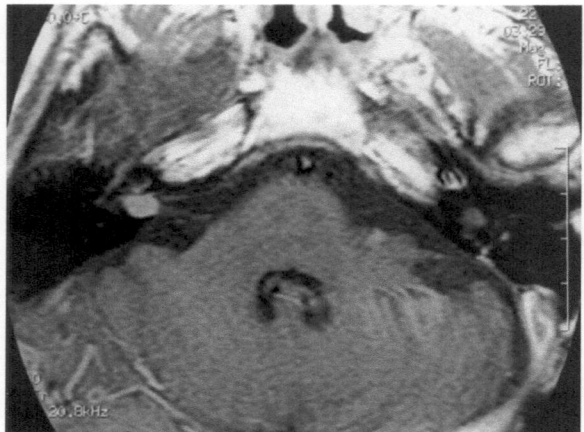

Fig. 13.11. Metastasis. Axial enhanced T1-weighted MR image demonstrating a small enhanced intracanalicular mass which appears indistinguishable from a small facial or acoustic neuroma. Pathological examination revealed an isolated metastasis from a primitive lung carcinoma

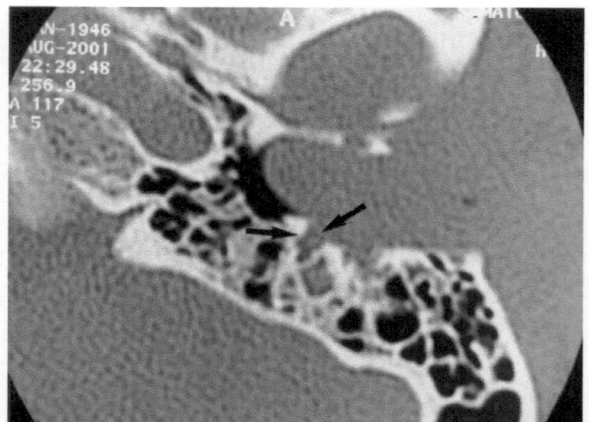

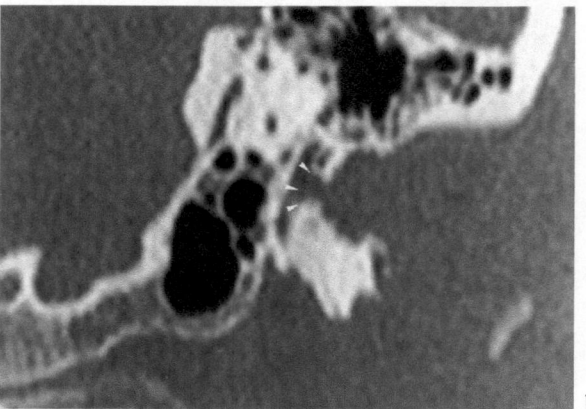

Fig. 13.12a, b. Epidermoid carcinoma. Axial (**a**) and coronal (**b**) CT scans demonstrating the erosive changes extending to the mastoid portion of the facial canal explaining the facial paralysis presented by the patient (*arrows*)

togenous spread of metastases (e.g., breast, lungs, prostate; Fig. 13.12). But clinical manifestations, such as facial paralysis, are rare and often late, contrary to the frequent post-mortem discovery of temporal metastases. Preoperative imaging is essential to show the CT lytic lesions, as well as the enhancing tumoral extension along the facial nerve, but also to depict the vascular carotid, jugular, and venous sinus permeability, the extent to the intracranial dura, the integrity of the cochleo-vestibular structures, etc.

Lastly, the facial nerve can be secondarily involved in parotid adenoid cystic carcinoma. The mastoid segment is predominantly affected due to the characteristic retrograde perineural extension of such a lesion. Magnetic resonance detects the irregular enhancing extension along the facial nerve as well as the extent to the neighboring structures and the cranial dura. More rarely, parotid metastases or other benign parotid lesions, such as adenoma or Warthin tumors, can be detected following facial palsy.

13.3
Infectious and Inflammatory Pathology

Actually, if neuroimaging is prominently dedicated to search for tumoral pathology, most facial palsies are related to the so-called Bell's palsy or idiopathic facial paralysis, or, more rarely, to herpetic (Ramsay-Hunt) facial palsies (Figs. 13.13, 13.14; GIRARD 1993; MARTIN-DUVERNEUIL et al. 1997). More seldom are

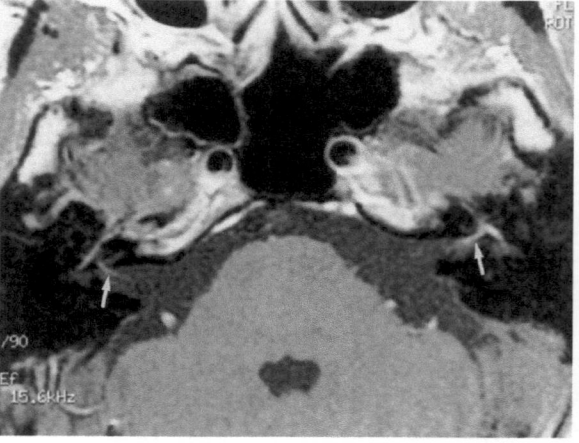

Fig. 13.13. Idiopathic bilateral facial paralysis. Axial enhanced T1-weighted MR image showing a bilateral linear enhancement of the geniculate ganglion areas pathologically extending to the distal intracanalicular segments of the facial nerve (*arrows*)

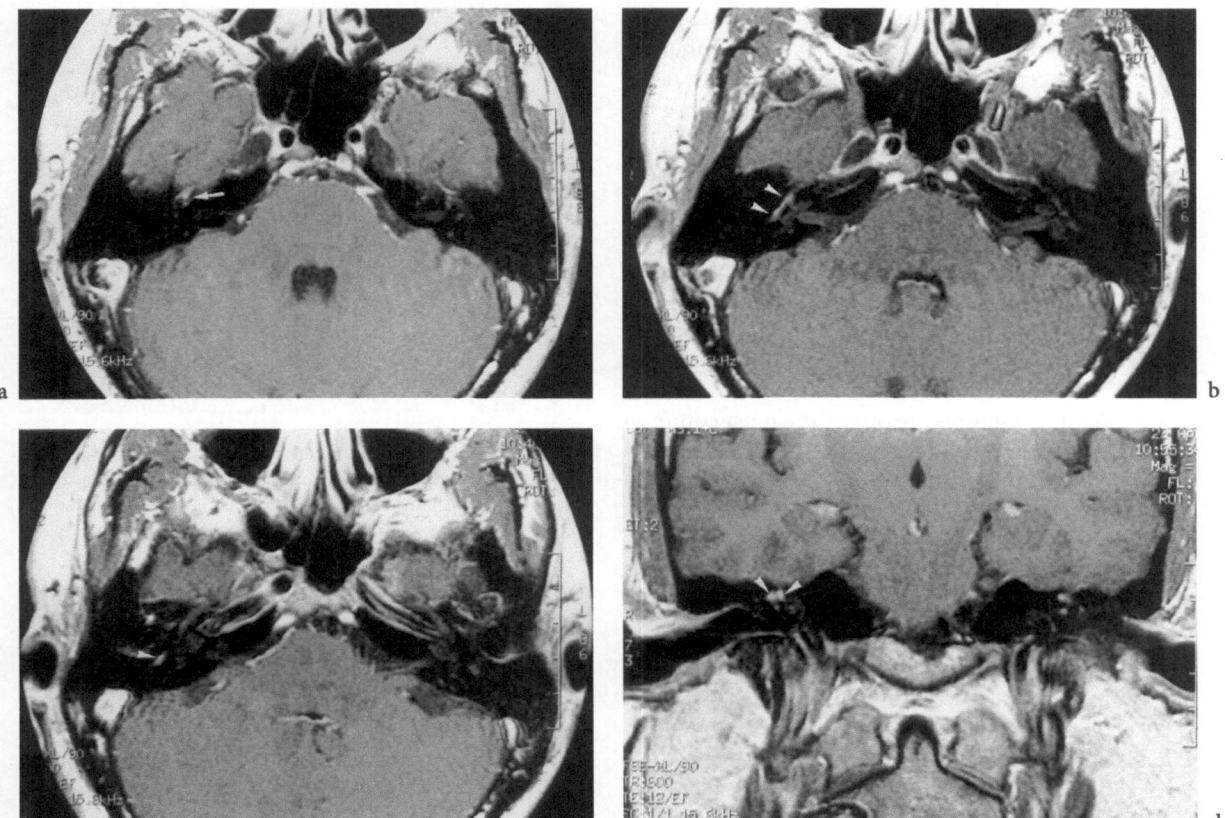

Fig. 13.14a–d. Left idiopathic facial paralysis. Axial enhanced (**a–c**) and coronal (**d**) T1-weighted MR images demonstrating a marked linear enhancement of the geniculate ganglion (**a, d**), the tympanic (**b**) and the mastoid (**c**) segment of the facial nerve (*arrows*). No extension to the intracanalicular segment was seen

the neuritis involving the facial nerve in AIDS. The probably autoimmune origin or the other associated clinical manifestations, such as an herpetic eruption involving the external acoustic meatus, tinnitus, vertigo, and/or a sensorineural hearing loss, orientate the diagnosis in most cases, and imaging is only required in some more difficult cases, when facial paralysis is incomplete, recurrent, nonregressive in less than 6–8 weeks, or associated with other clinical findings suggesting another underlying pathology. The CT scan is noncontributory. Pre- and postcontrast MR scan displays a variable linear nontumoral enhancement along the facial nerve that asks the question of the normal patterns of the facial nerve after contrast administration. Enhancement can be observed in the first days after the onset, as in chronic Bell's palsy, thus bringing only little help in predicting the outcome; it can also be absent. Duration of such enhancement is also quite variable but may persist for up to 7 months (GIRARD 1993). Enhancement is probably secondary to histopathological inflammatory involvement of the nerve

and/or its membranes which could lead to disruption of the blood–nerve barrier.

In fact, facial nerve also displays in daily routine imaging a significant linear enhancement corresponding to the facial circumneural arteriovenous plexus that circumscribes the facial nerve and predominates along the geniculate ganglion as well as the tympanic and the mastoid segments (GEBARSKI et al. 1992; MARTIN-DUVERNEUIL et al. 1997; SARTORETTI-SHEFFER et al. 1994). Enhancement is detected in at least one segment in 98% of cases, and never observed in the cisternal, canalicular, or parotid segments. Intensity of such enhancement is quite variable, the most intense findings being located in the geniculate ganglion and the tympanic segment as well as the frequently observed localized mild enhancing thickening of the nerve related to the thickness of the arteriovenous plexus which appears quite distinct from the nodular, focal-enhancing patterns of tumoral lesions (MARTIN-DUVERNEUIL et al. 1997). A right-to-left asymmetry is frequent.

Three criteria have been proposed to assess the pathological inflammatory nature of such enhancement: enhancement extending outside the facial canal; detection of an intense enhancement along the labyrinthine or the mastoid segments; and extension of this enhancement to the eighth nerve (MARTIN-DUVERNEUIL et al. 1997).

13.4
Posttraumatic Facial Palsy

Temporal bone fractures are one of the most common basilar fractures and are arbitrarily classified as longitudinal or transverse depending on the orientation of the fracture plane. Longitudinal fractures are the most common and are usually caused by a blow to the temporoparietal area. Facial nerve damage is observed in only 20% of the cases. The geniculate ganglion is the most frequently injured area. Immediate or complete facial palsy suggests laceration or compression by fracture, whereas delayed onset of facial palsy most likely evokes edema. Disruption of the ossicular chain with secondary facial palsy can also occur (Fig. 13.15). Transverse fractures are rarer, but facial palsies are most frequently observed (40–50% of cases) secondary to rupture or laceration of the facial nerve related to a fractured bone fragment (MAY and SCHAITKIN 2000; ZIMMERMAN et al. 2000).

At the time of presentation, facial palsy may be masked by an associated facial trauma. High-resolution thin-section CT is the technique of choice. Subtle bone fractures may be difficult to detect early because of the adjacent hemotympanum and/or otorrhea. Brain CT scan will search for associated brain injuries patterns. Magnetic resonance may display a linear posttraumatic enhancement similar to that of acute idiopathic facial palsy related to contusion or even compression of the facial nerve (Fig. 13.16; GIRARD 1993; ZIMMERMAN et al. 2000). Associated brain injuries are not rare; they are accurately depicted on complementary T2-weighted axial slices.

13.5
Essential Hemifacial Spasm

Essential hemifacial spasm or unilateral facial nerve hyperactive dysfunction is usually characterized by intermittent spasms in the orbicularis oculi muscle that increase in severity and frequency (MAY and

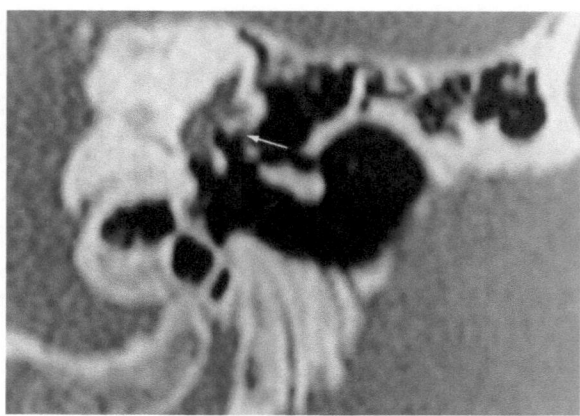

Fig. 13.15. Posttraumatic facial paralysis. Coronal CT scan showing the impacting extremity of the displaced incus through the tympanic segment of the facial canal (*arrow*)

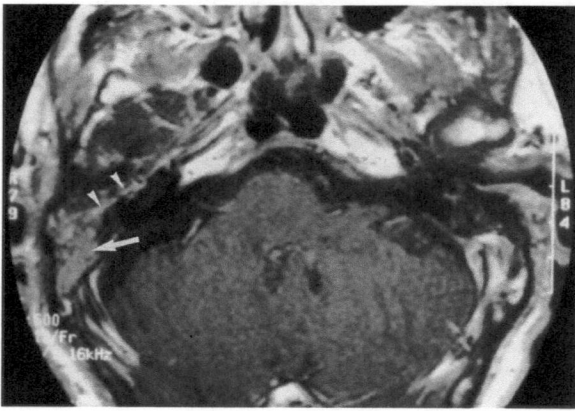

Fig. 13.16. Posttraumatic facial paralysis. Axial enhanced T1-weighted MR image demonstrating the marked enhancement of the tympanic segment of the facial nerve (*arrowheads*) adjacent to the hyperintense posthemorrhagic enhancement of the attico-antral cavity (*arrow*)

SCHAITKIN 2000). Neuroimaging aims primarily at ruling out a potential underlying cause such as tumors involving the facial nerve. Essential hemifacial spasm is presumed to be due to compression of the facial nerve at the root entry zone, the emergency area of the facial nerve from the brain stem, by a pulsating artery. These arterial compressions are related to the middle cerebellar artery (60%), the PICA (30%), and more rarely to a megadolicho vertebral artery (10%). Angio-MR sequences and/or 3D inframillimetric T2 sequences, such as constructive interference in steady state sequence, can simultaneously visualize the brain stem, the facial nerve, and these vascular structures (ADLER et al. 1992; TASH et al. 1991; USHIRO et al. 1993).

13.6
Conclusion

The facial nerve and its pathology remain complex, and the diversity and often small size of the tumoral pathology require an accurate and careful technique to allow an early detection of lesions involving the facial nerve. Both CT and contrast-enhanced MR are most often complementary techniques. Clinical presentation as well as intricate radioclinical correlations are thus essential to obtain the most accurate and early preoperative diagnosis of such lesions. Their rare occurrence should no longer lead to an often delayed diagnosis which impairs prognosis.

References

Adler CH, Zimmerman RA, Savino PJ et al. (1992) Hemifacial spasm: evaluation by magnetic resonance imaging and magnetic resonance tomographic angiography. Ann Neurol 32:502–506

Bartels L (1991) Facial nerve and medially invasive petrous bone cholesteatomas. Ann Otol Rhinol Laryngol 100:308–316

Conley J, Juarbe C, Patow CA et al. (1991) Metastatic melanoma to the facial nerve. Plast Reconstr Surg 87:341–345

Curtin HD, Wolfe P, May M (1987) "Ossifying" hemangiomas of the temporal bone: evaluation with CT. Radiology 64:831–835

Gao P, Osborn AG, Smirnotopoulos JG et al. (1992) Epidermoid tumor of the cerebellopontine angle. AJNR 13:863–872

Gebarski SS, Telian SA, Niparko JK (1992) Enhancement along the normal facial nerve in the facial canal: MR imaging and anatomic correlation. Radiology 183:391–394

Girard N, Poncet M, Chays A, Florence A, Gignac D, Magnan J, Raybaud C (1993) MRI exploration of the intrapetrous facial nerver. J Neuroradiol 20:226–238

Girard N, Raybaud C, Poncet M (1994) 3D-FT MRI of the facial nerve. Neuroradiology 36:462–468

Inoue Y, Tabuchi T, Hakuba A et al. (1987) Facial nerve neuromas: CT findings. J Comput Assist Tomogr 11:942–947

Ishii K, Takahashi S, Matsumoto K et al. (1991) Middle ear cholesteatoma extending into the petrous apex: evaluation by CT and MR imaging. AJNR 12:719–724

Iwanaga M, Yamamoto E, Fukumoto M et al. (1984) Facial nerve neurinoma: two cases located in the horizontal portion. Laryngoscope 94:938–941

Kienzle GD, Goldenberg MH, Just NWM et al. (1986) Facial nerve neurinoma presenting as middle cranial fossa mass: CT appearance. J Comput Assist Tomogr 10:391–394

Larson TL, Talbot JM, Wong ML (1995) Geniculate ganglion meningiomas: CT and MR appearances. AJNR 16:1144–1146

Latack JT, Gabrielsen TO, Knake JE et al. (1983) Facial nerve neuromas: radiologic evaluation. Radiology 149:731–739

Lidov M, Som PM, Stacy C et al. (1991) Eccentric cystic facial schwannoma: CT and MR features. J Comput Assist Tomogr 15:1065–1067

Lo W, Horn K, Carberry J et al. (1986) Intratemporal vascular tumors: evaluation with CT. Radiology 159:181–185

Lo W, Brackmann D, Shelton C (1989a) Imaging case study of the month: facial nerve hemangioma. Ann Otol Rhinol Laryngol 98:160–161

Lo W, Shelton C, Waluch V et al. (1989b) Intratemporal vascular tumors: detection with CT and MR imaging. Radiology 171:443–448

Mafee MF, Valvassori GE, Kumara A et al. (1988) Tumors and tumor-like conditions of the middle ear and mastoid: role of CT and MRI. Otolaryngol Clin North Am 21:349–375

Martin N, Sterkers O, Mompoint D et al. (1989) Cholesterol granulomas of the middle ear cavities: MR imaging. Radiology 172:521–525

Martin N, Sterkers O, Nahum H (1990) Chronic inflammatory diseases of middle ear cavities: Gd-DTPA-enhanced MR imaging. Radiology 176:399–405

Martin N, Lebras F, Krief O et al. (1992a) Anatomie IRM in vivo du paquet acoustico-facial. J Neuroradiol 19:88–97

Martin N, Sterkers O, Mompoint D et al. (1992b) Facial nerve neuromas: MR imaging. Neuroradiology 34:62–67

Martin N, Sterkers O, Nahum H (1992c) Haemangioma of the petrous bone: MRI. Neuroradiology 34:420–422

Martin-Duverneuil N, Sola-Martinez T, Miaux Y et al. (1997) Contrast enhancement of the facial nerve on MRI: normal or pathological? Neuroradiology 39:207–212

May M, Schaitkin BM (2000) The facial nerve, 2nd edn. Thieme, New York

Millen SJ, Daniels DL, Meyer GA (1990) Gadolinium-enhanced magnetic resonance imaging in facial nerve lesions. AJNR 102:26–33

Muhlbauer MS, Clark WC, Robertson JH et al. (1987) Malignant nerve sheath tumor of the facial nerve: case report and discussion. Neurosurgery 21:68–73

Phelps PD (1990) Glomus tumours of the ear: an imaging regime. Clin Radiol 41:301–305

Sartoretti-Schefer S, Wichmann W, Valavanis A (1994) Idiopathic, herpetic, and HIV-associated facial nerve palsies: abnormal MR enhancement patterns. AJNR 15:479–485

Sterkers JM, Corlieur P (1986) Paralysie faciale progressive par angiome caverneux de l'acqueduc de Fallope. Ann Otolaryngol 103:501–508

Sullivan MJ, Babyak JW, Kartush JM et al (1987) Intraparotid facial nerve neurofibroma. Laryngoscope 97:219–223

Tampieri D, Melanson D, Ethier R (1989) MR imaging of epidermoid cysts. AJNR 10:351–356

Tash R, Demerritt J, Sze G et al. (1991) Hemifacial spasm: MR imaging features. AJNR 12:839–842

Ushiro K, Yanagida M, Kumazawa T et al. (1993) MR imaging of vascular compressions in hemifacial spasm. Acta Otolaryngol (Stockh) 500:54–57

Veillon F (1991) Imagerie de l'oreille. Flammarion, Paris

Zimmerman RA, Gibby WA, Carmody RF (2000) Neuroimaging: clinical and physical principles. Springer, Berlin Heidelberg New York

The Clinician's View

I. DHOOGE

Abnormalities of the facial canal and nerve are in most cases associated with other congenital external and middle ear malformations. Correct identification and precise description of its course is extremely important when surgery is planned.

In recent years, the surgical management of severe ear malformations have shown interesting fluctuations in attitudes. Atresia repair surgery is worthwhile if proper patient selection is made by use of stringent audiological and radiological criteria and state-of-the-art surgery is performed. One of the major concerns in undertaking exploration of a congenital atresia is that in approximately 20% of these patients the facial nerve will have an abnormal course and is therefore liable to surgical damage.

Secondly, surgery in malformed ears has become increasingly more important with the dramatic changes in the indication for cochlear implantation and consequently in patient selection criteria since 1980s. Due to the continuous growth of knowledge in this field, and technical advances, implantation is no longer contraindicated in the malformed cochlea. In patients with malformation of any extent, complications must be expected. The facial nerve usually has an atypical course, and there is a risk of injury to it even during intra-operative monitoring; therefore, it is of great importance that the surgeon have a correct description of its course pre-operatively.

14 Postoperative Temporal Bone Imaging

Luc van den Hauwe

CONTENTS

14.1
Introduction

Postoperative changes can be very subtle, especially after ossicular chain reconstruction, or very complex as in middle ear and mastoid surgery for chronic middle ear disease, including cholesteatoma; therefore, comprehensive information regarding the surgical procedure(s) performed and the motivation for the examination should be addressed to the radiologist. Also, clinical information and the results of paraclinical testing [audiometry, auditory brain-stem responses (ABR), etc.] can be helpful in analyzing the postoperative changes in these patients. Preferably, previous pre- and/or postoperative examinations – sometimes realized in other institutions – should be available for comparison.

It is obvious that plain radiography and polytomography have become obsolete in the evaluation

Luc van den Hauwe, MD
Department of Radiology, AZ KLINA, Augustijnslei 100,
B-2930 Brasschaat, Belgium

of patients with conductive (CHL) or sensorineural hearing loss (SNHL), tinnitus, and vertigo. To confirm correct position of the electrode array after cochlear implantation, however, plain radiography and especially digital radiography are used routinely.

Computed tomography (CT) is the imaging modality of choice in the evaluation of the postoperative middle ear because of its widespread availability and its ability to depict discrete bony abnormalities, and to assess the re-aeration of the middle ear cleft. Intravenous injection of contrast medium is only useful when brain abscess formation is suspected. Helical CT (Hermans et al. 1995) and especially multidetector CT (MDCT) have been a breakthrough (Williams et al. 2000). Improved spatial resolution in the z-axis and scan speed result in fast, high-quality CT examinations. Sagittal and coronal reformattings as well as three-dimensional renderings of the MDCT data can be realized almost routinely. Endoluminal views of the tympanic cavity can be obtained and virtual endoscopy can be performed to exclude ossicular chain disruption (Klingebiel et al. 2001).

Magnetic resonance (MR) imaging is the imaging modality of choice in patients with vestibular schwannoma (VS), not only in the diagnostic workup of patients with SNHL, but also in the follow-up and after treatment surgery. The use of MR imaging has also been advocated to differentiate recurrent cholesteatoma from granulation tissue after mastoidectomy. Although early results seem to be very promising, higher spatial resolution, thinner slices, and less susceptibility artifacts are needed if MR imaging wants to replace second-look surgery in cholesteatoma patients.

Most prostheses are not a contraindication for MR imaging (Shellock and Schatz 1991). The presence of a functioning cochlear implant (CI) has been considered as an absolute contraindication to MR examination for many years and most radiologists remain reluctant when patients with a CI are referred for MR imaging. It has been demonstrated, however, that most of the electromagnetic interferences between the CI and the MR system remain within acceptable limits. But MR imaging should be performed only if there is a strong medical indication and after assessment of the relative risks involved (TEISSL et al. 1998).

14.2
Surgery in Chronic Middle Ear Disease

Chronic otitis media (COM) indicates irreversible middle ear pathology. Manifestations of COM include middle ear effusion, also known as secretory otitis media (SOM), tympanic membrane retractions, acquired cholesteatoma, granulation tissue, cholesterol granuloma, ossicular erosion, and ossicular fixation due to tympanosclerosis (SWARTZ and HARNSBERGER 1998). Often the mastoid is poorly pneumatized. Eustachian tube dysfunction with subsequent decreased intratympanic pressure is one of the elements responsible for COM. Tympanostomy tubes or transtympanic ventilating tubes can be placed to normalize intratympanic pressure and they are used in patients with recurrent acute otitis media and longstanding SOM. They are available in various types of plastics or stainless steel. Most of these tympanostomy tubes have a bobbin shape and their CT appearance is mostly characteristic

(Fig. 14.1; SWARTZ et al. 1983). The different surgical procedures performed in chronic middle ear disease have been well illustrated by MUKHERJI et al. (1994). Diagrams of the procedures are shown below, courtesy of the author. The purpose of middle ear and mastoid surgery in patients with cholesteatoma is to remove all diseased tissue while preserving as much of the normal structures, i.e., the ossicular chain and the bony wall of the external auditory canal (EAC).

14.2.1
Mastoidectomy

Mastoidectomy may be categorized into closed cavity (EAC wall maintained) and open cavity types (EAC wall resected). In closed cavity mastoidectomy, also known as canal-wall-up mastoidectomy, the posterior wall of the EAC is preserved; the mastoid air cells including Koerner's septum are removed. In this manner, communication of the surgically created cavity (mastoid bowl) with the antrum and epitympanum is established (Fig. 14.2).

In open cavity mastoidectomy, also known as canal-wall-down mastoidectomy, the posterosuperior wall of the EAC is removed, allowing communication

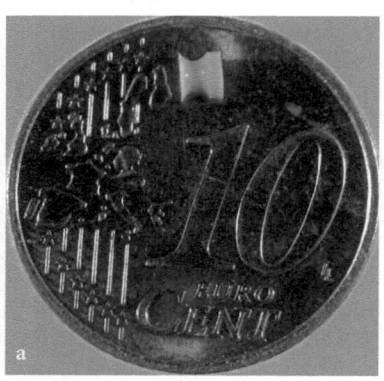

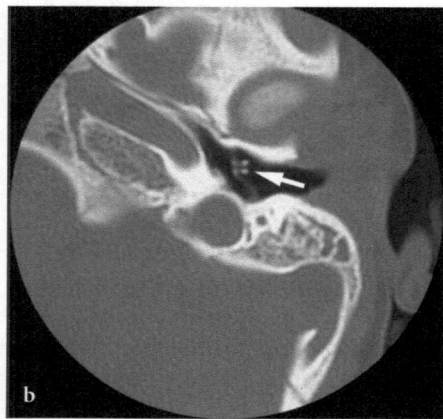

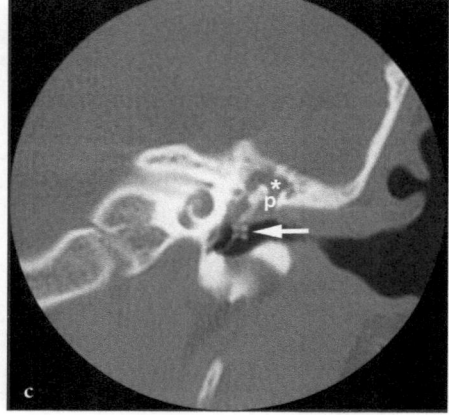

Fig. 14.1a–c. Tympanostomy tubes. **a** A nonmetallic tympanostomy tube, bobbin type, was inserted bilaterally. **b** Axial CT image of the left ear shows a normal appearance of the tympanostomy tube (*arrow*). **c** Coronal CT image confirms the presence of the ventilation tube (*arrow*). Opacification of the attic (*asterisk*) and Prussak's space (*p*) with medial displacement of the ossicular chain is noticed. No erosion of the scutum, ossicular chain, or tegmen tympani is observed, favoring the diagnosis of chronic otitis media

between the mastoid cavity and the EAC. Further access to the middle ear cavity is created, depending on the extent of disease encountered. If disease is limited to the epitympanum, only the scutum needs to be resected and the ossicular chain can be preserved (Fig. 14.3). When the ossicular chain is involved in the disease process, a radical mastoidectomy is performed. The tympanic membrane is detached from its annulus and the mastoid segment of the facial nerve canal is skeletonized allowing wide access to the middle ear cavity (Fig. 14.4); however, the stapes superstructure is left in place whenever possible.

14.2.2
Tympanoplasty–Ossicular Reconstruction

Tympanoplasty is a technique used to eradicate middle ear pathology and to reconstruct the conductive hearing system. Based on the degree of ossicular bypass, five types of tympanoplasty have been defined by Wullstein (SWARTZ and HARNSBERGER 1998). Routine postoperative imaging studies are not required after simple myringoplasty (type-I tympanoplasty); however, when

imaging is performed within the first weeks after the procedure, a thickening of the tympanic membrane can be noticed, as well as a middle ear effusion. In type-II tympanoplasty the malleus is bypassed and the graft connects directly to the body of the incus. In type-III tympanoplasty the graft attaches to the capitulum of the stapes; in type-IV tympanoplasty to the footplate of the stapes and in type-V tympanoplasty the graft attaches to the oval window.

Ossicular reconstructions are commonly performed in patients with extensive cholesteatoma with involvement of the ossicular chain, as well in patients with tympanosclerosis, otosclerosis, or congenital ossicular malformations. Initially, cartilage and temporalis fascia have been used, before the introduction of allografts. Allografts have gained wide acceptance, especially in Europe. The main reason for using allografts is their excellent biocompatibility; however, they require time and skill for sculpting and availability may be a problem. Moreover, they may harbor foci of cholesteatoma and a growing risk of transmitting infectious diseases, such as Creutzfeldt-Jakob and AIDS, have been mentioned (STONE et al. 2000). For all these reasons, synthetic prostheses have

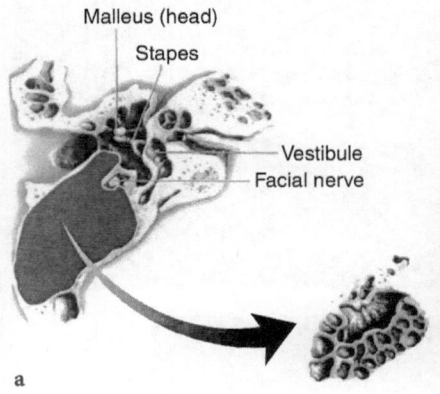

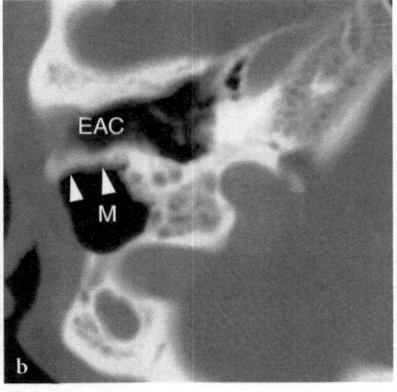

Fig. 14.2a, b. Canal-wall-up mastoidectomy. a Removal of the mastoid air cells with preservation of the posterior wall of the right external auditory canal (EAC). (From MUKHERJI et al. 1994) b Axial CT image at the level of the mesotympanum shows the residual mastoid bowl (*M*), which has been created by removal of the mastoid air cells. Posterior wall (*arrowheads*) of the EAC is preserved in this form of mastoid surgery

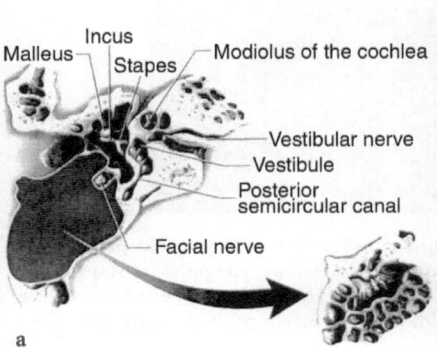

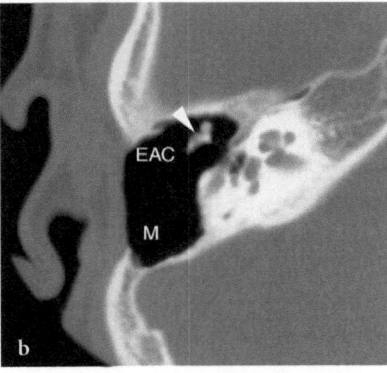

Fig. 14.3a,b. Canal-wall-down mastoidectomy with ossicular preser-va-tion. a Resection of both the mastoid air cells and posterior wall of the EAC (canal-wall-down) at the right side. The ossicles are preserved in this procedure. (From MUKHERJI et al. 1994) b Axial CT image at the level of the meso-tympanum shows the postoperative mastoid bowl (*M*), with preservation of the ossicles (*arrowhead*). In contrast with canal-wall-up mastoidectomy, the posterior wall of the EAC has been resected. Ossicular reconstruction was not required in this case

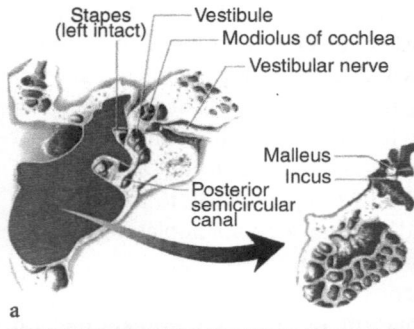

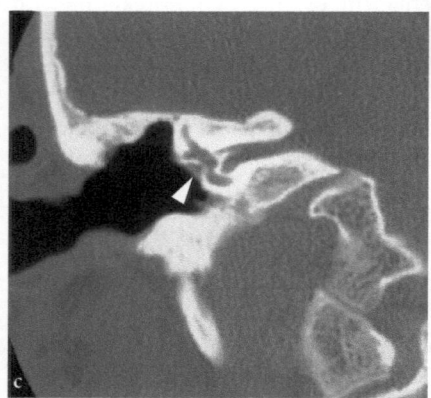

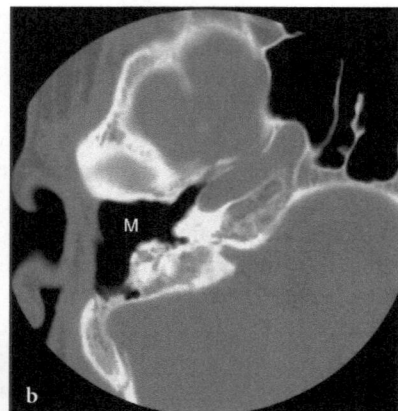

Fig. 14.4a–c. Canal-wall-down mastoidectomy with removal of malleus and incus. **a** Exenteration of the mastoid air cells, posterior wall of EAC, and incus. The stapes superstructure is preserved. (From MUKHERJI et al. 1994) **b** Axial CT image at the level of the mesotympanum demonstrates the mastoidectomy defect (*M*), with removal of the posterior wall of the EAC. Malleus and incus have been resected, with preservation of the stapes superstructure. **c** Coronal CT image obtained at the level of the oval window shows a small residual soft tissue component (*arrowhead*)

been developed. Prostheses most commonly used for ossicular reconstructions include stapes prostheses for otosclerosis (Fig. 14.5), incus interposition, auto- or homografts (Fig. 14.6), partial ossicular replacement prostheses (PORP), and total ossicular replacement prostheses (TORP; Fig. 14.7).

Otological evaluation of patients who have undergone ossicular reconstruction is often difficult. Computed tomography can be helpful in demonstrating prosthetic failure (recurrent cholesteatoma, granulation tissue, adhesions or mechanical problems) that may cause postoperative CHL and identify patients in whom revision surgery is considered (STONE et al. 2000).

14.2.3
Failure/Recurrence

A drawback of the closed cavity approach is that recurrent or residual disease cannot be seen otoscopically during postoperative follow-up, and therefore, "second look" surgery is mandatory (TIERNEY et al. 1999). An important role of imaging is attempting to differentiate recurrent cholesteatoma from postoperative granulation tissue in these patients.

The imaging findings of recurrent cholesteatoma have been described extensively (VEILLON et al.

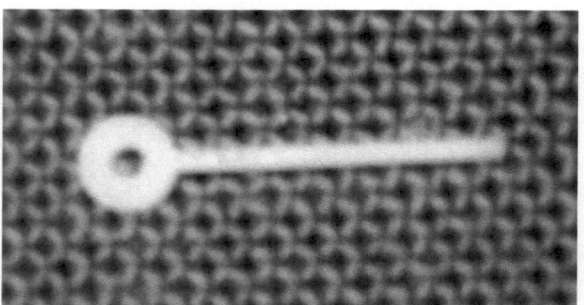

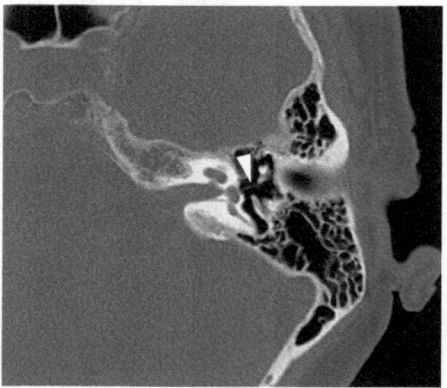

Fig. 14.5a, b. Stapes prosthesis in a 33-year-old patient with fenestral otospongiosis. **a** A Teflon-type polymer stapes prosthesis. **b** Axial CT image of the left ear, obtained at the level of the oval window, shows correct position of the prosthesis (*arrow*)

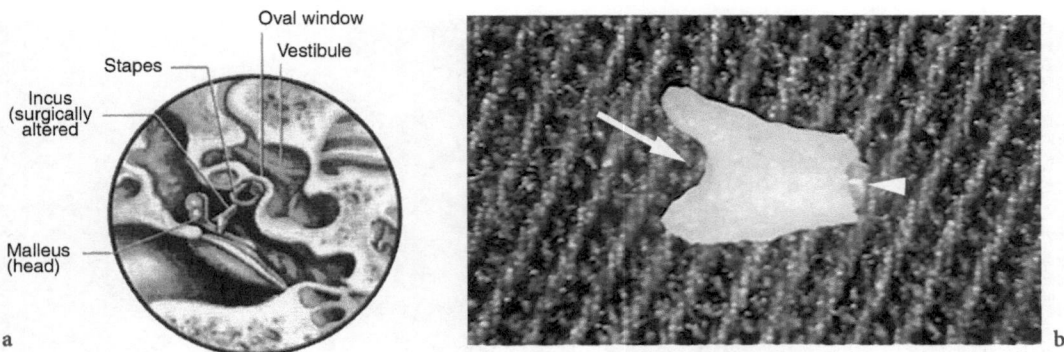

Fig. 14.6a, b. Incus interposition **a** A surgically altered incus that has been placed between the malleus and stapes in an attempt to maintain ossicular function. (From MUKHERJI et al. 1994). **b** An example of a sculptured autologous incus interposition graft. The notch (*arrow*) will fit under the handle of the malleus and the circular groove (*arrowhead*) will be placed on the head of the stapes

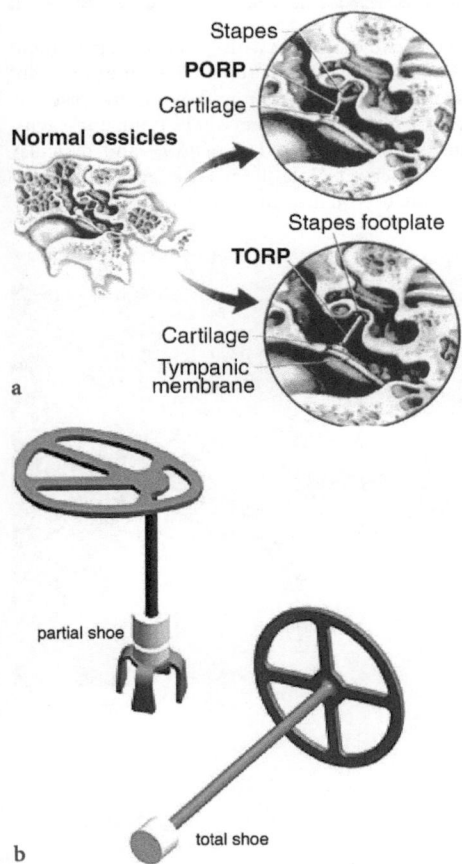

Fig. 14.7a, b. Ossicular replacement prostheses. **a** Two types of ossicular prostheses that are used for preserving ossicular function. Partial ossicular replacement prosthesis (PORP) involves placement of a synthetic prosthesis that articulates between the tympanic membrane and head of the stapes. Total ossicular replacement prosthesis (TORP) is used when the head and crura of the stapes have been resected. The prosthesis extends from the tympanic membrane to the stapes footplate. (From MUKHERJI et al. 1994). **b** Universal titanium prosthesis, which can be used both as a PORP (partial shoe) and as a TORP (total shoe). (Courtesy of Xomed, Medtronic Belgium)

1991). Computed tomography findings suggestive for recurrent cholesteatoma include a progressively enlarging focal mass associated with bone erosion (Fig. 14.8) or ossicular displacement (Fig. 14.9).

On MR, cholesteatoma is most often hyperintense on T2-weighted images, hypointense on T1-weighted images, and is unenhanced on postcontrast images (Fig. 14.10). A rim enhancement, however, can be seen around the cholesteatoma (Fig. 14.11; MARK and CASSELMAN 2002).

The use of CT and/or MR imaging to assess the cavity and to detect residual or recurrent disease has been evaluated in a number of small series. Computed tomography has low sensitivity and low specificity, not allowing to differentiate between recurrence, scar tissue, or inflammation (BLANEY et al. 2000). Poor radiosurgical correlation suggests that, at the present time, also MR imaging is not a valid alternative to a second-look surgical intervention in the case of cholesteatoma treated by canal-wall-up tympanoplasty (VANDEN ABEELE et al. 1999); therefore, second-look surgery remains the gold standard to diagnose recurrent or residual cholesteatoma (THOMASSIN and BRACCINI 1999).

In the future, diffusion-weighted MR images with a high diffusion sensitivity (b-1000) may be helpful in differentiating granulation tissue from cholesteatoma (MAHESWARI and MUKHERJI 2002). Cholesteatoma shows high signal intensity on the b-1000 diffusion images, where all other lesions, such as fluid, inflammatory tissue, cholesterol granuloma, etc., have a low signal intensity (Fig. 14.12). Early results are very promising, and this technique could eventually replace second-look surgery in cholesteatoma patients, but first higher spatial resolution and thinner slices are needed and susceptibility artifacts must be reduced (MARK and CASSELMAN 2002). The value of delayed

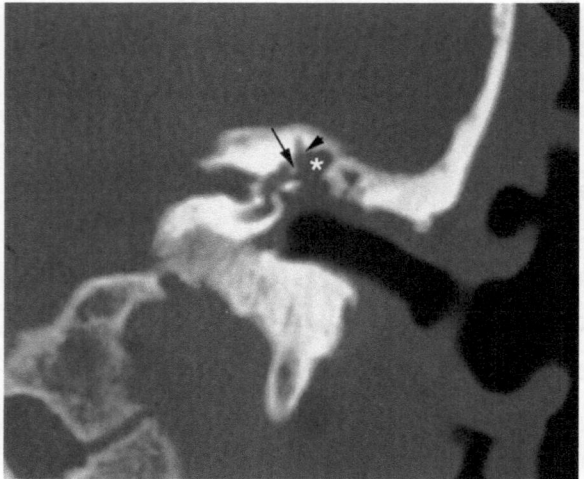

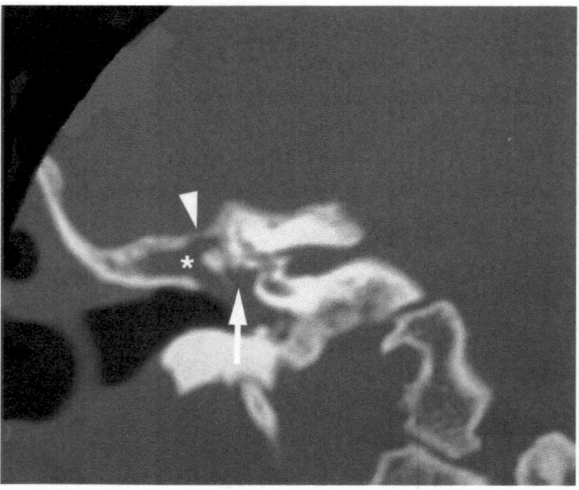

Fig. 14.8. Recurrent cholesteatoma with bony erosion. Postoperative coronal CT scan of the left ear after radical mastoidectomy shows a soft tissue mass in the attic, associated with erosion of the lateral (*arrow*) and superior (*arrowhead*) semicircular canals

Fig. 14.9. Recurrent cholesteatoma with ossicular displacement and bony erosion. Postoperative coronal CT scan of the right ear after canal wall up mastoidectomy shows a progressively enlarging mass (*asterisk*) filling the whole tympanic cavity. Erosion of the tegmen tympani (*arrowhead*) and ossicular chain (*arrow*) is observed. Note the mass effect with medial displacement of the ossicular chain (*arrow*)

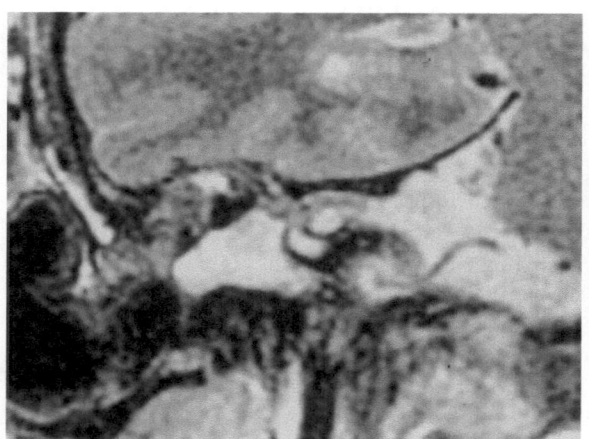

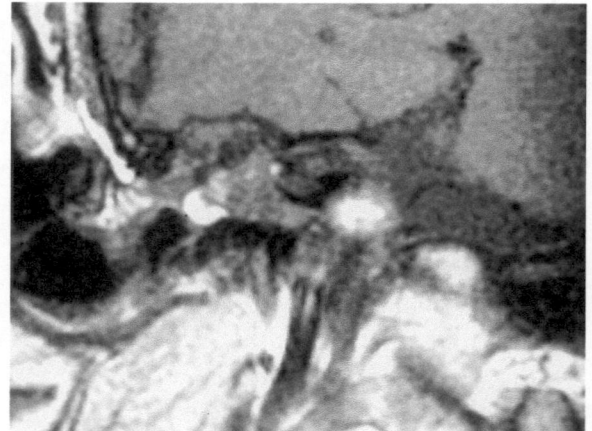

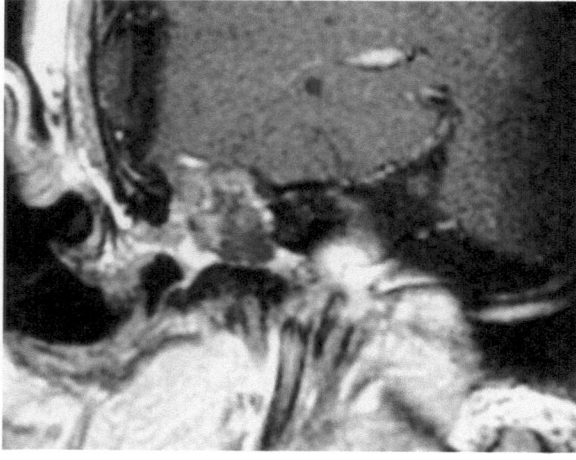

Fig. 14.10a–c. Characteristic MR features of cholesteatoma. **a** Coronal T2-weighted image shows almost total obliteration of the tympanic cavity with the presence of a hyperintense mass lesion in the meso- and hypotympanum. **b** Coronal T1-weighted image displays the lesion as having low signal. **c** Same coronal image, after gadolinium-injection. No obvious enhancement is discerned

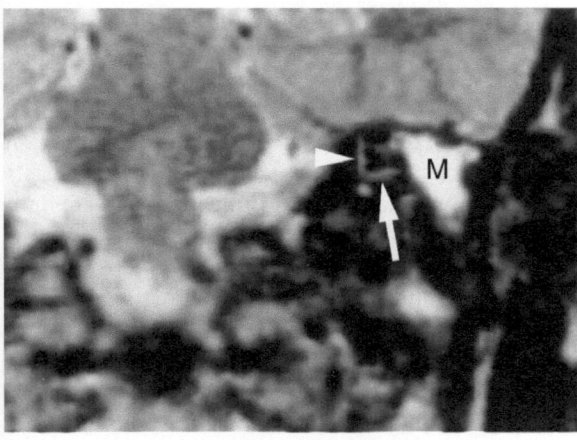

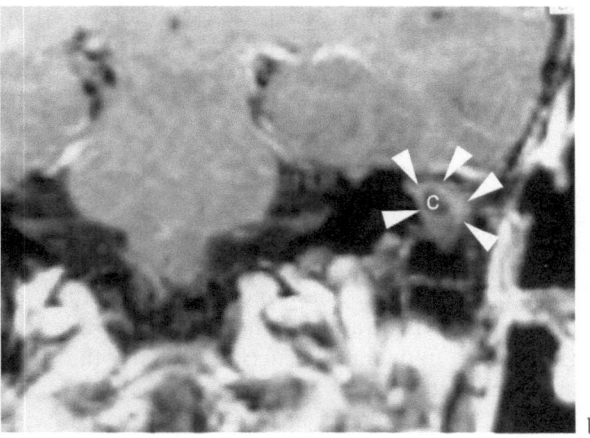

a   b

Fig. 14.11a, b. Rim enhancement in recurrent cholesteatoma after gadolinium injection. **a** Coronal T2-weighted image shows high signal intensity in the left mastoid cavity (*M*). Note the normal appearance of the lateral (*arrow*) and superior semicircular canals (*arrowhead*). **b** Coronal T1-weighted image after Gd-injection shows a hypointense central area (*C*) with peripheral contrast enhancement (*arrowheads*). Diagnosis was confirmed during surgery. (Courtesy of D. Vanden Abeele, Antwerp)

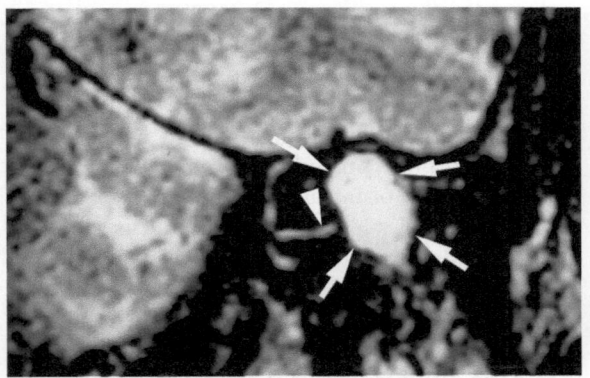

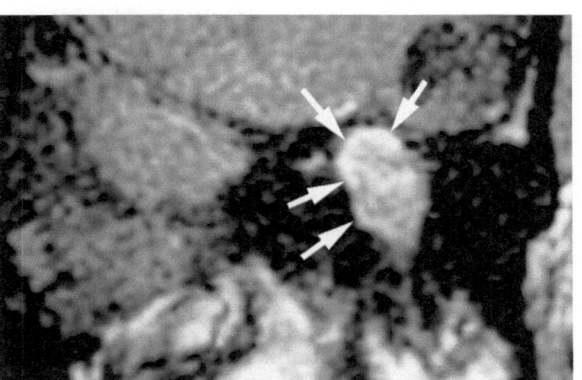

a   b

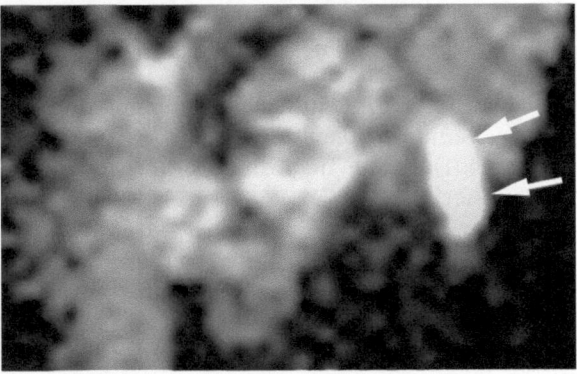

c

Fig. 14.12a–c. Diffusion-weighted MR imaging in a patient surgically treated for atticoantral cholesteatoma of the left ear. Computed tomography (not shown) demonstrated complete obliteration of the middle ear cavity and mastoid. **a** Coronal T2-weighted image shows a hyperintense mass in the mastoid area (*arrows*), extending anteriorly to the level of the posterior branch of the lateral semicircular canal (*arrowhead*). **b** On the Gd-enhanced T1-weighted image, the lesion remains hypointense. Only some subtle rim enhancement can be seen around the lesion (*arrows*). **c** The lesion has a high signal intensity on the B-1000 diffusion image (*arrows*), which is typical for a cholesteatoma. All other lesions, such as fluid, inflammatory tissue, cholesterol granuloma, etc., have a low signal intensity. (Courtesy of B. De Foer and J.W. Casselman, Antwerp and Bruges)

contrast-enhanced T1-weighted images needs to be further evaluated in larger series. In a small number of patients, WILLIAMS et al (2003). were able to reduce their number of false-positives cases using this technique. Scar tissue was clearly hyperintense on delayed enhanced images, whereas it appeared hypointense on early contrast-enhanced images.

14.3
Stapes Surgery in Otosclerosis Patients

Many diseases and dysplasias can affect the osseous components of the temporal bone. Some diseases, such as otosclerosis, are limited to the temporal bone and do not occur elsewhere in the body (HASSO et al. 1996). The term "otosclerosis" was introduced by Adam Politzer, who described the histopathological findings in 1894 (DECLAU et al. 2001). Otosclerosis occurs in two phases: an early, active phase, during which bone resorption occurs (otospongiotic stage); and a later, inactive phase (sclerotic stage). Diagnosis of otosclerosis is based on clinical findings, audiometric testing, and family history, but medical imaging is often demanded to confirm the diagnosis (NOWÉ et al. 2003). The typical clinical features of otosclerosis are gradually increasing hearing loss (HL), most frequently occurring between the third and fifth decades. Although usually both ears are affected, often there is an asymmetry in HL with one ear showing a greater conductive impairment. Tinnitus is a common symptom and it may become louder as the HL progresses. The origin of the tinnitus is not clear, but it may be the result of cochlear degeneration or an abnormal degree of vascularity within the labyrinthine capsule. Vertigo is rare and is probably the effect of toxic enzymes on the vestibular labyrinth (DE BRUIJN 2000). In otosclerosis, three major patterns of involvement are discerned: fenestral; retrofenestral; and mixed. Firstly, there is a purely fenestral type, which involves the oval window, most commonly the anterior aspect in the approximate location of the embryologic fissula ante fenestram. The second type is a retrofenestral (cochlear) form, primarily involving the cochlea, with SNHL as a result. Both types of otosclerosis may coexist in one patient, resulting in mixed HL (D'ARCHAMBEAU et al. 1990).

Although stapes surgery is presently considered the treatment of choice, hearing aids or BAHA may be a good alternative in those cases where surgery is not desirable or possible (RAUT et al. 2002). The administration of sodium fluoride, to stabilize cochlear deterioration, remains a matter of controversy, partly due to the unknown toxic effect of long-term medication (DE BRUIJN 2000).

Currently, stapes surgery consists of the traditional stapedectomy, introduced by SHEA in 1958, in which the footplate is totally or near-totally removed, and stapedotomy in which a small fenestra is made through the central portion of the footplate. Small fenestra stapedotomy, first popularized by MARQUET et al. (1972), is the operation of choice since this technique has less early complications, including vertigo and reparative granuloma formation.

A variety of different prostheses (pistons) is available. They differ in size, shape, and weight. Biomaterials most often used for prostheses are a Teflon-type polymer, stainless steel, titanium, and platinum. Teflon is still the most favored piston in the UK, although combinations with platinum and stainless steel are increasingly being used in some centers (RAUT et al. 2002). The main differences in the design of stapes prostheses are at the point of connection with the incus. The attachment to the incus consists of either a loop that surrounds the incus or a cup into which the lenticular process fits.

In the majority of cases (more than 90%), postoperative results are good and no further imaging studies are required; however, unsuccessful outcomes (persistent or recurrent CHL, vertigo, and fluctuating SNHL) may be observed. Control CT examination is performed in these patients to demonstrate abnormalities that may require re-intervention. Abnormal findings on CT to identify are incorrect stapes prosthesis position, inflammatory changes, perilymphatic fistula (PLF), and regrowth of otosclerosis (WILLIAMS et al. 2000).

According to CAUSSE et al. (1983), three categories of complications after otosclerosis surgery can be discerned: intraoperative complications; immediately postoperative complications; and delayed postoperative complications. Vertigo immediately after the surgical procedure can be explained by the sudden drop of intralabyrinthine pressure while opening the oval window, especially in cases of pre-existing hydrops. Other causes of vertigo include intraoperative contamination of the labyrinth with blood and compression of the saccule when the shaft of the prosthesis enters the vestibule (Fig. 14.13). Prosthesis displacement is the most common cause of CHL recurrence or persistence after surgery.

Computed tomography visualization of the prosthesis depends on its material (Fig. 14.14; CHAKERES and MATTOX 1985). Thin metallic or Teflon prostheses may be more difficult to identify (KÖSLING and BOOTZ 2001). Prosthetic position in the middle ear can be determined with HRCT, especially when helical or, even better, MDCT is used (RANGHEARD et al. 2001). Conventional CT is limited by the obliquity of the prosthesis relative to the conventional scan planes. Helical CT yields high-resolution reformatting in oblique planes along the main axis of the prosthesis, allowing a more accurate depiction of the prosthesis status. Multiplanar reconstructions provided by helical CT acquisition greatly improve imaging accuracy by showing the full length of the prosthesis on single axial or coronal reformatted images. Nevertheless, the resolution of reformatted images remains insufficient to determine the type of surgical procedure that has been performed (WILLIAMS et al. 2000). The dislocation of the prosthesis of the stapes footplate may

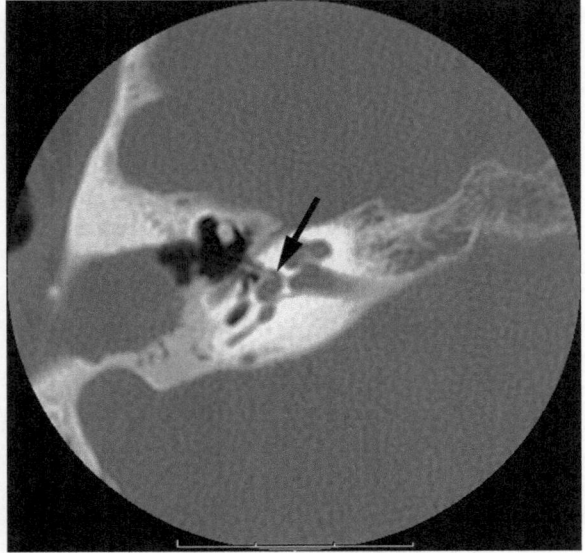

Fig. 14.13. Protrusion of the prosthesis into the vestibule. Axial control CT examination in a patient with vertigo immediately after stapes surgery. The tip of the prosthesis (*arrow*) is protruding more than 2 mm into the vestibule with compression of the saccule

be limited to an inframillimetric gap between the footplate plane and the tip of the prosthesis. In such cases the medial end of the prosthesis may appear to be in the correct position on conventional CT, but oblique multiplanar reconstructions accurately show the abnormal location of the prosthesis.

Fixation of the prosthesis can be caused by postoperative fibrous adhesions. The CT scan shows a soft tissue mass around the prosthesis or the ossicles and may cover the oval window. The PLF is a more serious complication that counts for 10% of all stapedectomy failures. Fluctuation of hearing and vertigo are the most common clinical symptoms associated with PLF. Tiny air bubbles at the end of the stapes prosthesis detected with CT are indicative of a pneumolabyrinth, which is the most important indirect sign of PLF; however, a pneumolabyrinth cannot be expected in all patients with PLF (KÖSLING et al. 1995). Computed tomography may also identify small fluid collections immediately outside the oval window and abnormal fluid collections in the middle ear and the mastoid cells in these patients (PICKUTH et al. 2000). Proliferation of

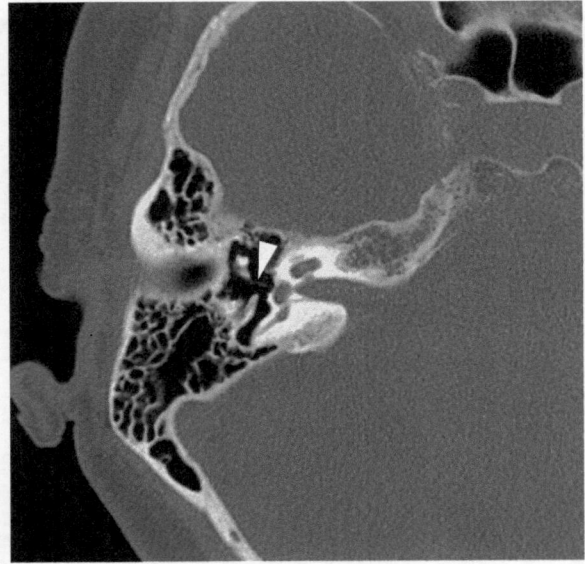

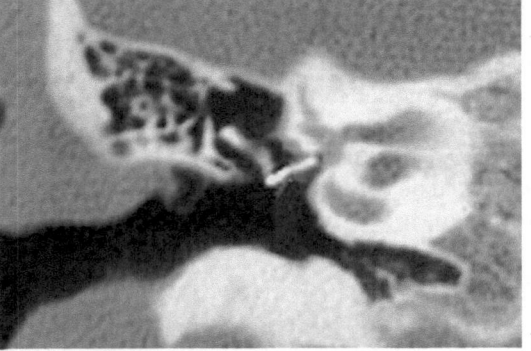

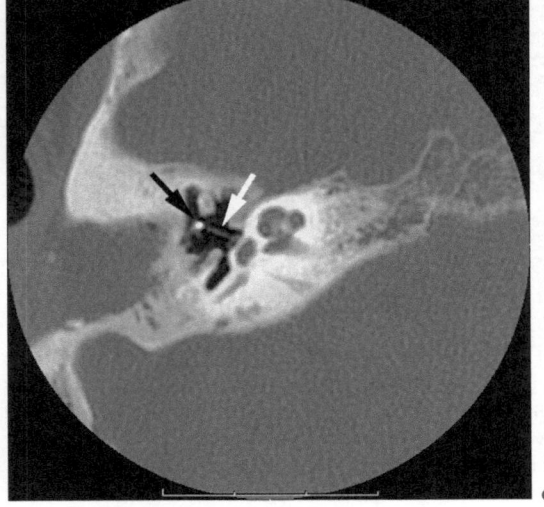

Fig. 14.14a–c. Computed tomography visualization of the prosthesis is material dependent. **a** A thin Teflon-type polymer prosthesis (*arrowhead*) is less conspicuous when compared with **b** golden (*arrowhead*) or **c** combined Teflon–platinum prostheses (platinum component: *black arrow*; Teflon-type polymer component: *white arrow*)

the otosclerotic focus may cause the impairment of a correctly located prosthesis. A slightly hyperdense calcified space-occupying mass in the oval window niche, surrounding the medial end of the prosthesis, may be observed in these patients.

Acute labyrinthitis and secondary endolymphatic hydrops are two other causes of vertigo after stapes surgery. These conditions have no pathognomonic CT manifestations (PICKUTH et al. 2000); therefore, if CT is not contributive as to the origin of SNHL and vertigo, MR imaging may be helpful in demonstrating reparative intravestibular granuloma, intralabyrinthine hemorrhage, and labyrinthitis. High signal intensity of the labyrinth on T1- and T2-weighted is indicative for postoperative hemorrhage. A combination of low signal intensity on T2-weighted images and strong enhancement after injection of gadolinium is noticed in patients with fibrous obliteration of the labyrinth as in reparative granuloma and suppurative labyrinthitis (Fig. 14.15; RANGHEARD et al. 2001). Labyrinthine – and especially cochlear – enhancement may also be a possible sign of PLF (MARK and FITZGERALD 1993).

The attachment of the prosthesis to the long process of the incus plays an important role concerning the gain in hearing and the development of late complications such as incus erosion and necrosis (KWOK et al. 2002).

Decreased thickness of the long process of the incus as seen on coronal CT scans may indicate incus necrosis. This is a late complication of stapes surgery and generally occurs after 3 or more years (KÖSLING and BOOTZ 2001).

14.4
Treatment Options in Vestibular Schwannoma

Vestibular schwannoma (VS), frequently also referred to as acoustic schwannoma, is a benign tumor of the vestibulocochlear nerve (N. VIII). From a pathological point of view, the term VS is more correct as these tumors are composed of Schwann cells and typically involve the vestibular rather than the acoustic division of the eighth cranial nerve (ELDRIDGE and PARRY 1992).

They constitute approximately 7–8% of all primary intracranial neoplasms and approximately 90% of the cerebellopontine angle (CPA) tumors. Symptoms of VS are variable and are related to the site of origin – internal auditory canal (IAC) vs CPA – and on the size of the tumor. Symptoms related to VS include SNHL, tinnitus, vestibular dysfunction, and other symptoms that are related to compression of the cranial nerves in the CPA cistern, or brain stem. Magnetic resonance imaging replaced CT for the detection of VS in the early 1990s, when the use of gadolinium made MR the most sensitive method to demonstrate these lesions (MULKENS et al. 1993). Careful analysis of the high-resolution T2-weighted images (CISS, GRASS, DRIVE, etc.) may allow in some cases to determine from which branch of the vestibulocochlear nerve the tumor is arising (SARTORETTI-SCHEFER et al. 2000) and virtual endoscopy may demonstrate the anatomical relationships of the tumor with the facial nerve (Fig. 14.16; NOWÉ et al. 2003).

Once the diagnosis of VS is made on MR, different treatment options are available. Surgery, radiation

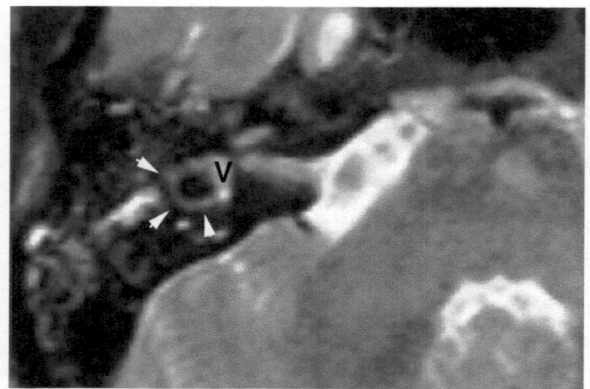
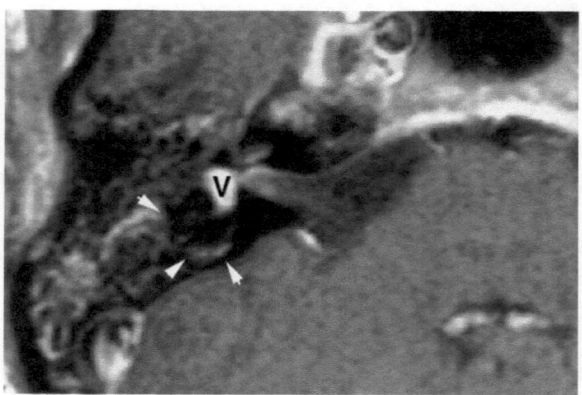

a   b

Fig. 14.15a,b. Fibrous obliteration of the membranous labyrinth following otosclerosis surgery of the right ear. **a** Axial T2-weighted image shows loss of signal at the level of the lateral semicircular canal (*small arrows*) and in a lesser extent also in the vesytibule (*V*), when compared to the other side. **b** Axial T1-weighted image after injection of gadolinium shows strong enhancement not only of the vestibule (*V*) and lateral semicircular canal (*small arrows*), but also at the level of the basal turn of the cochlea and in the internal auditory canal.

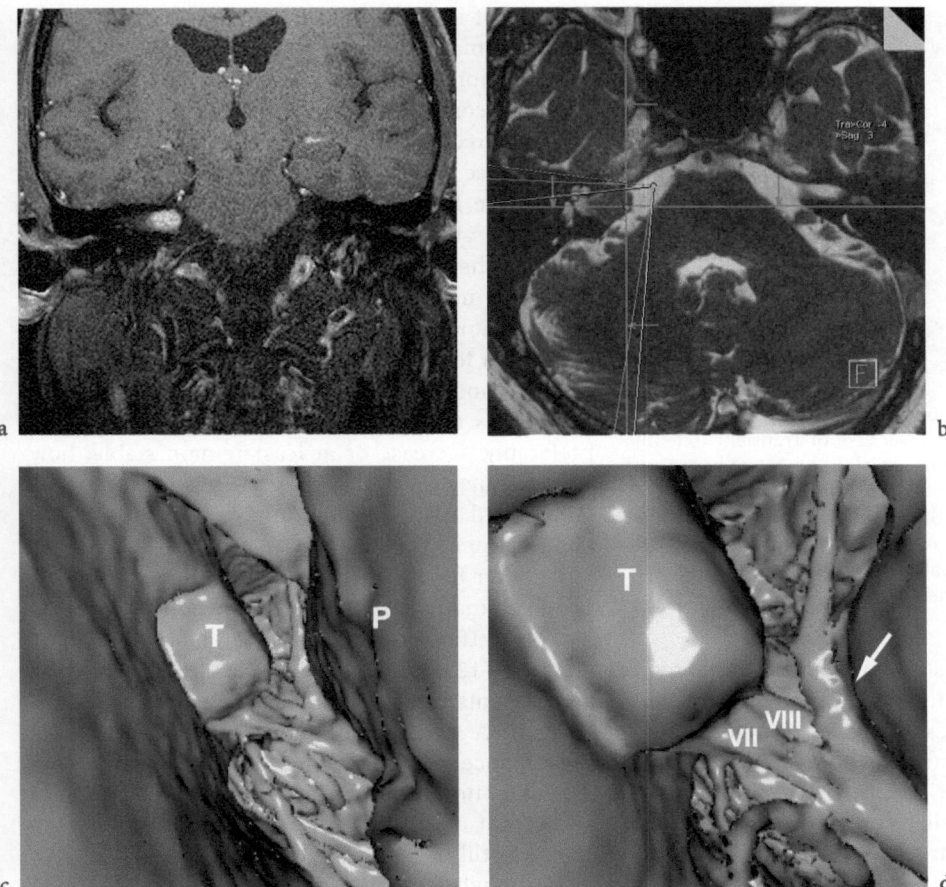

Fig. 14.16a–d. Virtual endoscopy in right vestibular nerve schwannoma (*VS*). **a** Coronal Gd-enhanced T1-weighted image with fat saturation shows an enhancing lesion in the right internal auditory canal, bulging into the right cerebellopontine angle cistern (*CPA*). **b** Axial thin-section CISS image (0.6-mm slice thickness). The fly-through volume is displayed as a pyramid, representing the field of vision of the virtual camera with the imaginary viewpoint at the top (A P and M L projection). **c, d** Virtual endoscopy images. The tumor (*T*) bulges into the right CPA cistern. The anatomical relationship of the tumor with the facial (*VII*) and vestibulocochlear (*VIII*) nerves is well seen. The curvature of the pons is readily identified (*P*). A blood vessel (*arrow*) loops across the facial-vestibulocochlear nerve bundle. (Courtesy of V. Nowé and P.M. Parizel, Antwerp)

therapy, or a conservative approach can be chosen, depending on patients' health and age, hearing status, facial nerve function, and other factors. Also, MR imaging features may influence the decision of the surgeon; therefore, size, location, and growth of the tumor, extension of VS into the fundus, signal intensity of the cerebrospinal fluid (CSF) in the IAC distal to the tumor, and intralabyrinthine signal intensity on T2-weighted images should be evaluated carefully (CASSELMAN 2001).

14.4.1
Conservative Management

Several publications have shown that VS are slowly growing tumors with an annual growth rate of 1–2 mm/year (CHARABI et al. 1998); therefore, some authors consider conservative management – "wait and scan" – a reasonable option for selected patients instead of radiation or surgery, especially in elderly patients (Fig. 14.17; HOISTAD et al. 2001); however, an increased number of newly diagnosed small tumors has been observed (CHARABI et al. 1998). Besides an increased awareness of otolaryngologists and earlier

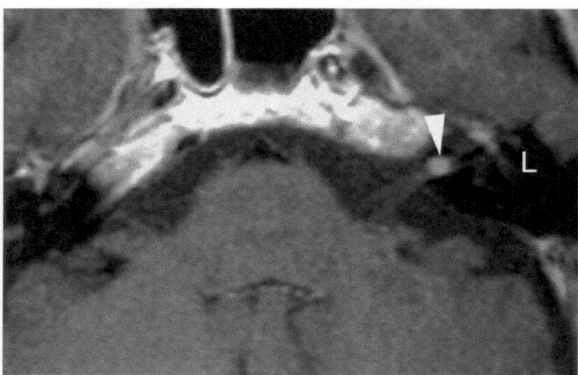

Fig. 14.17. "Wait-and-scan" policy in a 54-year-old man who was admitted to the hospital because of transient ischemic attacks (TIAs). An MR examination of the brain was performed to rule out ischemic disease. Axial gadolinium-enhanced T1-weighted image shows a small VS (*arrowhead*) as an incidental finding, since there were no related complaints, such as SNHL, vertigo, tinnitus, or facial palsy. Annual follow-up MR shows no increase in tumor volume

screening with ABR, this is above all due to the more widespread use of MR imaging. These patients with small VS have a significantly better change of hearing preservation after surgery (IRVING et al. 1995). It has been published that adopting the wait-and-scan policy, these tumors will grow and candidates for hearing preservation surgery will lose their eligibility (CHARABI et al. 1998). On the other hand, many VSs followed by periodic MR imaging studies do not grow (FUCCI et al. 1999); therefore, close follow-up in these patients is mandatory, and if tumor growth is observed on repetitive MR studies, patients should be operated on (P.H. Van de Heyning, personal communication). Evaluation of tumor volume on serial MR examinations can be done with 1-mm-thick contrast-enhanced T1-weighted gradient-echo images (MPRAGE, FSPGR, 3D TFE, etc.). Surface measurements in square millimeters, performed on all images on which the VS can be seen, will eventually allow calculation of the tumor volume (CASSELMAN 2001).

14.4.2
Radiosurgery

Gamma knife therapy has been considered as a safe and effective management for VSs, especially in preventing facial function and hearing. It can be applied as primary treatment in selected patients (e.g., patients in poor clinical condition with a growing VS), but is also an option as additional treatment for regrowing residual VS (BERTALANFFY et al. 2001). The purpose of irradiation in patients with VS is to provide maximal local tumor control while minimizing complications such as cranial nerve injuries. Excellent local control can be obtained when treatment is administered in moderate doses and reduction in the tumor dose may increase the hearing preservation rate in the future (BUSH et al. 2002). The possible induction of secondary neoplasia in the treatment field and the possibility of malignant transformation of benign neoplasia, even after 30–40 years, should not be ignored (MALIS 2000).

Regular follow-up MR examinations are to be performed, most often at 6-month intervals. The tumor volume, as evaluated on serial MR studies, should preferably decrease or at least remain stable; however, a transient volume increase has been reported and should not be confounded with tumor growth and treatment failure (PRASAD et al. 2000).

Another feature that has to be evaluated on serial MR examinations is tumor enhancement. A central loss of contrast enhancement is frequently observed within 6–12 months after radiosurgery; probably it represents central radiation necrosis (PRASAD et al. 2000). A significantly higher incidence of central nonenhancement has been observed in tumors that exhibited an early increase in size (Fig. 14.18; PRASAD et al. 2000). The true significance of these changes still needs to be established, since, interestingly enough, facial and vestibulocochlear nerve deficiency occur after this same time interval.

14.4.3
Surgery

Familiarity with the anatomic alterations of each surgical procedure makes it easier for the radiologist to interpret the postoperative findings. Most common approaches in VS surgery include a translabyrinthine (TL) approach, a retrosigmoid (RS) suboccipital craniotomy, and middle fossa temporal (MFT) craniotomy. There is a great deal of controversy about the ideal approach for the removal of VS (HABERKAMP et al. 1998). In addition to personal favors and experience of the surgeon, factors determining the surgical approach include patients' health and age, size of tumor, hearing status, and location of tumor in the IAC and the CPA. Careful reporting of the MR examination by the radiologist may help the surgeon in this perspective. If fluid is still present between the VS and the fundus of the IAC, a RS suboccipital or MFT approach can be used. If no fluid is left, a TL approach is preferred, leaving, however, the patient

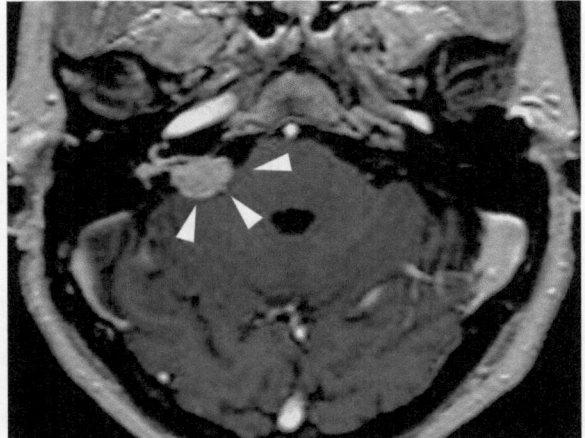

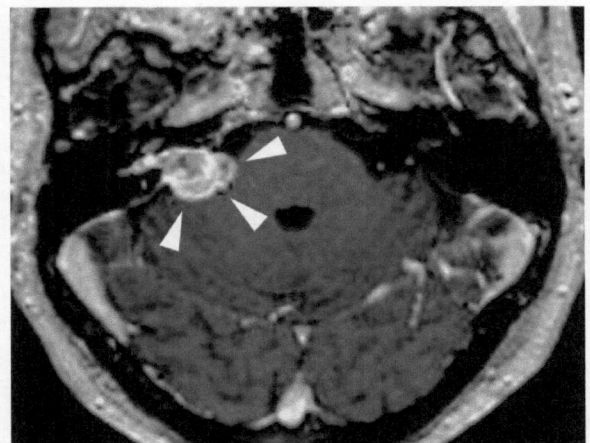

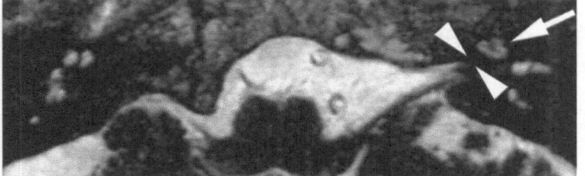

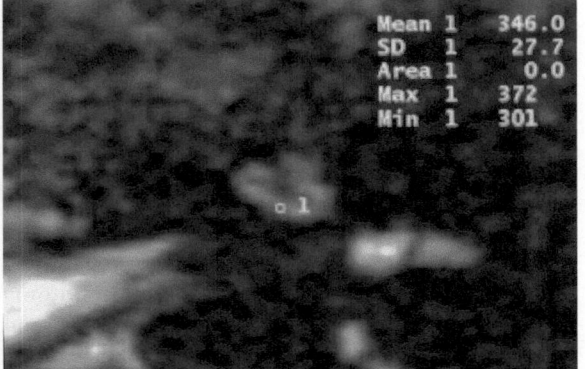

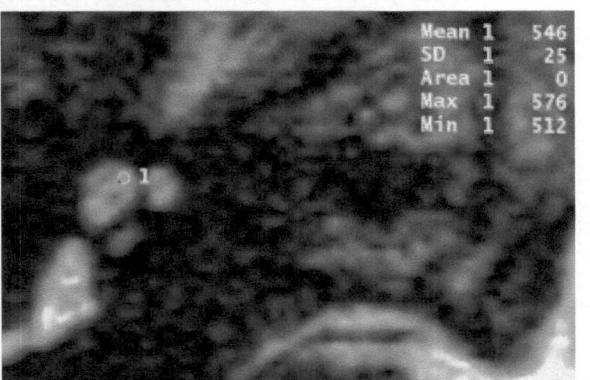

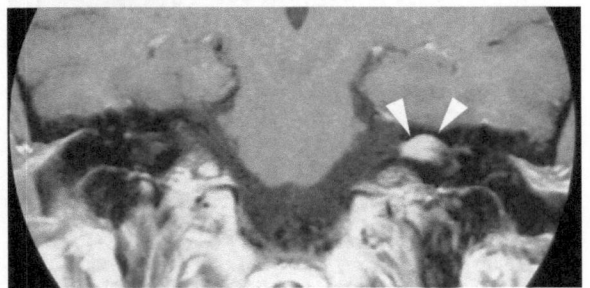

Fig. 14.18a, b. Gamma knife therapy for a right-sided VS (*arrowheads*) in a 61-year-old man. **a** Pre-treatment axial gadolinium-enhanced T1-weighted image. **b** Comparable MR image, 6 months after therapy. A transient volume increase and a central loss of contrast enhancement is observed after radiosurgery. This probably represents central radiation necrosis. (Courtesy of P. David and B. Balériaux, Brussels)

deaf (SOMERS et al. 2001). Another important sign is the signal intensity on T2-weighted images of the CSF between the VS and the fundus, and the signal intensity of the intralabyrinthine fluid (CASSELMAN 2001). Hearing preservation is achieved four times more often when normal signal intensity of these fluids is found than when the signal intensity of the fluid is decreased (SOMERS et al. 2001). It should, however, be noted that this signal changes on T2-weighted images only have been described with the 3DFT-CISS sequence (Siemens, Erlangen, Germany) at present time (Fig. 14.19). Similar ultra-thin heavily T2-weighted sequences provided by other manufacturers, such as GRASS (General Electric, Milwaukee, Wis.), or DRIVE (Philips, Best, The Netherlands) do not show these signal alterations (CASSELMAN 2002).

Fig. 14.19a–d. Intralabyrinthine signal intensity changes in a 43-year-old woman, presenting with left-sided SNHL. **a–c** Axial 0.7-mm-thick gradient-echo T2-weighted images at the level of the IAC show an intracanalicular mass lesion at the left side, extending into the fundus of the IAC (*arrowheads*). Loss of signal of the intralabyrinthine fluid in the left cochlea is observed (*arrow*) **a** Signal intensity of the intralabyrinthine fluid of the **b** right and **c** left cochlea can be measured using a small circular region of interest. A significant loss of signal at the left side can be observed. **d** Coronal T1-weighted image after injection of gadolinium shows strong and homogeneous enhancement of the mass (*arrowheads*) favoring the diagnosis of VS

14.4.3.1
Translabyrinthine Approach

The TL approach, the most direct route to the CPA, allows wide opening of the IAC for complete gross tumor removal and early identification of the facial nerve at the lateral limit of the IAC, with little or no cerebellar retraction (BRACKMANN 1992). Indications for TL resection are lesions of the IAC and CPA which are not amenable to hearing preservation, or intracanalicular tumors without serviceable hearing. A TL approach to the IAC is a transtemporal labyrinthectomy; it provides complete exposure of the IAC including the fundus, which facilitates tumor removal but destroys any residual hearing (Fig. 14.20; MCELVEEN et al. 1993). The mastoidectomy cavity and the translabyrinthine craniotomy can be secured with fat to prevent cerebrospinal fluid leaks. Also the eustachian tube and aditus ad antrum can be packed with temporalis muscle, oxidized regenerated cellulose (Surgicel), or both. On high-resolution T2-weighted images, the high signal from the normal fluid-filled membranous labyrinth may be (partially) absent. A large area of high signal on T1-weighted images from the fat filling the mastoidectomy may be the clue to the radiologist to determine which procedure has been performed.

14.4.3.2
Retrosigmoid Suboccipital Craniotomy

The RS approach of the IAC, is a frequently used technique to remove VS when hearing preservation is the issue. A suboccipital craniotomy is performed just behind the sigmoid sinus (Fig. 14.21). The cerebellum is gently pushed away to reach the pontocerebellar cistern. To reach the most lateral portion of the tumor, the posterior wall of the IAC is progressively drilled away (P.H. VAN DE HEYNING, personal communication). It has been described in the literature that this technique is hampered by the fact that final tumor removal is done without direct visualization of the fundus, with potential for tumor recurrence, and that therefore, close follow-up is mandatory when nodular or mass-like enhancement is noticed on postoperative MR studies in these patients (HABERKAMP et al. 1998). Once again, it is noted that postoperative results depend in large part on the experience of the surgeon.

14.4.3.3
Middle Fossa Temporal Craniotomy

Deep extension of the tumor into the IAC can make hearing preservation difficult when a retrosigmoid craniotomy is used; therefore, an MFT approach

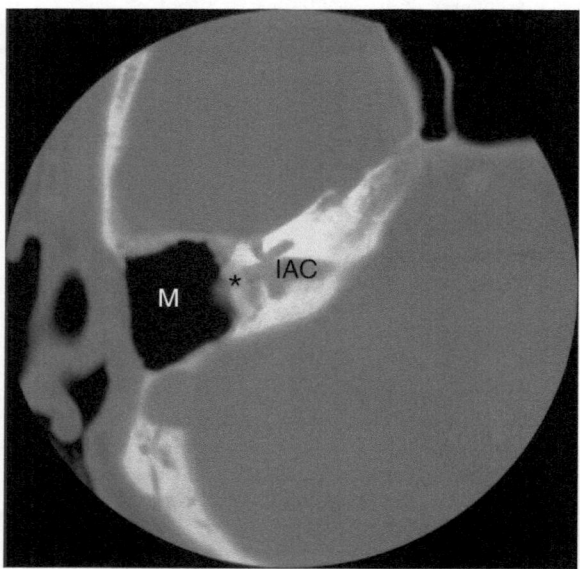

Fig. 14.20. Translabyrinthine approach for VS in a 53-year-old woman. Axial CT scan at the level of the mesotympanum shows the mastoid bowl (*M*) with partial removal of the cochlea and vestibule

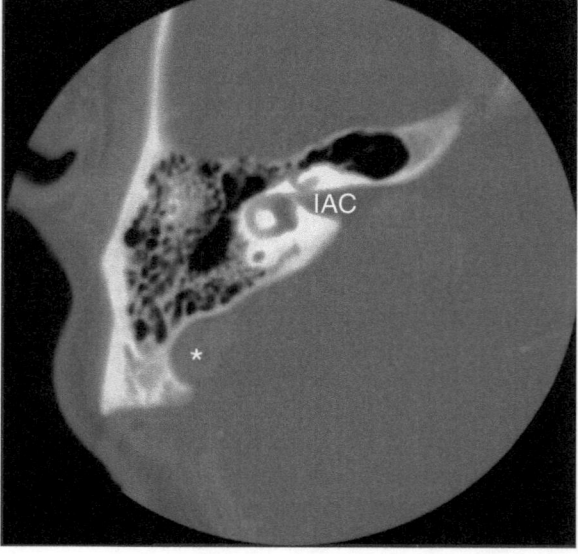

Fig. 14.21. Retrosigmoid approach for VS in a 59-year-old man. Axial CT scan at the level of the internal auditory canal (IAC) shows a retrosigmoid (*asterisk* indicates sigmoid sinus) suboccipital craniotomy

has been advocated (SELESNICK et al. 2001). Also in patients with small tumors and normal or nearly normal hearing, this approach can be considered. Almost complete exposure of the IAC, including the fundus, can be obtained performing a craniotomy at the level of the temporal squamosa. The operative defect that is created is closed with fascia, muscle, or both. A scar in the subcutaneous fat above the EAC is noticed on MR. Intense linear enhancement along the roof of the IAC indicates the use of a fascia graft to close the bony defect. Although the exposure of the fundus of the IAC is likely greater through the middle fossa approach, this factor may potentially lead to recurrences, particularly when the tumor arises from the inferior vestibular nerve (HABERKAMP et al. 1998).

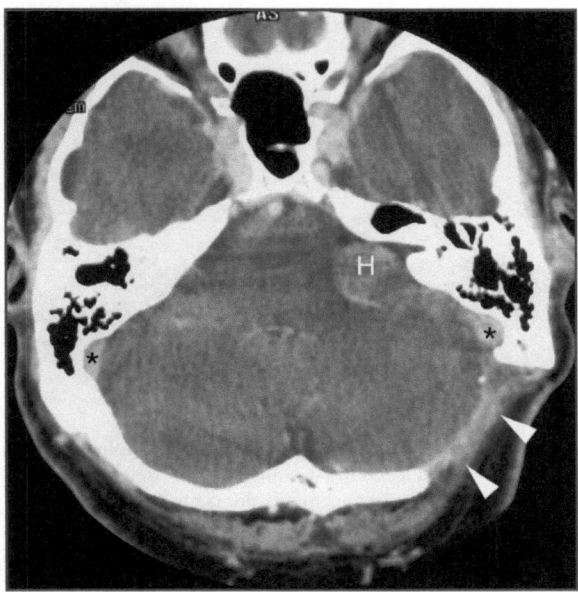

Fig. 14.22. Routine immediate postoperative CT within 24 h following resection of a VS to rule out complications. A retrosigmoid approach (*arrowheads*; *asterisk* indicates sigmoid sinus) has been chosen to gain access to the left cerebellopontine angle cistern. A hematoma (*H*) can be observed. There is no significant mass effect on the brain stem

14.4.4
Complications–Recurrences

14.4.4.1
Complications

Reported complications of VS surgery in the literature include facial nerve paresis, CSF leak, meningitis that may be associated with a CSF leak, injury to the anterior inferior cerebellar artery (AICA), posterior fossa hemorrhage, and hematoma at the CPA which may cause hydrocephalus due to fourth-ventricle compression. Uncommon complications include late cerebellar abscess, supratentorial subcortical white matter hemorrhages, and incomplete tumor removal if the tumor is densely adherent to the AICA or to the brain stem (WIET et al. 1992). In practice, routine immediate postoperative CT is performed within 24 h following resection to rule out hemorrhage (Fig. 14.22; HOROWITZ et al. 1996).

14.4.4.2
Recurrences

Tumor recurrences large enough to re-operate are rare, since re-growth after removal is rare and residual tumor tends to grow slowly (LYE et al. 1992). Tumor growth after surgery is presumed to represent residual rather than recurrent tumor, since microscopic foci of tumor may be left inadvertently or deliberately to preserve facial nerve function or hearing (CASS et al. 1991).

Intracranial enhancement after various neurosurgical procedures has been described in up to 100% of postoperative patients (MILLEN and DANIELS 1994).

It may be the result of disruption of the blood-brain barrier (blood-nerve barrier), chemical meningitis from subarachnoid hemorrhage, development of granulation tissue, and inflammation around resorbable surgical materials (e.g., absorbable gelatin powder and sponge, etc.). CASS et al. 1991 admitted that it is difficult to distinguish postoperative changes from residual tumor. WEISSMAN et al. (1997) described four different patterns of enhancement in the IAC after VS surgery: thin and thick linear enhancement; nodular enhancement; and mass-like enhancement. Thin and thick linear enhancement in the IAC is probably normal after surgery (Fig. 14.23); however, it may be difficult to differentiate thick linear enhancement from nodular enhancement; thickened leptomeninges may retract over time creating a nodular appearance that could mimic recurrent tumor (Fig. 14.24). Mass-like enhancement is difficult to interpret (Fig. 14.26); therefore, nodular and mass-like enhancement require close followup to monitor growth of residual tumor. Especially nodular enhancement in the fundus on postoperative studies after RS craniotomy merits special attention.

Also the membranous labyrinth may show postsurgical alterations. High signal on T1-weighted

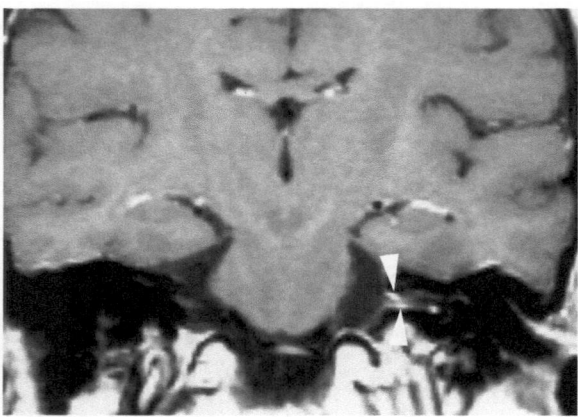

Fig. 14.23. Linear enhancement in the IAC following VS resection. Coronal contrast-enhanced T1-weighted image shows thin linear enhancement along and within the IAC (*arrowheads*), 6 months after surgery. No residual tumor can be observed

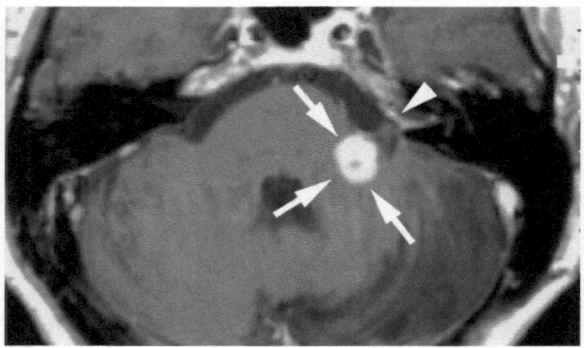

Fig. 14.25. Mass-like pattern of enhancement. Control MR examination, 2 years after resection of a VS shows clearly a residual tumor

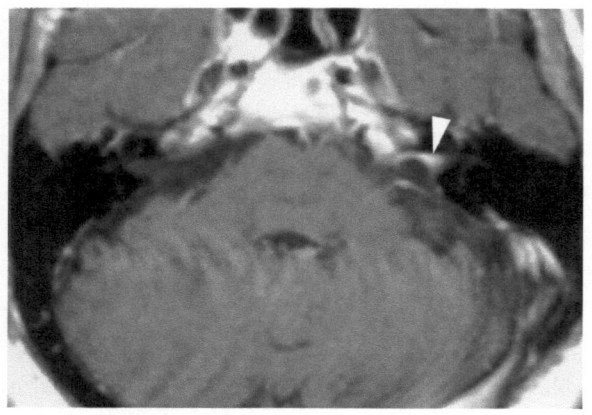

Fig. 14.24. Small nodular enhancement in the IAC following VS resection. Axial contrast-enhanced T1-weighted image shows small nodular enhancement in the IAC. Follow-up MR examinations (not shown) showed no evolution

images from the labyrinth, most frequently observed in the cochlea, is frequently encountered and may reflect blood metabolites (e.g., extracellular methemoglobin; WEISSMAN et al. 1997).

Hearing preservation surgery is often not possible, and the surgeon cannot always rely on subjective accounts of hearing loss or changes in the audiogram to monitor growth of potential residual tumor; therefore, MR imaging is indispensable in the postoperative management of VS patients. There are currently no uniform guidelines concerning the timing of postoperative MR studies. WEISSMAN et al. (1997) developed a postoperative imaging algorithm: within 6 months after surgery – but

no sooner than 1 month – a first MR examination that may serve as a baseline study is performed. If the baseline study shows only linear enhancement, MR examination is repeated after 1 year and subsequently after 3 years when no intervening changes appear. Nodular or mass-like enhancement on the baseline study warrants closer follow-up at intervals of 6 months. If the enhancement regresses, the interval may be increased to 1 year (WEISSMAN et al. 1997).

14.5
Role of Imaging After Cochlear Implantation

Cochlear implantation has become a standard treatment for profound deafness in adults and children who are born deaf, or become deaf early in life (RAMSDEN and GRAHAM 1995).

In most cases, deafness is the result from degeneration of the hair cells located within the organ of Corti. Conventional hearing aids only amplify the sound and are therefore of limited use to these patients. A cochlear implant (CI) is an artificial hearing device designed to produce useful hearing sensations by direct stimulation of residual functioning spiral ganglion cells of the cochlear nerve, bypassing the hair cells.

Multichannel devices have been shown to have significant advantages over a single-channel implant since they provide more complex sound analysis

(COHEN et al. 1993); therefore, these multichannel devices are preferred.

The multichannel CI consists of both surgically implanted and externally worn components (Fig. 14.26). The implanted components include the receiver/stimulator and the electrode array (Fig. 14.27). The receiver/stimulator is placed beneath the postauricular soft tissues. The electrode array is inserted into the scala tympani through the round window or through a cochleostomy, which is drilled into the cochlear promontory ±1 mm anterior and inferior to the round window (Fig. 14.28). The externally worn components include the speech processor and the headset. Recently, ear-level speech processors that are worn behind the ear became available (Fig. 14.29).

The hearing process using a CI is illustrated in Fig. 14.30. The speech processor does not just make sounds louder as does a hearing aid. Instead, it selects out the most significant sound information in the speech signal and then produces a pattern of electri-

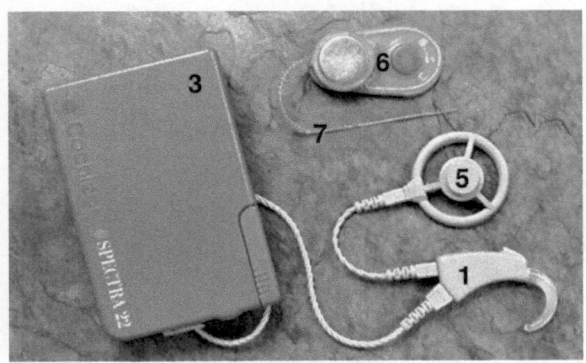

Fig. 14.26. Components of the multichannel cochlear implant (Med-El Combi 40+). The multichannel CI consists of both externally worn and surgically implanted components. The externally worn components include the headset and the speech processor. The implanted components include the receiver/stimulator and the electrode array

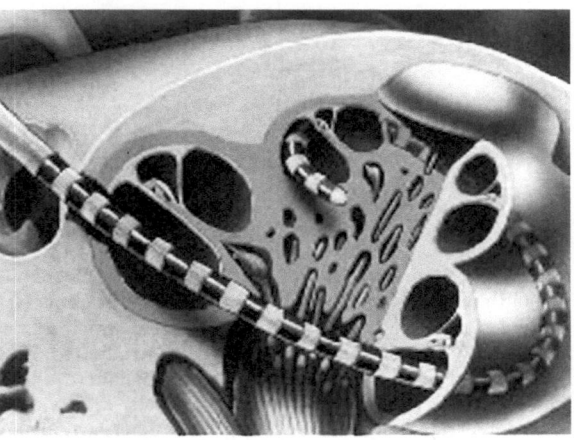

Fig. 14.28. The electrode array is inserted into the scala tympani through the round window or through a cochleostomy, which is drilled into the cochlear promontory

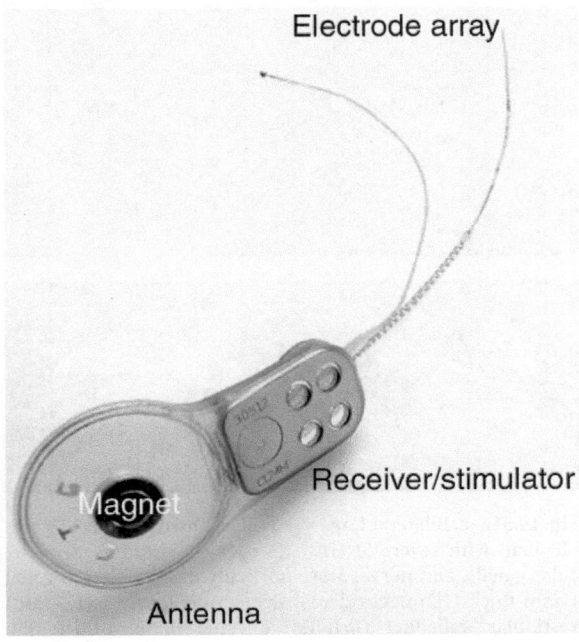

Fig. 14.27. The internal components of the cochlear implant

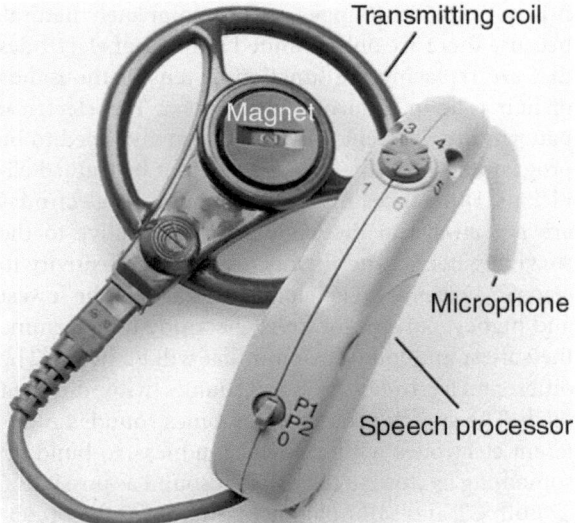

Fig. 14.29. ESPrit, cochlear limited, integrated speech processor, which is worn behind the ear, contains both a microphone and speech processor. The transmitter coil is magnetically coupled to the receiver/stimulator, which is placed beneath the postauricular soft tissues

the bony structures for surgical planning, such as the bony borders of the malformed labyrinth, thickness of the parietal or occipital bone, and pneumatization of the mastoid cells (WESTERHOF et al. 2001). Magnetic resonance imaging is superior for analyzing congenital malformations of the inner ear such as Mondini malformation and large vestibular aqueduct (Fig. 14.31), which is the most frequent con-

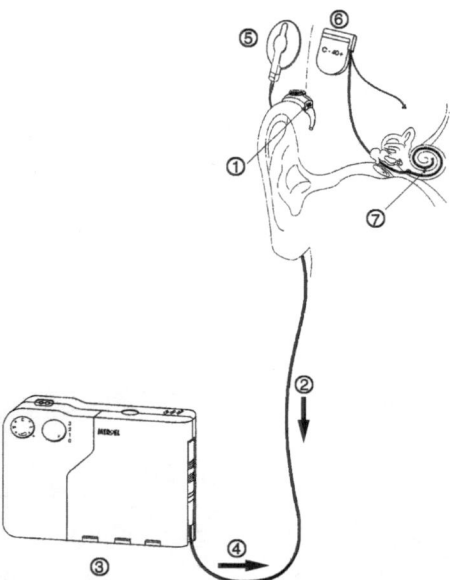

Fig. 14.30. Drawing illustrates the hearing process using a CI. Speech and other sounds are picked up by the microphone (*1*) and sent (*2*) to the speech processor (*3*). The processor translates the sounds into an electrical signal which is sent via a cable (*4*) to the transmitting coil (*5*). The radiofrequency transmission passes through the skin to the implant (*6*) which transforms this signal again into electrical pulses sent via the electrode array to stimulate hearing nerve fibers within the cochlea (*7*)

cal pulses in the patient's ear. This pattern is selected to match as close as possible to the original speech. It is not possible to make sounds completely natural, because there are only a limited number of electrodes that are replacing the function of tens of thousands of hair cells in a normal hearing ear. The electrical patterns are different for each person and need to be programmed into the speech processor by trained clinicians. Differences may arise because the electrodes are not always in the same position relative to the surviving nerves and the nerves vary in sensitivity to electrical currents. The clinician measures the lowest and highest current for every electrode to determine the softest and loudest sound that will be heard. The different electrodes produce sounds with different pitch. The speech processor combines sounds on different electrodes with different loudness, to build up something as close to the original sound as possible.

Both CT and MR imaging play a role in the preoperative workup of these patients. Not only the origin of the SNHL may be found, but also the likelihood of success of the procedure and the best side for implantation may be determined (HARNSBERGER et al. 1987). Computed tomography is superior to study

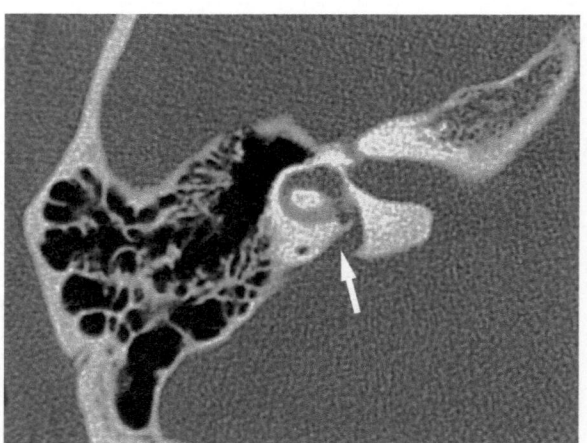

a

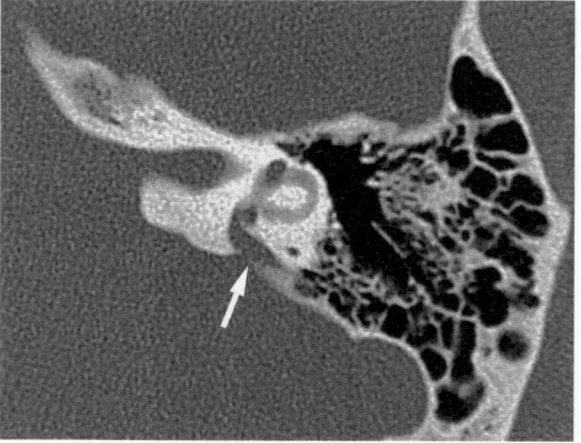

b

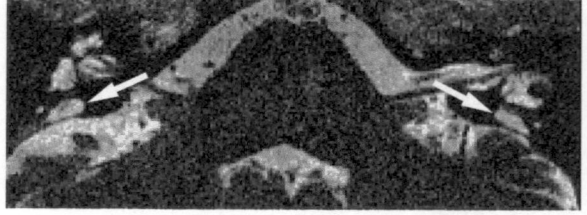

c

Fig. 14.31a–c. Bilateral large vestibular aqueduct in a 32-year-old man with severe SNHL. The cochlea, vestibule, semicircular canals, and nerves were normally developed. **a, b** Axial 1-mm-thick CT images demonstrate an enlarged (>1.5-mm) vestibular aqueduct (*arrows*). **c** Axial 0.7-mm-thick T2-weighted gradient-echo (3DFT-CISS) image demonstrates an enlarged endolymphatic duct (*arrows*)

genital anomaly causing SNHL (CASSELMAN et al. 1996). The most important malformations that MR imaging alone can identify are hypoplasia or aplasia of the vestibulocochlear nerve, since complete absence of the eighth nerve excludes the possibility of cochlear implantation (CASSELMAN et al. 1997). A positive brain-stem evoked potential predicts a functional nerve, but a negative test does not distinguish between a functional, damaged, or undeveloped nerve (BROWN et al. 1994)

Obliteration of the intralabyrinthine spaces, replacing the intralabyrinthine fluid, should also be reported to the clinician, since this may also preclude cochlear implantation. Fibrous obliteration, e.g., after trauma, inner ear surgery, after labyrinthitis/meningitis, or in autoimmune disease (Cogan's syndrome), can only be

detected on ultrathin T2-weighted images. Differentiation with ossification (Fig. 14.32; labyrinthitis ossificans) is only possible when both CT and MR imaging are performed (CASSELMAN 2001).

Early postoperative radiological evaluation is performed to confirm satisfactory intra-cochlear electrode placement. Electro-physiological examination by electrode mapping does provide information regarding electrode position but is not so precise and is not normally performed until around 1 month after surgery (LAWSON et al. 1998). This evaluation of CI can be performed with CT (Fig. 14.33); however, the best overview and assessment of insertion depth of the electrode array is probably obtained with plain films (Fig. 14.34; SHPIZNER et al. 1995). The number of active electrodes that have been inserted can be determined

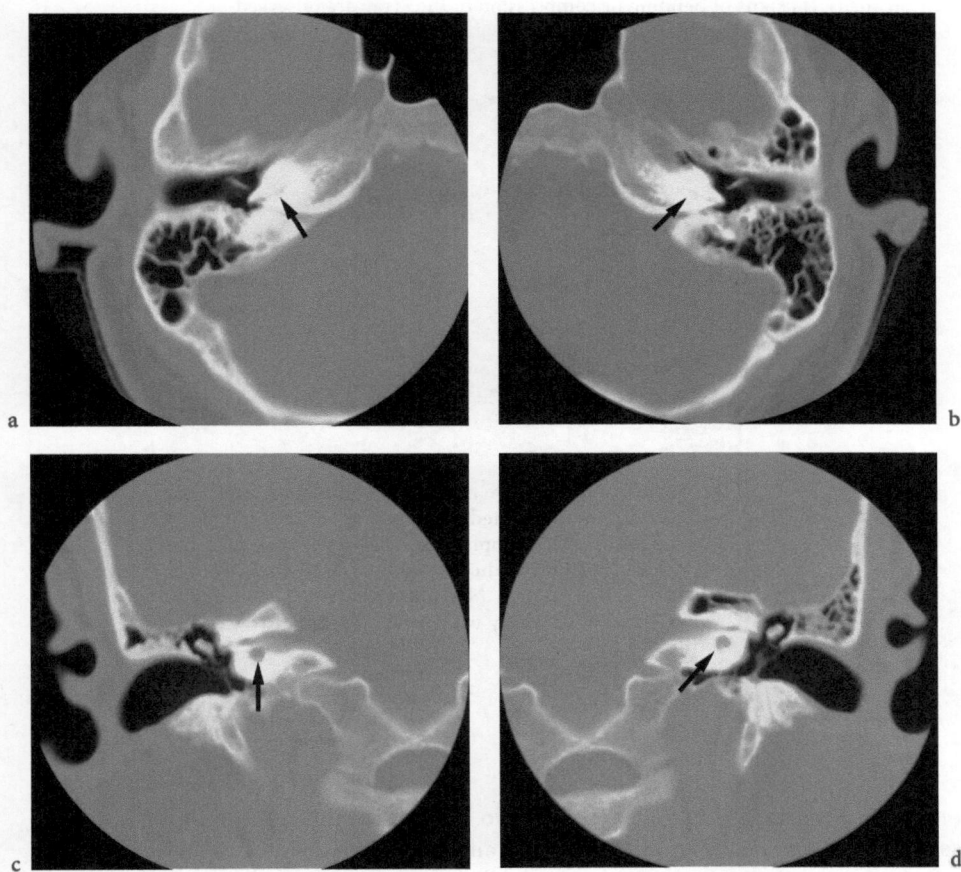

Fig. 14.32a–d. Bilateral labyrinthine ossification of the cochlea in a 30-year-old woman presenting with progressive SNHL. Diagnosis of chronic meningogenic labyrinthitis or labyrinthitis ossificans was made. **a, b** Axial 1.5-mm-thick CT images demonstrate an almost total bony obliteration of the basal, middle, and apical turn of the cochlea (*arrows*). **c, d** Coronal 1.5-mm-thick CT images confirm bony obliteration of the middle turn of the cochlea. Faint ossific changes are seen at the level of the apical turn of the cochlea which has been relatively spared (*arrows*). Note the normal aspect of the tympanic cavities, making the diagnosis of tympanogenic labyrinthitis less probable

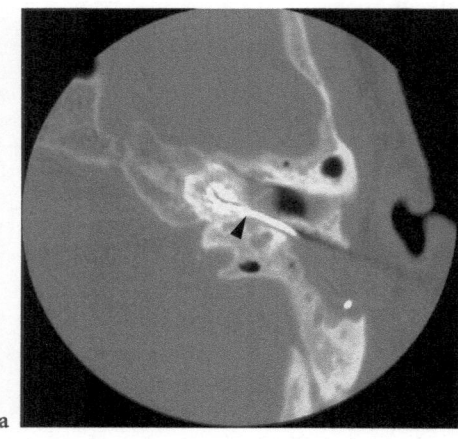 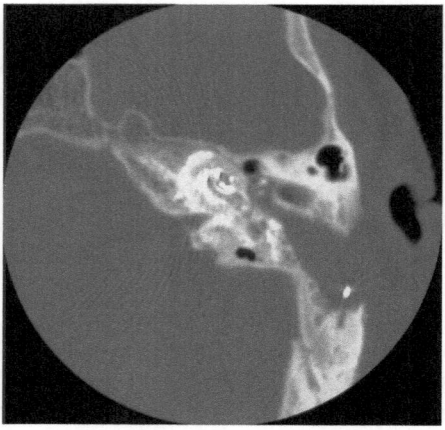

Fig. 14.33a, b. Postoperative CT after cochlear implantation in a 65-year-old man with bilateral profound mixed hearing loss as a result of combined cochlear and fenestral otospongiosis. **a** Axial 1-mm-thick CT image at the level of the round window demonstrates intracochlear position of the electrode array, inserted through the round window (*arrowhead*). Full insertion of all electrodes in the cochlea is observed. **b** Axial CT image 1 mm below **a**. The normally inserted electrode array follows a gentle curve within the different cochlear turns. No signs of bending or compression of the array are observed

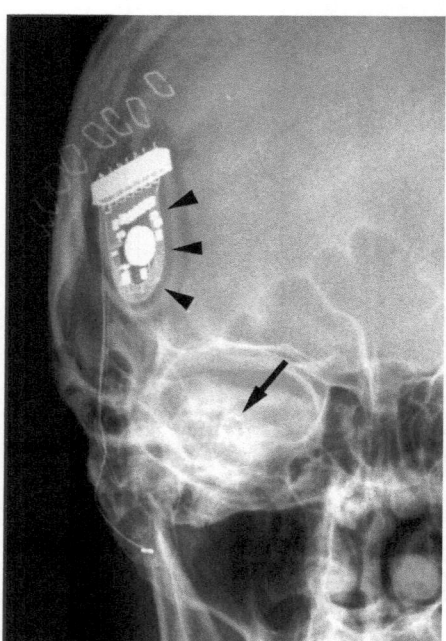

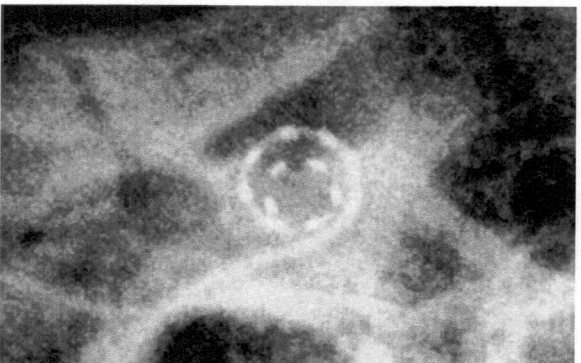

Fig. 14.34a, b. Postoperative transorbital anteroposterior view demonstrates all implanted components of a right-sided multichannel cochlear implant. **a** The *arrow* indicates the intracochlear position of the electrode array, the *arrowheads* the receiver/stimulator. **b** Magnification view shows gentle curving of the of the array with regular spacing between the electrodes

and possible complications, such as electrode kinking or slippage, can be assessed. Conventional radiography with a modified Stenver's projection is performed (MARSH et al. 1993). A vertical line along the axis of the superior semicircular canal passes through the vestibule and bisects the electrode at the round window region where the cochleostomy is sited and defines the lateral margin of the cochlea. Due to the improved contrast resolution, digital radiography enables each electrode to be identified in relation to the inner ear structures and the number of intra-cochlear electrodes can be readily determined. Radiation exposures are less for the digital technique (±120 μGy) when compared with conventional radiography (±470 μGy) or CT scanning (±950 μGy). This technique can also be used intraoperatively (LAWSON et al. 1998).

The presence of a functioning cochlear implant (CI) has been considered as an absolute contraindication to MR examination for many years. It has been demonstrated, however, that most of the electromagnetic interferences between the CI and the MR system remain within acceptable limits under certain conditions (Teissl et al. 1998). Nevertheless, force, torque, and fixation are risks that must be considered. The radiologist together with the clinician, after assessment of the relative risks involved, must judge whether the MR examination should be performed. Various models of CI exist and possible interactions are dependent on MR equipment and procedures that are used. It is therefore recommended to consult the manufacturer of a CI to determine whether the particular MR imaging procedure intended to be performed is considered safe (Teissl et al. 1998).

14.6
Conclusion

When otoscopic examination and audiological findings fail to demonstrate the reason why surgery has been unsuccessful, patients are often sent to the radiologist for imaging of the temporal bone. Motivation for the examination, comprehensive information regarding the surgical procedure, and previous examinations for comparison are indispensable to allow correct analysis of the imaging findings.

Helical CT or MDCT is the imaging modality of choice in the evaluation of patients who had middle ear surgery for COM and otosclerosis. The use of MR imaging, including diffusion-weighted images, may be an alternative to second-look surgery, if recurrent cholesteatoma can be distinguished from granulation tissue. Also rare complications after stapes surgery may require further MR imaging, when CT is not contributive.

Magnetic resonance imaging is the imaging modality of choice in the follow-up and after surgery in patients with VS.

Plain (digital) radiography is used to confirm correct position of the electrode array after cochlear implantation. In patients with a functioning cochlear implant, MR imaging should be performed only if there is a strong medical indication.

Acknowledgements. The author acknowledges his colleagues P.M. Parizel, J.W. Van Goethem, and O. d'Archambeau, Department of Radiology, Universitair Ziekenhuis Antwerpen–University of Antwerp, for their kind readiness to share their imaging files. Thanks also to P. H. Van de Heyning, Department of ENT Surgery, Universitair Ziekenhuis Antwerpen–University of Antwerp, for his clinical input.

References

Bertalanffy A, Dietrich W, Aichholzer M et al. (2001) Gamma knife radiosurgery of acoustic neurinomas. Acta Neurochir (Wien) 143:689–695

Blaney SP, Tierney P, Oyarazabal M et al. (2000) CT scanning in „second look" combined approach tympanoplasty. Rev Laryngol Otol Rhinol 121:79–81

Brackmann DE (1992) Middle fossa approach for acoustic tumor removal. Clin Neurosurg 38:603

Brown CJ, Abbas PJ, Fryauf-Bertschy H et al. (1994) Intraoperative and postoperative electrically evoked auditory brain stem responses in nucleus cochlear implant users: implications for the fitting process. Ear Hear 15:168–176

Bush DA, McAllister CJ, Loredo LN et al. (2002) Fractionated proton beam radiotherapy for acoustic neuroma. Neurosurgery 50:270–273

Cass SP, Kartush JM, Wilner HI et al. (1991) Comparison of computerized tomography and magnetic resonance imaging for the postoperative assessment of residual acoustic tumor. Otolaryngol Head Neck Surg 104:182–190

Casselman JW (2001) MRI aids evaluation of temporal bone disease. Diagn Imaging March/April:60–65

Casselman JW (2002) High resolution MR of the inner ear with the DRIVE sequence. Presented at the meeting of the Neuroradiology Section of the Royal Belgian Association of Radiology (KBVR-SRBR)

Casselman JW, Kuhweide R, Ampe W et al. (1996) Inner ear malformations in patients with sensorineural hearing loss: detection with gradient-echo (3DFT-CISS) MR imaging. Neuroradiology 38:278–286

Casselman JW, Offeciers FE, Govaerts PJ et al. (1997) Aplasia and hypoplasia of the vestibulocochlear nerve: diagnosis with MR imaging. Radiology 202:773–781

Causse JB, Causse JR, Wiet RJ et al. (1983) Complications of stapedectomies. Am J Otol 4:275–280

Chakeres DW, Mattox DE (1985) Computed tomographic evaluation of non-metallic middle-ear prostheses. Invest Radiol 20:596–600

Charabi S, Thomsen J, Tos M et al. (1998) Acoustic neuroma/vestibular schwannoma growth: past, present and future. Acta Otolaryngol 118:327–332

Cohen NL, Waltsman SB, Fisher SG (1993) Prospective randomised study of cochlear implants. N Engl J Med 328:233–237

D'Archambeau O, Parizel PM, Koekelkoren E et al. (1990) CT diagnosis and differential diagnosis of otodystrophic lesions of the temporal bone. Eur J Radiol 11:22–30

De Bruijn AJG (2000) Clinical and audiological aspects of stapes surgery in otosclerosis. PhD thesis, Amsterdam University

Declau F, Van Spaendonck M, Timmermans JP et al. (2001) Prevalence of otosclerosis in an unselected series of temporal bones. Oto Neurotol 22:596–602

Eldridge R, Parry D (1992) Vestibular schwannoma (acoustic neuroma). Concensus development conference. Neurosurgery 30:962–964

Fucci MJ, Buchman CA, Brackmann DE et al. (1999) Acoustic

tumor growth: implications for treatment choices. Am J Otol 20:495–499

Haberkamp TJ, Meyer GA, Fox M (1998) Surgical exposure of the fundus of the internal auditory canal: anatomic limits of the middle fossa versus the retrosigmoid transcanal approach. Laryngoscope 108:1190–1194

Harnsberger HR, Dart DJ, Parkin JL et al. (1987) Cochlear implant candidates: assessment with CT and MR imaging. Radiology 164:53–57

Hasso AN, Opp RL, Swartz JD (1996) Otosclerosis and dysplasias of the temporal bone. In: Som PM, Curtin HD (eds) Head and neck imaging, 3rd edn. Mosby Year-Book, St. Louis, pp 1432–1448

Hermans R, Marchal G, Feenstra L et al. (1995) Spiral CT of the temporal bone: value of image reconstruction at submillimetric table increments. Neuroradiology 37:150–154

Hoistad DL, Melnik G, Mamikoglu B et al. (2001) Update on conservative management of acoustic neuroma. Otol Neurotol 22:682–685

Horowitz SW, Leonetti JP, Azar-Kia B et al. (1996) Postoperative radiographic findings following acoustic neuroma removal. Skull Base Surg 6:199–205

Irving RM, Beynon GJ, Viani L et al. (1995) The patient's perspective after vestibular schwannoma removal: quality of life and implications for management. Am J Otol 16:331–337

Klingebiel R, Bauknecht HC, Kaschke O et al. (2001) Virtual endoscopy of the tympanic cavity based on high-resolution multislice computed tomographic data. Otol Neurotol 22:803–807

Kösling S, Woldag K, Meister EF et al. (1995) Value of computed tomography in patients with persistent vertigo after stapes surgery. Invest Radiol 12:712–715

Kösling S, Bootz F (2001) CT and MR imaging after middle ear surgery. Eur J Radiol 40:113–118

Kwok P, Fisch U, Strutz J et al. (2002) Stapes surgery: How precisely do different prostheses attach to the long process of the incus with different instruments and surgeons? Otol Neurotol 23:289–295

Lawson JT, Cranley K, Toner JG (1998) Digital imaging: a valuable technique for the postoperative assessment of cochlear implantation. Eur Radiol 8:951–954

Lye RH, Pace-Balzan A, Ramsden RT et al. (1992) The fate of tumour rests following removal of acoustic neuromas: an MRI Gd-DTPA study. Br J Neurosurg 6:195–202

Maheshwari S, Mukherji SK (2002) Diffusion-weighted imaging for differentiating recurrent cholesteatoma from granualtion tissue after mastoidectomy: case report. AJNR 23:847–849

Malis L (2000) Gamma surgery for vestibular schwannoma (letter). J Neurosurg 92:892–894

Mark AS, Casselman JW (2002) Anatomy and disease of the temporal bone. In: Atlas SW (ed) Magnetic resonance imaging of the brain and spine, 3rd edn. Lippincott, Williams and Wilkins, Philadelphia, pp 1363–1432

Mark AS, Fitzgerald DC (1993) Segmental enhancement of the cochlea on contrast-enhanced MR: correlation with the frequency of hearing loss and possible sign of perilymphatic fistula and autoimmune labyrintihtis. AJNR 14:991–996

Marquet J, Greten WL, Van Camp KJ (1972) Considerations about the surgical approach in stapedectomy. Acta Otolaryngol 74:406–410

Marsh MA, Xu J, Blarney PJ et al. (1993) Radiologic evaluation of multichannel intracochlear implant insertion depth. Am J Otol 14:386–391

McElveen JT Jr, Wilkins RH, Molter DW et al (1993) Hearing preservation using the modified translabyrinthine approach. Otolaryngol Head Neck Surg 108:671–679

Millen SJ, Daniels DL (1994) The effect of intracranial surgical trauma on gadolinium-enhanced magnetic resonance imaging. Laryngoscope 104:804–813

Mukherji SK, Mancuso AM, Kotzur IM et al. (1994) CT of the temporal bone: findings after mastoidectomy, ossicular reconstruction, and cochlear implantation. AJR 163:1467–1471

Mulkens TH, Parizel PM, Martin J-J et al. (1993) Acoustic schwannoma: MR findings in 84 tumors. AJR 160:395–398

Nowé V, Verstreken M, Wuyts FL et al. (in press) Enhancement of the otic capsule in active retrofenestral otosclerosis AJR

Pickuth D, Brandt S, Berghaus A et al. (2000) Vertigo after stapes surgery: the role of high resolution CT. BJR 73:1021–1023

Prasad D, Steiner M, Steiner L (2000) Gamma surgery for vestibular schwannoma. J Neurosurg 92:745–759

Ramsden R, Graham J (1995) Cochlear implantation. Br Med J 311:1588

Rangheard AS, Marsot-Dupuch K, Mark AS et al. (2001) Postoperative complications in otospongiosis: usefulness of MR imaging. AJNR 22:1171–1178

Raut VV, Toner JG, Kerr AG et al. (2002) Management of otosclerosis in the UK. Clin Otolaryngol 27:113–119

Sartoretti-Schefer S, Kollias S, Valavanis A (2000) Spatial relationship between vestibular schwannoma and facial nerve on three-dimensional T2-weighted fast spin-echo MR images. AJNR 21:810–816

Selesnick SH, Rebol J, Heier LA et al. (2001) Internal auditory canal involvement of acoustic neuromas: surgical correlates to magnetic resonance imaging findings. Otol Neurotol 22:912–916

Shea JJ Jr (1958) Fenestration of the oval window. Ann Otol Rhinol Laryngol 67:932–951

Shellock FG, Schatz CJ (1991) Metallic otologic implants: in vitro assessment of ferromagnetism at 1.5 T. AJNR 12:279–281

Shpizner BA, Holliday RA, Roland JT et al. (1995) Postoperative imaging of the multichannel cochlear implant. AJNR 16:1517–1524

Somers T, Casselman J, de Ceulaer G et al. (2001) Prognostic value of magnetic resonance imaging findings in hearing preservation surgery for vestibular schwannoma. Otol Neurotol 22:87–94

Stone JA, Mukherji SK, Jewett BS et al. (2000) CT evaluation of prosthetic ossicular reconstruction procedures: What the otologist needs to know. Radiographics 20:593–605

Swartz JD, Harnsberger HR (1998) The middle ear and mastoid. In: Swartz JD, Harnsberger HR (eds) Imaging of the temporal bone, 3rd edn. Thieme, New York, pp 47–169

Swartz JD, Wolfson RJ, Russell KB et al. (1983) High resolution computed tomography of the middle ear and mastoid, part III. Surgically altered anatomy and pathology. Radiology 148:461–464

Teissl C, Kremser C, Hochmair ES et al. (1998) Cochlear implants: in vitro investigation of electromagnetic interference at MR imaging – compatibility and safety aspects. Radiology 208:700–708

Thomassin JM, Braccini F (1999) Role of imaging and endoscopy in the follow up and management of cholesteatomas operated by closed technique. Rev Laryngol Otol Rhinol (Bord) 120:75–81

Tierney PA, Pracy P, Blaney SP et al. (1999) An assessment of the value of the preoperative computed tomography scans prior to otoendoscopic "second look" in intact canal wall mastoid surgery. Clin Otolaryngol 24:274–276

Vanden Abeele D, Coen E, Parizel PM et al. (1999) Can MRI replace a second look operation in cholesteatoma surgery? Acta Otolaryngol 119:555–561

Veillon F, Charneau D, Le Guennec P et al. (1991) Imagerie tomodensitométrique des récidives post-opératoires des cholestéatomes. In: Veillon F (ed) Imagerie de l'oreille. Flammarion Médecine-Sciences, Paris, pp 153–170

Weissman JL, Hirsch BE, Fukui MB et al. (1997) The evolving MR appearance of structures in the internal auditory canal after removal of an acoustic neuroma. AJNR 18:313–323

Westerhof JP, Rademaker J, Weber BP et al. (2001) Congenital malformations of the inner ear and the vestibulocochlear nerve in children with sensorineural hearing loss: evaluation with CT and MRI. J Comput Assist Tomogr 25: 719–726

Wiet RJ, Teixido M, Liang JG (1992) Complications in acoustic neuroma surgery. Otolaryngol Clin North Am 25:389–412

Williams MT, Ayache D, Elmaleh M et al. (2000) Helical CT findings in patients who have undergone stapes surgery for otosclerosis. AJR 174:387–392

Willliams MT, Ayache D, Alberti C et al. (2003) Detection of postoperative residual cholesteatoma with delayed contrast-enhanced MR imaging: initial findings. Eur Radiol 13:169–174

The Clinician's View

I. Dhooge

Postoperative temporal bone imaging can be helpful in clarifying early postoperative complications (CSF leak, facial nerve problems, dislocation of a prosthesis, etc.) and late complications (brain herniation, ossicular problems, etc.).

Postoperative imaging can also be a tool for follow-up after removal of a tumor in the temporal bone or in the cerebello-pontine angle or the internal auditory canal.

In the management of cholesteatoma, it would be very helpful if imaging could differentiate between residual cholesteatoma, cholesterol granuloma or effusion, granulation tissue, or scar formation. Then, the second-stage exploratory tympanotomy could in some cases be omitted.

In cochlear implant surgery, postoperative imaging can confirm the integrity and correct positioning of the implant. Information about insertion length and angle, and distance from the modiolus, may be useful for managing frequency mapping and optimizing speech-coding strategies.

15 Virtual Endoscopy of the Middle and Inner Ear

E. Neri, C. Cappelli, S. Berrettini, D. Caramella, C. Bartolozzi

CONTENTS

15.1
Introduction

Virtual endoscopy is a technique developed for providing a simulation of fiberoptic endoscopy, and is obtained by processing CT, MR, or US data sets (Rubin 1996; Yuh 1999). Using dedicated computer programs it is possible to fly through or around 3D objects; the anatomical structure to display from the inside is selected by means of a data-set segmentation obtained with 3D processing techniques based on surface or volume rendering.

Vining first reported the application of virtual endoscopy in the study of bronchi (1993) and colon (1994); however, virtual endoscopy can also be applied to the study of multiple organs (i.e., larynx and trachea, paranasal sinuses, brain ventricles, vessels, biliary tract, urinary tract, joints). Among these, the study of the middle and inner ear has peculiar and distinctive aspects. In fact, the direct exploration of the middle ear cavity requires in vivo the perforation of the tympanic membrane, and it is usually per-

E. Neri, MD; C. Cappelli, MD; D. Caramella, MD;
C. Bartolozzi, MD
Division of Diagnostic and Interventional Radiology, Department of Oncology, Transplants, and Advanced Technologies in Medicine, University of Pisa, Via Roma 67, 56100 Pisa, Italy
S. Berrettini
Division of Otolaryngology, Department of Neuroscience, University of Pisa, Via Roma 67, 56100, Pisa, Italy

formed during surgery; inversely, virtual endoscopy displays the middle ear cavity simply by processing CT data sets and obviously is not invasive.

Another advantage of virtual endoscopy is to simplify the interpretation of high-resolution computed tomography (HRCT), data of which are commonly presented with axial and coronal planes. The display of complex anatomy with 3D perspectives is of specific aid for otolaryngologists in planning surgery.

Actually, virtual endoscopy is the only uninvasive method which generates 3D views of the anatomical component of the middle and inner ear, closely resembling otoendoscopic images. This chapter reviews the technical approach to virtual endoscopy of the middle and inner ear, and covers the potential clinical applications of the technique.

15.2
Technical Approach to Virtual Endoscopy

15.2.1
Image Acquisition

The first application of virtual endoscopy to the study of the middle ear was carried out by Pozzi Mucelli (1997), who reported the use of conventional CT images for the generation of 3D reconstructions. In further and succeeding experiences (Neri 2000a, 2001a; Klingebiel 2001a; Nakasato 2001) virtual endoscopy was obtained with single or multislice spiral CT, which provided a direct volumetric acquisition at millimetric or sub-millimetric resolution.

With regard to imaging parameters, our group has proposed the following protocol with single-slice spiral CT (Neri 2000a): axial and coronal acquisitions; beam collimation 1 mm; pitch 1 and 0.5 mm reconstructions spacing; bone algorithm; tube rotation 1 s; tube current 160 mA with 120 kVp; field of view 16 cm.

Caldemeyer (1999) performed a study in 19 patients comparing axial 0.5 mm thickness and 0.2 mm reconstructions spacing helical protocol with direct axial and coronal 1 mm thickness conventional CT. The experience showed that helical CT with 3D coronal reconstruction produces diagnostic images comparable with or superior to conventional 1-mm technique because helical CT can obtain thinner slices. Recently, KLINGEBIEL (2001a) reported that the anatomical details of the middle ear, with specific regard to the stapes superstructure, seems to be better displayed using the multislice technology, because of an improved spatial resolution and an increased scan speed, which reduces motion-related artifacts; therefore, 3D rendering of high-resolution multislice CT data of the petrous bone may be expected to provide endoluminal views of superior image quality. The protocol proposed by KLINGEBIEL (2001b) includes 0.5-mm slice thickness, 0.2-mm reconstruction interval, pitch factor 0.75, and tube current 50 mA with 120 kV.

Using a fixed matrix multislice CT with detector width 1.25 mm, two detectors can be enrolled permitting each to contribute for the half of the width, equal to 0.63 mm. The reconstruction spacing can be variable but equal to or less than 0.63 mm. With such protocol, used in our institution, coronal images are created with multiplanar reconstructions in order to reduce the examination time and the patient dose. The necessity to generate coronal images derives from the lack of gantry angulation in multislice CT (KLINGEBIEL 2001a). In such condition direct coronal acquisition is difficult to obtain even positioning the patient in a forced hyperextension of the neck.

15.2.2
Technical Basis of Virtual Endoscopy

Virtual endoscopy provides an endoscopic-like view from a given point within the ear. The perspective is reached by using a so-called ray-casting reconstruction algorithm (ROTH 1982), which projects virtually parallel rays toward the target field of view from a source point (the eye of the observer, which is the point in which the endoscope is positioned). These rays traverse the acquired volume along a divergent direction, and applying surface or volume rendering algorithms the encountered voxels are classified and displayed.

In normal patients the classification process of the middle ear structures can be done in optimal conditions since the density of bone is easy to differentiate from the air content of the tympanic cavity. Inversely, the presence of abundant fluid or tissue, like in otitis media or cholesteatoma, make difficult the separation between air, bone, and the conditions themselves.

The reconstruction of the bone is quite simple for any image processing software, whether surface or volume rendering based. In the first case the edge line between bone and other tissues is identified at a density threshold of 160–200 HU. Again below this value, the mucosal layer of the tympanic cavity can be found and represented if the threshold value is reduced dramatically to identify the passage between mucosa and air, as –500 HU (POZZI MUCELLI 1997).

The knowledge of these segmentation values is extremely important to determine whether or not the reconstructed images correspond to reality. For this a comparison between real anatomy and 3D reconstructed endoluminal views from seven formalin-fixed anatomical specimens was performed by our group (NERI 2000a). We found a 100% agreement between the observations for endoluminal views and anatomical sections, even if in 2 cases the complete visualization of the middle ear cavity could not be initially obtained for the presence of tissue remnants within the external auditory meatus.

15.3
Study of the Middle Ear

The middle ear is an aerated space difficult to access by direct human vision. External otoendoscopy allows a partial visualization of the tympanic cavity. In general, it fails to demonstrate the epitympanum because of the superimposition of the ossicular chain. The unique possibility to display the cavity is to create a tympanic perforation, essentially motivated by the need of surgical guidance. The technique is called "trans-tympanic" endoscopy. ZINI (1967) first tried to visualize the middle ear using a system of micromirrors which allowed the exploration of the retrotympanum. This method, called indirect microtympanoscopy, is still used in clinical practice. MER (1967) was the first to introduce the fiberoptic endoscope into the tympanic cavity through a perforation of the tympanic membrane, and more later the middle ear cavity was visualized with a needle, rigid otoscope by NOMURA (1982).

Modern endoscopes are based on Hopkins' optic system with variable diameter (minimum 1 mm in diameter), and length and angle variable on the basis of the region to explore. The application of trans-tympanic endoscopy is almost reserved to the guidance of otosurgical procedures through a transtympanic access.

As mentioned above Pozzi Mucelli (1997) firstly tried to generate virtual endoscopic images of the tympanic cavity and obtained excellent results in visualizing the ossicular chain.

Virtual endoscopy of the middle ear can be obtained by creating a virtual empty space within the tympanic cavity with surface- or volume-rendering techniques. In both cases the inner wall of the tympanic cavity is displayed (Fig. 15.1). The majority of software available in commerce allow to point with the computer mouse within the air space and generate an endoscopic view of the cavity. The virtual endoscope can be inserted into any space of the middle ear and directed to look toward specific structures or anatomical regions.

In recent work carried out by our group (Neri 2001a), a virtual endoscopic analysis of the tympanic cavity was performed by following the traditional imaging proper of transtympanic endoscopy.

Creating an endoscopic perspective from the external auditory canal to look toward the middle ear, the tympanic cavity has been divided into four regions: retrotympanum (posterior); epitympanum (superior); protympanum (anterior); and hypotympanum (inferior; Fig. 15.1a, b).

The anatomy of the middle ear, as it is displayed by virtual endoscopy, is hereby described according to this anatomical partition.

The retrotympanum represents more than half of the posterior part of the tympanic cavity and includes the oval and round windows (Parlier-Cuau 1998). In this region virtual endoscopy displays its typical eminences and depressions, represented by pyramidal and styloid eminences (looking as smoothed elevations of the medial wall of the tympanic cavity), pyramidal ridge, ponticulus, subiculum, and eminence of tympanic portion of the facial nerve (Fig. 15.1c, b).

On the basis of such ridges, eminences, and depressions, the retrotympanum can be divided into four regions: superomedial or *posterior sinus tympani*; inferomedial or *sinus tympani*; superolateral or *facial sinus*; and inferolateral or *fossula of Grivot* (Guerrier 1976; Espinoza 1989).

The posterior sinus tympani can be visualized under the eminence of the facial nerve canal and posteriorly to the oval window. The sinus tympani appears as a parietal depression the landmarks of which are given by the ponticulus (superior), the subiculum (inferior–anterior), the pyramidal crest and eminence (posterior–lateral), and the promontory (anterior; Pickett 1995). Thomassin (1994) described three types of sinus tympani on the basis

of the sinus visibility at transtympanic endoscopy. The same evaluation is feasible at virtual endoscopy: sinus tympani of *easy exploration* is characterized by a simple depression of the tympanic wall; sinus tympani of *difficult exploration* is represented by a depression of the wall that continues into a deep canal through the tympanic wall and opens into the retrotympanum with a little orifice; and the *intermediate* sinus tympani has a deep but large canal.

The promontory appears as an eminence with a smooth surface that covers the round window. This opens from the tympanic cavity into the scala tympani of the cochlea.

The protympanum represents the anterior part of the tympanic cavity that includes the pharyngo-tympanic tube. The superior border of the tube divides the protympanum from the sinus epitympani. The inferior border separates the tube from the internal carotid artery.

The hypotympanum represents the floor of the tympanic cavity, separated from the mesotympanum by a horizontal plane crossing through the inferior border of the external meatus. The floor is characterized by many osseous crests the development of which is related to the dimensions of the sub-labyrinthic cells.

The epitympanum represents the superior part of the tympanic cavity the posterior landmark of which is given by the aditus ad antrum, the anterior by the supratubal recess, the lateral by the scutum, and the medial by the wall of the labyrinth at the level of the second portion of the facial nerve. The superior landmark is represented by the tegmen tympani. A significant advantage of virtual endoscopy in the exploration of the epitympanum is the demonstration of the entire incudo-malleolar joint obtained after the electronic removal of ligaments and soft tissues (Fig. 15.1d).

The ossicular chain can be entirely evaluated with multiple perspectives, because the endoscope can be positioned in any virtual space of the middle ear. From the external auditory canal, the long process of incus, the stapes, and the handle of malleus can be visualized (Fig. 15.1b). Meanwhile, from a point of view located within the hypotympanum virtual endoscopy can easily display the stapes, the lenticular process of incus (incudostapedial joint), and the long process of incus (Fig. 15.1e); however, the visualization of stapes superstructure is difficult to obtain for the partial-volume effects of CT acquisition. Multislice CT can improve the visualization of anatomic details such as the anterior and posterior crus of the stapes, because of its higher spatial resolution (Klingebiel 2001b).

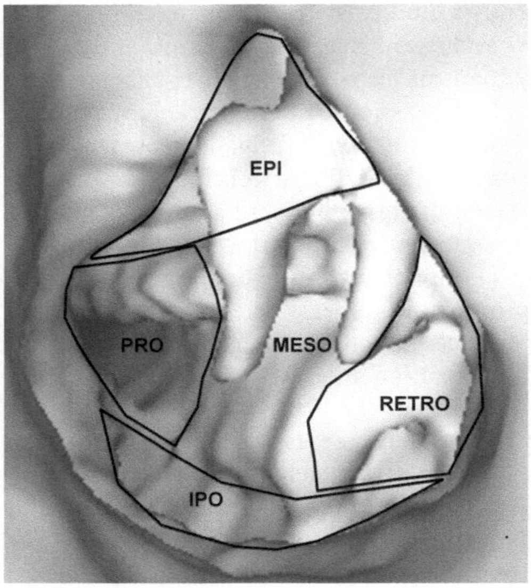

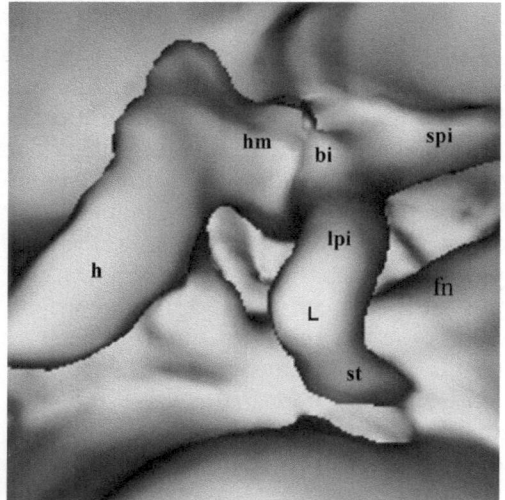

Fig. 15.1a–e. Multislice CT virtual endoscopy of the middle ear. **a** A typical virtual endoscopy perspective obtained from the external auditory canal (*EAC*) demonstrates the anatomical partition of the tympanic cavity: retrotympanum (*RETRO*), epitympanum (*EPI*), protympanum (*PRO*), hypotympanum (*IPO*) and mesotympanum (*MESO*). **b** The same endoscopic view displays the head of malleus (*hm*) and the handle (*h*), the body (*bi*), the long process of incus (*lpi*), the pyramidal eminence (*pe*), the promontory (*prom*), and the pharyngo-tympanic tube (*ptt*). **c** Detailed perspective of the retrotympanum, showing an intermediate-type sinus tympani (*st*), the round window fossa (*rwf*), the styloid (*se*), and pyramidal (*pe*) eminences. **d** Detailed perspective of the epitympanum created from the aditus ad antrum. The incus and the incudo-malleolar joint are visible, as well as the eminence of the lateral semicircular canal (*lsc*) and tegmen tympani (*tt*). The perspective resembles those obtained during a mastoidectomy. **e** Endoscopic view obtained positioning the virtual endoscope within the hypotympanum looking toward the epitympanum. The entire ossicular chain is visualized, including the short process of incus (*spi*) the lenticular process (*L*), and the stapes (*st*). In the medial wall the eminence of the tympanic portion of the facial nerve is well delineated (*fn*)

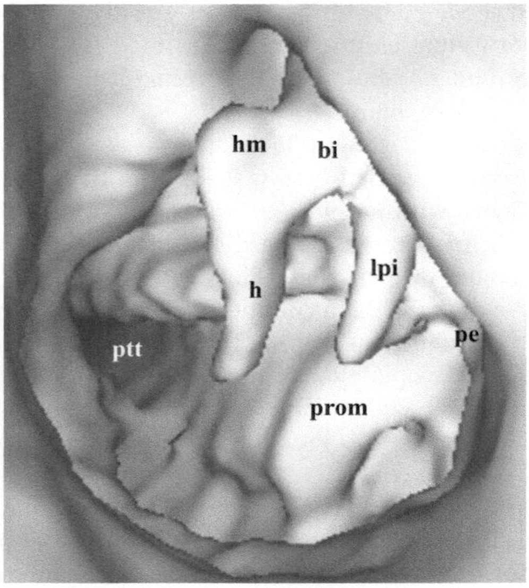

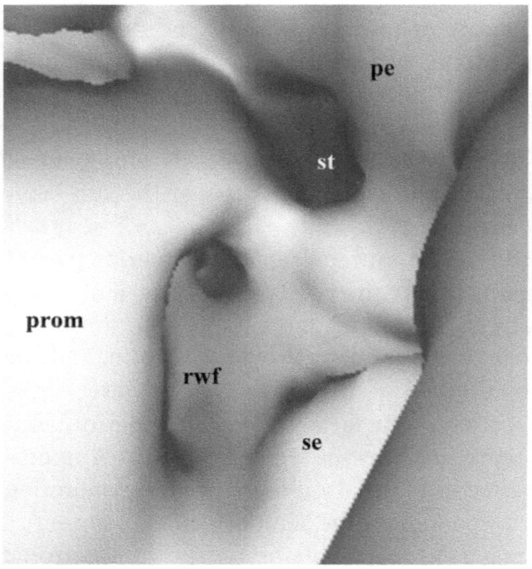

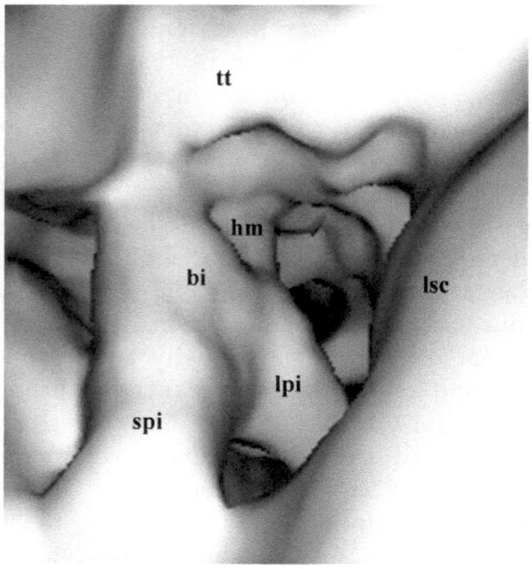

In the study of the middle ear the role of virtual endoscopy is still unclear. One potential advantage could be the preoperative display of patient's specific anatomy, helping surgeons to avoid damaging important structures such as the facial nerve. In the case of pathological conditions affecting the middle ear, and in particular space-occupying lesions, such as cholesteatoma, the endoscopic perspective is obstructed by the filling tissue. A careful removal of the tissue allows demonstration of the damage of the ossicular chain (Fig. 15.2). Another example is in the evaluation of large otosclerotic plaques which involves the medial wall of the tympanic cavity. In this case virtual endoscopy allows quantification of their extension (Fig. 15.3).

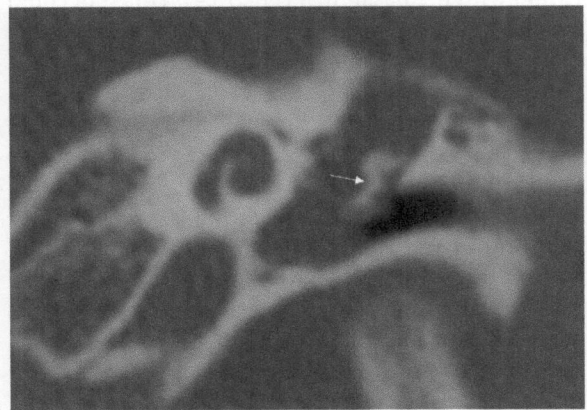

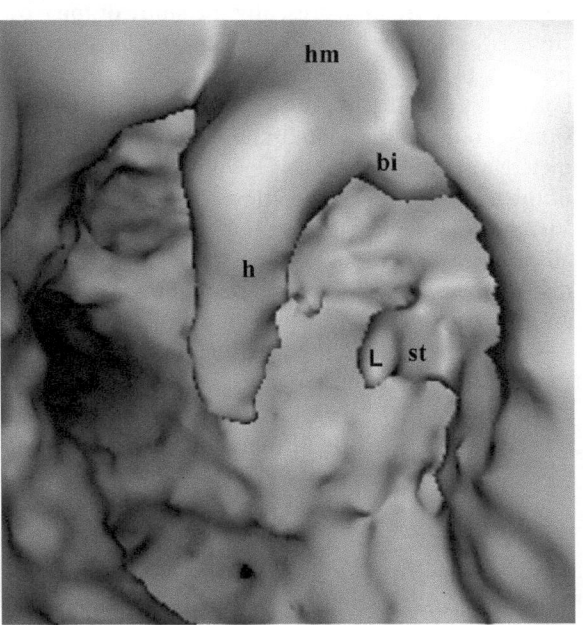

Fig. 15.2a, b. Computed tomography of the left petrous bone in cholesteatoma. **a** The coronal CT crossing through the handle of malleus (*arrow*) shows the complete filling of the tympanic cavity by soft tissue. **b** Virtual endoscopy obtained after electronic removal of the tissue demonstrates the erosion of the long process of incus and the residues of body (*bi*), lenticular process (*L*), and stapes (*st*)

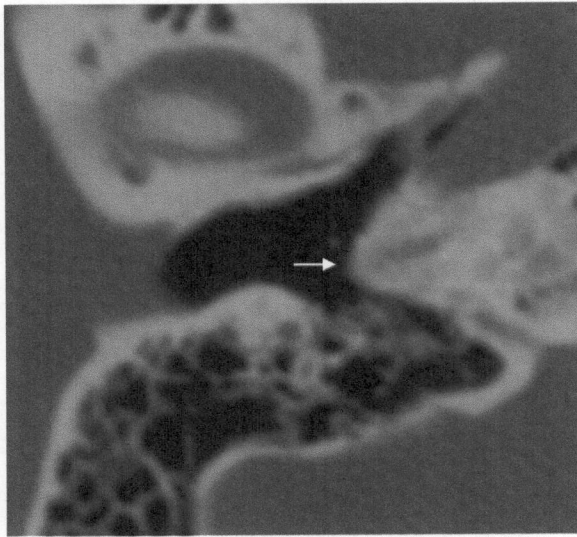

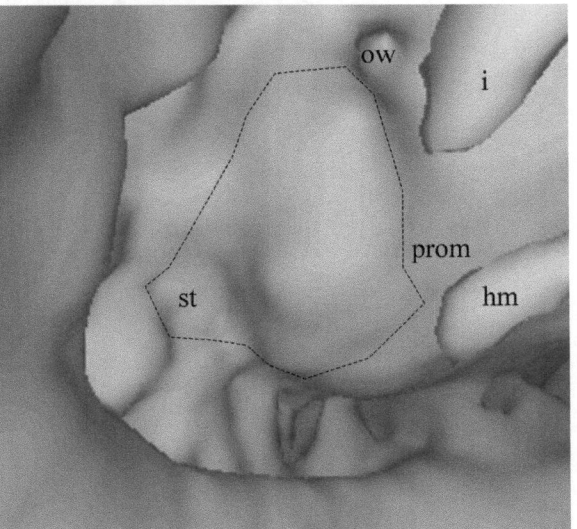

Fig. 15.3a, b. Computed tomography of the right petrous bone in otosclerosis. **a** The axial CT crossing through the basal turn of the cochlea shows otospongiotic changes in the bone labyrinth and the wide ossification of the round window fossa. **b** A CT virtual endoscopy of the retrotympanum demonstrates the complete coverage of the round window fossa by the otosclerotic plaque, with consequent occlusion of the round window. The sinus tympani is involved as well

15.4
Study of the Inner Ear

Computed tomography is the modality of choice for study of the osseous structures of the inner ear. The imaging protocol is the same used for middle ear imaging, because the study must be performed for both these anatomical regions; however, if we exclude conditions such as retrocochlear otosclerosis or petrous bone trauma, presently the study of the labyrinth is essentially managed by magnetic resonance imaging (MRI). Virtual endoscopy can be applied to both CT and MRI. With CT (Neri 2000a) it is possible to remove the membranous labyrinth allowing the creation of a virtual space within the bone spaces of the inner ear for the positioning of the endoscope. Virtual endoscopy of the bone labyrinth provides visualization of the vestibule from which it is possible to display the orifice of the basal turn of the cochlea, the ampulla, the openings of the semicircular canals, and the oval and round windows (located, respectively, in the lateral wall and on the floor of the vestibule).

To generate 3D data sets of the labyrinth with MRI it is necessary to use dedicated sequences, such as 3D fast spin-echo and constructive interference in steady state sequence, heavily T2-weighted for a selective visualization of the endolymph. The acquisition should also be done at high-resolution (0.5- or 1-mm partition thickness), in order to display the cochlea turns or the course of semicircular canals. In parallel to CT, virtual endoscopy of MRI data sets provides a direct view of the inner wall of the vestibule, of the openings of semicircular canals, and of the communication with the basal turn (Fig. 15.4). This tool could be of potential advantage in evaluating the patency of the basal turn of the cochlea, which is important when a cochlear implantation is planned.

As an alternative to virtual endoscopy, volume rendering can also provide external views of the labyrinth in both the cases of CT and MRI. With the method proposed by Tomandl (2000) for CT, after selection of the volume of interest, the application of the direct volume rendering produces 3D semitransparent representations of the cochlea, vestibule, semicircular canals, and labyrinthine segments of the facial canal. In order to obtain the selective visualization of these structures and reduce the superimposition of other bony walls (such as the medial wall of

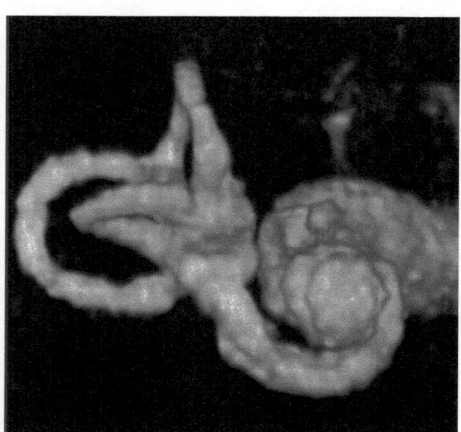

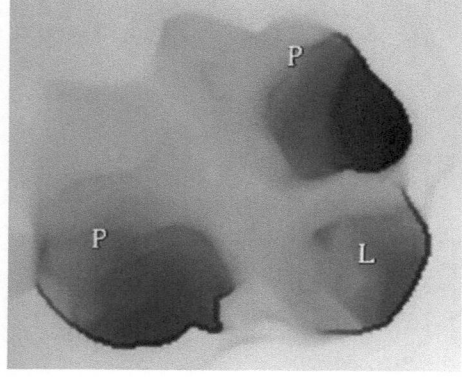

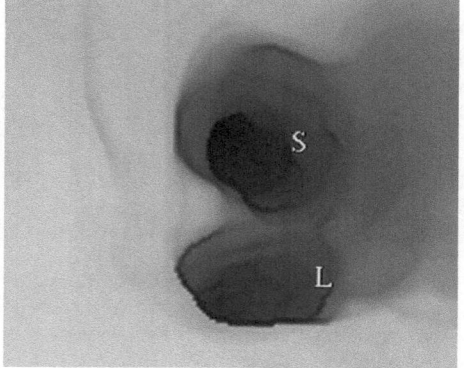

Fig. 15.4a–c. An MR virtual endoscopy of the right inner ear. **a** An MR volume rendering of the right labyrinth (lateral view) from high-resolution MRI data set. **b** An MR virtual endoscopy generated from the vestibule displays the two openings of the posterior semicircular canal (*p*) and the medial opening of the lateral semicircular canal (*l*). **c** A similar perspective shows the contralateral opening of the lateral semicircular canal (*l*) in relationship with the opening of the superior semicircular canal (*s*)

the tympanic cavity), different cut planes may be helpful.

Our group (NERI 2001b) has experienced the use of CT volume rendering in the follow-up of patients who underwent cochlear implantation. Volume rendering was helpful to display the path of cochlear electrode and to establish the length of the portion inserted in the cochlea.

In the case of MRI, volume rendering displays external 3D reconstruction of the endolymph which has a high signal intensity on T2-weighted images (NERI 2000). From the same data sets virtual endoscopy can generate endoluminal views from the vestibule, showing the communication with semicircular canals and the basal turn of the cochlea (BOOR 1999).

15.5
Conclusion

From the technical point of view visualization of the middle ear cavity, or the inner ear spaces, are quite simple with virtual endoscopy, and are not time-consuming. The major concern still regards the usefulness of this technique in clinical practice. To date, the main advantage of virtual endoscopy seems to be in the correlation between virtual and real anatomy, which could help surgeons in recognizing the patient's specific anatomical features prior to surgical interventions.

References

Boor S (1999) Virtual endoscopy of the inner ear and the auditory canal. Neuroradiology 42:543–547

Caldemeyer KS (1999) Temporal bone: comparison of isotropic helical CT and conventional direct axial and coronal CT. AJR 172:1675–1682

Espinoza J (1989) Surgical anatomy of the retrotympanum: on 25 temporal bones. Rev Laryngol Otol Rhinol 110: 507–515

Guerrier Y (1976) Topographic and surgical anatomy of the petrous bone. Acta Otorhinolaryngol Belg 30:22–50

Klingebiel R (2001a) High-resolution petrous bone imaging using multi-slice computerized tomography. Acta Otolaryngol 121:632–636

Klingebiel R (2001b) Virtual endoscopy of the tympanic cavity based on high-resolution multislice computed tomographic data. Otol Neurotol 22:803–807

Mer SB (1967) Fiberoptic endoscope for examining the middle ear. Arch Otolaryngol 85:387–393

Nakasato T (2001) Virtual CT endoscopy of ossicles in the middle ear. Clin Imaging 25:171–177

Neri E (2000a) Virtual endoscopy of the middle and inner ear with spiral computed tomography. Am J Otol 21:799–803

Neri E (2000b) High-resolution magnetic resonance and volume rendering of the labyrinth. Eur Radiol 10:114–118

Neri E (2001a) Virtual endoscopy of the middle ear. Eur Radiol 11:41–49

Neri E (2001b) Outcome of cochlear implantation: assessment by volume rendered spiral CT. Eur Radiol 11:256

Nomura YA (1982) Needle otoscope (an instrument of otoendoscopy of the middle ear). Acta Otolaryngol (Stockh) 93:73–79

Parlier-Cuau C (1998) High-resolution computed tomographic study of the retrotympanum. Anatomic correlations. Surg Radiol Anat 20:215–220

Pickett BP (1995) Sinus tympani: anatomic considerations, computed tomography, and a discussion of the retrofacial approach for removal of disease. Am J Otol 16:741–750

Pozzi Mucelli RS (1997) Virtual endoscopy of the middle ear with computed tomography. Radiol Med 94:440–446

Roth SD (1982) Ray casting for solid modelling. Comput Graph Image Proc 18:109–144

Rubin GD (1996) Perspective volume rendering of CT and MR images: applications for endoscopic imaging. Radiology 199:321–330

Thomassin JM (1994) La chirurgie sous guidage endoscopique des cavitée de l'oreille moyenne. Springer, Berlin Heidelberg New York

Tomandl BF (2000) Virtual labyrinthoscopy: visualization of the inner ear with interactive direct volume rendering. Radiographics 20:547–558

Vining DJ (1993) Virtual bronchoscopy: a new perspective for viewing the tracheobronchial tree. Radiology 189:438

Vining DJ (1994) Virtual colonoscopy. Radiology 193:446

Yuh EL (1999) Virtual endoscopy using perspective volume-rendered three-dimensional sonographic data: technique and clinical applications. AJR 172:1193–1197

Zini C (1967) La microtympanoscopie indirecte. Rev Laryngol Otol Rhinol 88:736–738

16 Functional MR Imaging of Hearing

S. Sunaert

CONTENTS

16.1
Introduction

Functional magnetic resonance imaging (fMRI) enables mapping of neuronal activity throughout the brain in individual healthy subjects and patients in a non-invasive way. In the auditory system it can be used to study auditory processing from brain stem to cortex, and has the potential to provide considerable new insight into the auditory neurophysiology.

At present, the application of fMRI in the auditory system is still at an early stage. Contrary to the explosive growth of fMRI studies in other sensory and motor modalities (mainly vision, somatosen-

S. Sunaert, MD, PhD
MR Research Center, Department of Radiology, University
Hospitals K.U. Leuven, Herestraat 49, 3000 Leuven, Belgium

sory, and motor), fMRI in the auditory system has been hindered by the acoustic MRI scanner noise, mainly originating from the gradient switching of the MR scanner, which interacts with the functional activation of the auditory system induced by the experimental acoustic stimuli. Many efforts have been undertaken – with success – in order to overcome the former technical difficulty. Since then, new information concerning central auditory function and dysfunction has emerged.

We first review the state-of-the-art fMRI technical principles necessary to study auditory processing. We primarily discuss the effects of scanner-generated acoustic noise and the approaches to overcome this problem. We then review the normal functional anatomy of the auditory system, from brain stem to auditory cortical regions. Finally, we review the applicability of fMRI to subjects with auditory disorders.

16.2
FMRI Technique

Functional MRI utilizes the physiological changes in oxy- and deoxyhemoglobin concentration in small cortical blood vessels upon neuronal activation without the need for radiation or the administration of contrast media or radioactive tracers. The spatial accuracy of the technique is of the order of millimeters and the temporal resolution of the order of 1 s, or even sub-second in case of event-related fMRI. This chapter describes the basic technical principles of fMRI and the specific methodological aspects when studying the auditory system.

16.2.1
Brain Activation and Cerebrovascular Physiology: Neurovascular (Un)Coupling

Activation of a brain area (Fig. 16.1) produces an increase in the metabolism of its neuronal and glial

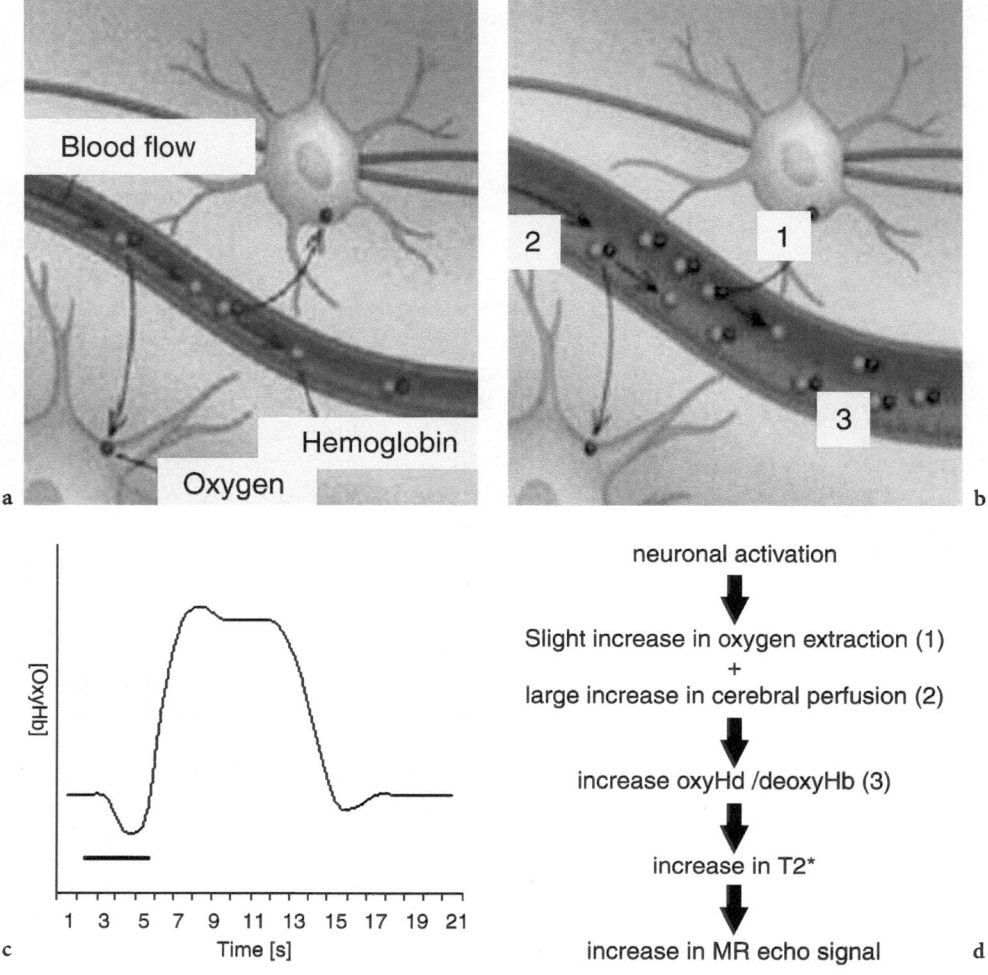

Fig. 16.1a–d. Brain activation and cerebrovascular (un)coupling. **a** Situation at rest, and **b** during neuronal activation. **c** Time course of the change of oxyhemoglobin concentration upon regional neuronal activation (during horizontal bar). **d** Sequence of cerebrovascular changes leading to increased T2* and MR signal

cell populations, accompanied by an increase in the regional cerebral blood flow (rCBF) in that area. This coupling between rCBF and neuronal metabolism has been under investigation ever since Roy and Sherrington introduced the concept of neurovascular coupling in 1890 (for a review, see VILLRINGER and DIRNAGL 1995). The fact that rCBF varies with local neuronal activity has allowed the study of brain function in vivo, via the measurement of rCBF by positron emission tomography and single photon emission computed tomography techniques. The function of this activation-dependent coupling seems logical: it has to maintain an adequate supply of oxygen and glucose available to the brain for varying levels of neuronal metabolism. The real-

ity, however, is more complicated: the amount of supplied oxygen does not seem to follow the actual consumption. As expected, the oxygen level of the blood initially slightly drops during the first second(s) of brain activation (the "early response"), indicating an increase in cerebral metabolic rate of oxygen ($CMRO_2$); however, this event is followed by a huge increase in the oxygen concentration (the "late" response) since the increase in blood flow overcompensates the metabolic demand for oxygen (Fig. 16.1c). An uncoupling between rCBF and oxidative metabolism thus takes place and leads to a local increase of blood oxygenation during brain activation. This late response reaches its maximum 3–9 s after onset of the neuronal activation.

16.2.2
Blood Oxygen Level Dependent Image Contrast

The described neurovascular (un)coupling between brain activation and cerebrovascular physiology leads to three effects that can contribute to the fMRI signal: an increase in the blood flow velocity, in the blood flow volume, and in the blood oxygenation level. Using carefully chosen MR imaging parameters, the contribution of blood flow velocity and blood flow volume can be minimized, while maximizing the blood oxygenation dependency of the fMRI signal. The thus obtained fMRI contrast was therefore called "blood oxygenation level dependent (BOLD) contrast." The first MR images which were sensitive to the level of blood oxygenation were presented by OGAWA et al. (1990): dark lines, coinciding with blood vessels, could be seen in gradient-echo images of anoxic rat brain, but not when the rat was breathing 100% oxygen. Initial fMRI experiments (BANDETTINI et al. 1992; FRAHM et al. 1992; KWONG et al. 1992) confirmed the possibility of mapping brain function following sensory stimulation. The BOLD imaging contrast finds its basis in the observation of THULBORN et al. (1982) who observed that the transverse relaxation time of water protons in the blood provides information about the oxygenation state of the blood. The magnetic state of the iron contained in the oxygen-carrying molecule hemoglobin (Hb) is dependent on the amount of oxygen that is present in Hb: it is paramagnetic when Hb is depleted of oxygen (deoxyhemoglobin), whereas it is diamagnetic when the Hb molecule is saturated (oxyhemoglobin).

Susceptibility-weighted images – T2* images – are very suited to measure the change in BOLD contrast upon neuronal activation.

In summary (Fig. 16.1), increase in neuronal activity leads to an increase in oxyHb concentration, i.e., a decrease in local susceptibility, that results mainly in an increase of the MR echo signal of the active brain tissue.

16.2.3
MRI Acquisition

The most widely used fMRI scan technique is ultrafast echo-planar imaging (EPI; MANSFIELD and MAUDSLEY 1977). This technically challenging method makes it possible to form a single-slice MR image in as little as 70–100 ms. Multiple adjacent slices, e.g., 30 slices, are acquired covering the complete brain in approximately 2000–3000 ms. In a blocked fMRI experiment two or more cognitive or sensorimotor tasks (conditions) are alternated resulting in an experiment that lasts several minutes during which the acquisition will be sequentially repeated during the course of the fMRI experiment (Fig. 16.2). In such a block-design fMRI experiment, tasks are generally alternated every 20–40 s.

16.2.4
Specific Constraints
When Performing Auditory fMRI

When a block-design fMRI scheme is applied to auditory studies, subjects undergo continuous stimulation by the scanner noise plus an alternate stimulation by experimental sound stimuli. The acoustic MRI scanner noise, mainly originating

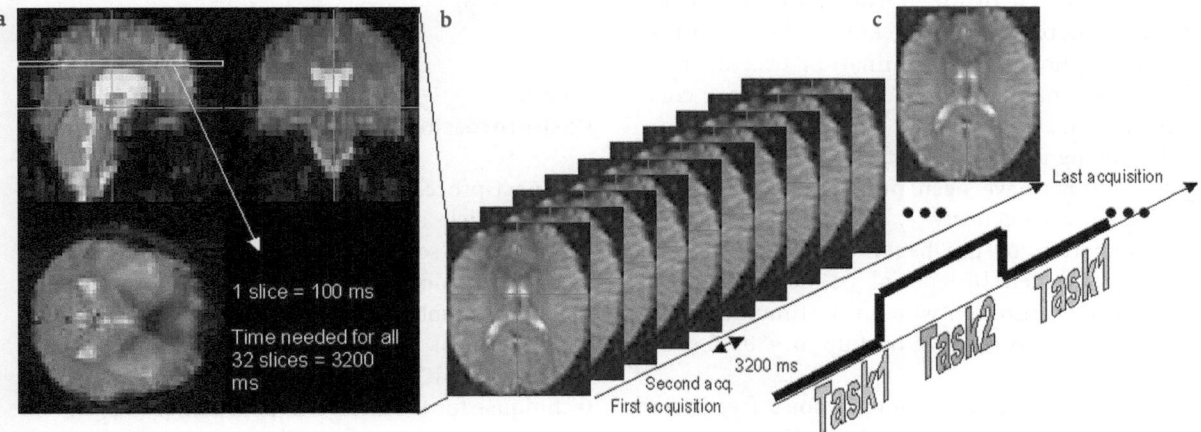

Fig. 16.2a–c. An fMRI acquisition. **a** A stack of 32 gradient-echo echo-planar-imaging (EPI) slices are acquired in 3200 ms. **b** This stack of 32 slices is being sequentially acquired. **c** In a blocked fMRI design two (or more) tasks are alternated every ten acquisitions

from the gradient switching of the EPI scans, may interact with the functional activation of the auditory system induced by the experimental acoustical stimuli. The amplitude of the gradient scanner noise of an EPI sequence, depending on MR system and scan parameters used, can in the "worst case" reach sound pressure levels up to 110 dB (HEDEEN and EDELSTEIN 1997). Furthermore, the MRI scanner sound is not a simple broadband noise, but an amplitude-modulated periodic sound with a complex spectrum. Fourier analysis of this noise reveals energy peaks at specific sound frequency spectrums.

It is therefore likely that some kind of interaction between the background scanner noise and the experimentally delivered stimuli will occur, which depends on the overlap of spectral components of the stimuli and the scanner noise. Moreover, subjects may be engaged in processes different from simple auditory perception because they have to extract the stimulus from the background MR-generated noise.

Indeed, several studies have shown that the scanner noise in fact interferes with the auditory activation of the brain revealed by the fMRI (CHO et al. 1998; ELLIOTT et al. 1999; SHAH et al. 1999). It has been shown that scanner noise itself causes brain activation especially in the primary auditory cortex (BANDETTINI et al. 1998; ULMER et al. 1998). Due to its loud and complex nature, the activity can be strong and might lead to a partial saturation of the vascular BOLD response, thus obscuring the activation pattern caused there by other sounds. ELLIOTT et al. (1999) showed that auditory activation elicited by modulated tones in high noise condition results in a smaller number of activated voxels than that in low noise condition. Furthermore, an increase of the background scanner noise during a phonetic discrimination task decreases the hemodynamic response in the auditory cortex (SHAH et al. 1999).

In solving the problem of the gradient noise, several solutions have been proposed, however, none completely satisfactorily.

Attenuation of the background scanner noise can be obtained by special padded headphones and earplugs, through which the stimuli are delivered; these can provide at best up to ~30 dB overall attenuation.

At the acquisition side, longer noise-free periods during acoustic paradigms have been suggested to be helpful (HALL et al. 1999). As the amount of noise depends on the number of slices in one acqui-

sition volume and on the time between two consequent volumes (TR, repetition time), reducing the number of slices and increasing the repetition time would be beneficial; however, this would reduce the amount of acquired information and increase the measurement time. Different modifications of "sparse" temporal sampling have been suggested (ELLIOTT et al. 1999; EDEN et al. 1999). One of them is sparse acquisition that utilizes the physiological delay between neuronal activity and the related hemodynamic response registered by the fMRI. In sparse acquisition, acoustic stimulation is presented in the period of silence between two consecutive periods of the fMRI data acquisition (Fig. 16.3). These spare experimental designs permits a more detailed insight and has been proven to result in better detection of auditory cortex activation compared with conventional block-design acquisitions (DI SALLE et al. 2001; SCHEFFLER et al. 1998; BILECEN et al. 1998a; HALL et al. 1999; BELIN et al. 1999).

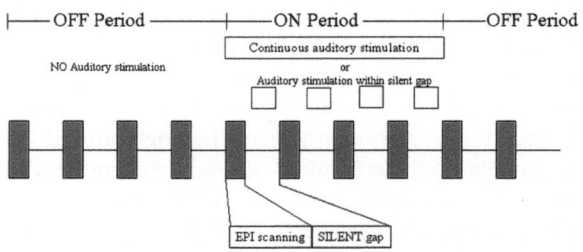

Fig. 16.3. Timing of acoustic stimulation and fMRI measurements in a "sparse" temporal sampling fMRI acquisition. *Gray bars* indicate EPI measurements followed by a resting period (silent gap). During the "on" period acoustic stimulation is switched on either continuously, or pulsed (within the silent gap)

16.2.5
Post-Processing of fMRI Data

The post-processing of fMRI falls outside the scope of this article and is discussed in detail elsewhere (for a review see, for example, TURNER et al. 1998). Briefly, the processing of functional MR brain images involves a number of steps which include correction techniques for head motion, spatial normalization to a standard brain, spatial smoothing, statistical techniques for the reliable separation of the relevant fMRI signal change from the noise, and visualization techniques for localizing activation foci on the anatomy of individual subjects.

16.3
Functional Anatomy of the Auditory System

16.3.1
Anatomy of the Auditory Cortex

Auditory signals are transmitted both ipsilaterally and contralaterally by a chain of neurons extending from the cochlea to the primary auditory cortex (Fig. 16.4), also referred to as Heschl's gyrus on the supratemporal plane along the depth of the Sylvian fissure. BRODMANN (1909) labeled this patch of cortex as area 41. On imaging, Heschl's gyrus is an arch-like gyrus located entirely in the Sylvian fissure. It is oriented oblique within the supratemporal plane and runs from the level of the subcentral region lat-erally to the retroinsular level medially. This relation is best seen on transverse MRI cuts (Fig. 16.5). On sagittal and coronal MR cuts, the transverse temporal gyrus is easily recognized as a "knob" oriented dorsally from the supratemporal plane (Fig. 16.5). Sometimes, two gyri of Heschl are found in the right hemisphere, and are thus called the anterior and posterior transverse temporal gyri, whereas in the left hemisphere one gyrus can generally be found. Heschl's gyrus is limited anteriorly and posteriorly by transverse supratemporal sulci: the anterior one separates Heschl's gyrus from the planum polare, and the posterior one from the planum temporale.

The belt of cortex that forms an arc around area 41 corresponds to the auditory association cortices, and was labeled by BRODMANN (1909) as areas 42 and 22.

16.3.2
FMRI of Monaural and Binaural Auditory Stimulation

There have been several studies depicting auditory activation (BINDER et al. 1994; MILLEN et al. 1995; ZATORRE 1997; STRAINER et al. 1997). In general, simple auditory stimuli (e.g. a noise burst) activate the primary auditory cortex, whereas more complex stimuli activate auditory areas more broadly. A gross map of the auditory activation in response to binaural musical stimulation can be seen in Fig. 16.6. As expected with more complex stimuli, the activity is localized symmetrically in the primary auditory and auditory association cortices.

When auditory stimulation is delivered in one ear only (monaural stimulation), the activation of the auditory cortex is bilateral but highly lateralized to the contralateral side. Using fMRI, SCHEFFLER et al. (1998) reported that the mean lateralization ratios (left volumes to right volumes for right-sided monaural stimulation and right to left for left-sided monaural stimulation) were 3.4 and 5.2, respectively, using 1-kHz pure-tone monaural stimulation. No difference is apparent in regions activated between right and left ear stimulation. The bilateral projection from the cochlea to the cortex (Fig. 16.4) enables highly specialized neurons to determine the time difference should a sound source be farther from one ear than from the other, allowing a sound source to be located. The auditory input in one ear projects predominantly via the contralateral superior olivary complex to the contralateral auditory cortex (Fig. 16.4).

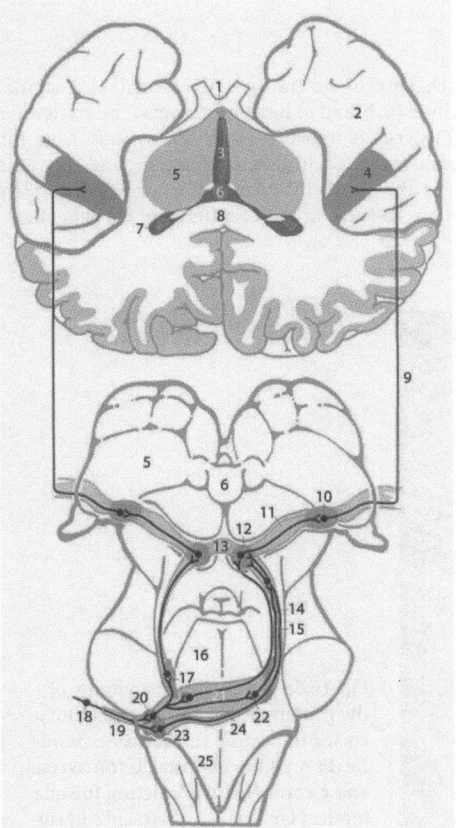

Fig. 16.4. The auditory sensory cortex receives its main afferents from the auditory projections originating in the cochleae, as pre-processed in multiple subcortical nuclei. Fibers pass in the acoustic nerve (cranial nerve VIII) (19) to the brainstem. Nuclei along the ascending auditory pathways lie in the anterior (20) and posterior (23) cochlear nuclei, trapezoid body (22) superior olivary complexes (17), lateral lemnisci (15), inferior colliculi (12), and medial geniculate bodies (10). (Adapted from KRETSCHMANN and WEINRICH 1998)

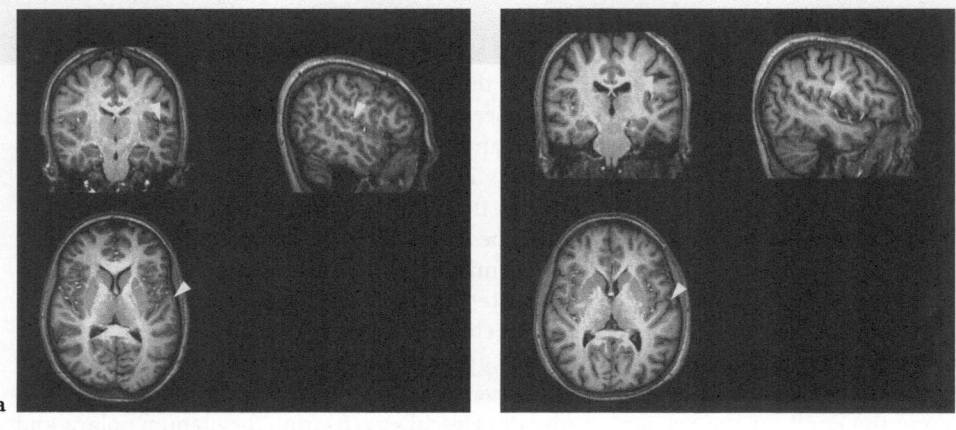

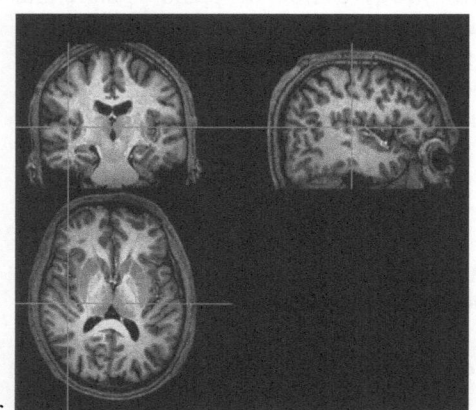

Fig. 16.5. Anatomy of Heschl's gyrus on transversal, coronal, and sagittal T1-weighted MRI cuts in three (**a, b,** and **c**) healthy subjects. The transverse temporal gyrus or Heschl's gyrus is indicated with *arrowheads.* Note the oblique orientation of Heschl's gyrus within the supratemporal plane, as seen on transverse cuts, and the „knob-like" formation oriented dorsally from the supratemporal plane, as seen on both sagittal and coronal cuts

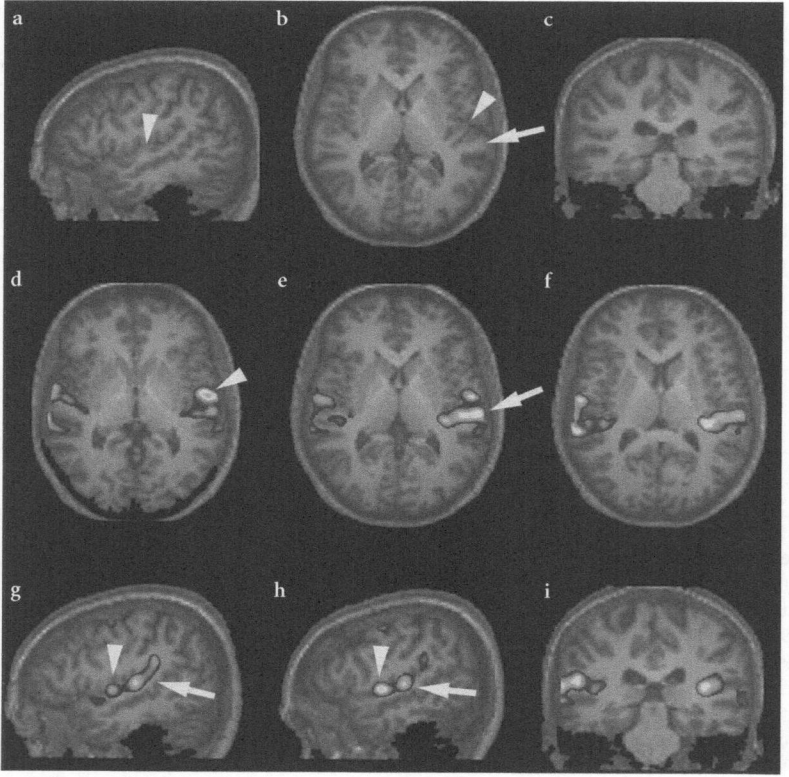

Fig. 16.6a–i. Functional anatomy of the primary and secondary auditory cortex in healthy subject. **a** Anatomical T1-weighted sagittal, **b** transversal, and **c** coronal cuts, depicting the anatomical landmarks of Heschl's gyrus (*arrowhead*) and the planum temporale (*arrow*). **d–f** FMRI activation obtained during binaural musical stimulation vs no stimulation acquired with a sparse temporal sampling fMRI acquisition scheme, overlaid on **g** transverse, **h** sagittal, and **i** coronal cuts. Both primary auditory cortex (Heschl's gyrus; *arrowhead*) and secondary auditory cortices (*arrow*) are activated bilaterally

16.3.3
Tonotopy

Characteristic for the functional anatomy of Heschl's gyrus is its tonotopic organization, which is the spatial organization of frequencies (Fig. 16.7). Similar to the somatotopic organization of the sensorimotor cortex (the typical spatial organization of the sensorimotor cortex for specific body parts, i.e., the homunculus of Penfield), or the retinotopic organization of the visual cortex (i.e., each location in the visual field corresponds to a particular region within the primary visual cortex), the primary auditory cortex contains a tone-frequency specific map. Furthermore, multiple tonotopically organized maps also exist in the surrounding auditory association cortices. Recent fMRI studies have been able to demonstrate this tonotopic organization within Heschl's gyrus, depending on the frequency of pure tone stimuli (Fig. 16.7): responses elicited for tones in the lower frequencies predominated in the lateral transverse temporal gyrus, whereas those for higher frequencies appear localized in the medial part (WESSINGER et al. 2001; TALAVAGE et al. 2000; STRAINER et al. 1997; BILECEN et al. 1998b).

16.3.4
FMRI of Subcortical Auditory Pathway Structures

From neurophysiological measurements in animals it is clear that the tonotopic organization is the major organizational principle throughout the complete ascending auditory system, from the cochlea, over the subcortical nuclei, until the level of the primary and association auditory cortices (Fig. 16.4). It remains to be shown whether the fMRI technique will be able to depict tonotopy in humans at the subcortical levels. Thus far, fMRI data on the human pontine auditory pathway available from the literature are confined to a communication by MELCHER et al. (2000) who detected (non-tonotopic) activation of the cochlear nuclei ipsilateral to the monaural presentation of a musical stimulus, and by HESSELMANN et al. (2001) who visualized activation in the cochlear nuclei and the superior olivary nucleus in response to periodic click stimulation. There are also several articles that deal with the activation of the inferior colliculi and the medial geniculate body (GUIMARAES et al. 1998; MELCHER et al. 2000). We also managed to visualize activation of these structures during presentation of a musical stimulus on a 3-T imager (Fig. 16.8).

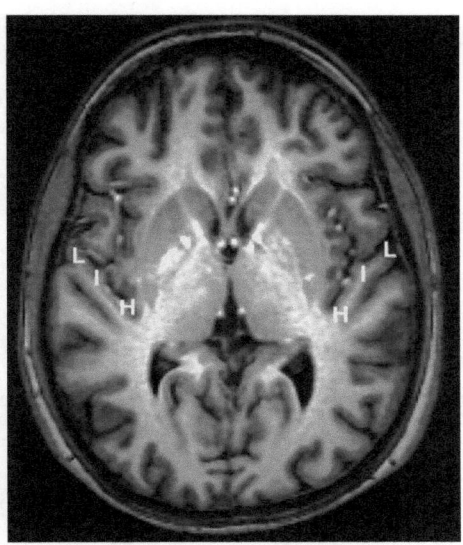

Fig. 16.7. The tonotopic organization of the primary auditory cortex located in Heschl's gyrus. *H* denotes highest tone frequency, *I* intermediate, and *L* lowest tone frequency

16.3.5
Auditory Speech Perception and Language Areas

Specific auditory cortical areas are associated with processing stimuli that have the quality of human voice: BINDER et al. (1996) suggested that the (left) planum temporale is more involved in the processing of higher acoustical features and speech. Additional data (BELIN et al. 2000) demonstrated activation in the superior temporal sulci for passive listening to single words. Sentential as compared with single-word processing seems to involve additional association cortices (MULLER et al. 1997).

16.4
FMRI in Patient with Auditory Disorders

16.4.1
Unilaterally Deaf Subjects

As described above, normal-hearing subjects stimulated monaurally produce approximately three to five times more extensive cortical activation contralaterally than ipsilaterally to the stimulated ear. In contrast to this physiological finding are the data that were acquired in unilateral deaf patients. SCHEFFLER et al. (1998) demonstrated that unilaterally deaf

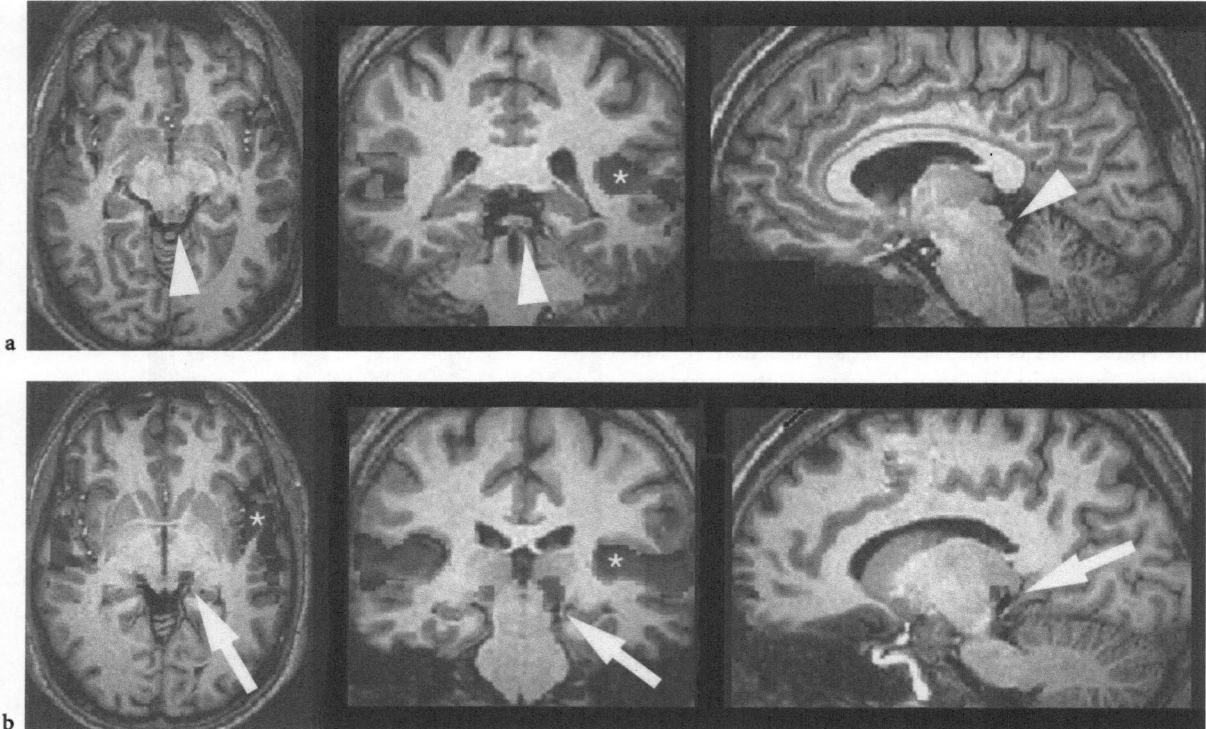

Fig. 16.8. Auditory activation in response to binaural musical stimulation obtained on a 3-T imager (significant at $p<0.05$ corrected for multiple comparisons). Note the activation in the superior colliculi bilaterally (*arrowhead*), the medial geniculate bodies (*arrow*), and the primary and secondary auditory cortices (*asterisk*)

patients stimulated in the functioning ear have less disparity in the activation extent of contralateral vs ipsilateral; in some patients the activation was almost symmetrical. These data are in line with magnetoencephalographic studies (VASAMA and MAKELA 1995) and animal lesion data (SCHWABER et al. 1993) and suggest a functional reorganization of the central auditory system after unilateral damage.

The work of BILECEN et al. (Fig. 16.9; 2000) explored the development of this phenomenon over time. They had the rare opportunity to repeatedly measure fMRI signals in response to auditory stimulation in an initially normal-hearing subject who had lost hearing after an acoustic neurinoma resection (Fig. 16.10). This patient had been studied 1 month before surgery (then normal hearing) and 1, 5, and 55 weeks after surgery (then unilaterally deaf). One week after surgery, unilateral stimulation of the intact left ear yielded a response that was strongly contralateral (left/right ratio: 1/4.8). Five weeks after surgery, less disparity was found (left/right ratio: 1/3.6), and 1 year later the response was almost bilaterally balanced (left/right ratio: 1/1.3). This progressive balancing of activity was largely a result of increasing ipsilateral activity rather than decreasing contralateral activity. A progressing compensatory reorganization with bilateral representation of unilateral acoustic stimulation was thus observed over a period of approximately 1 year. The exact mechanism and sites of this reorganization are largely unknown but might be due to the abundant presence of ipsilateral connections in the ascending auditory pathway (Fig. 16.4). These ipsilateral connections, which are normally suppressed, might become disinhibited when contralateral inhibitory inputs are removed. The biological significance of the cortical reorganization remains to be elucidated, but clearly fMRI, given its complete non-invasiveness and safety, quickly becomes the tool of choice to longitudinally study these reorganizations.

16.4.2
Cochlear Implants

Cochlear implants have proved to be effective and reliable listening devices in profoundly deaf adults and congenitally profoundly deaf children. It involves

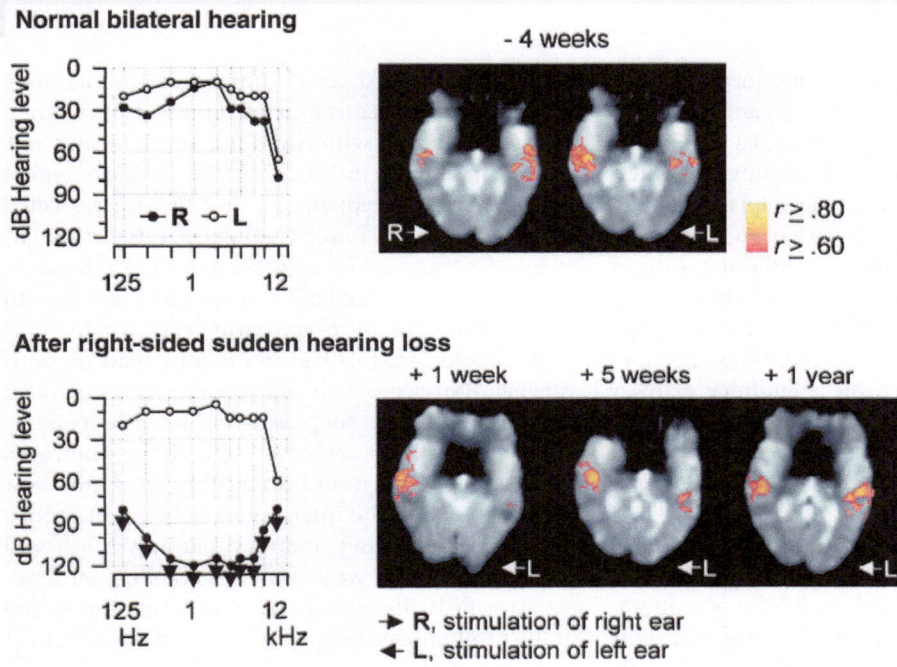

Normal bilateral hearing

− 4 weeks

$r ≥ .80$
$r ≥ .60$

After right-sided sudden hearing loss

+ 1 week + 5 weeks + 1 year

→ R, stimulation of right ear
← L, stimulation of left ear

Fig. 16.9. Pure tone audiometry 1 week before and 3 months after acoustic nerve resection. FMRI activity in the primary auditory cortex after stimulation with a 1-kHz sine tone at 95 dB SPL. Before surgery, a chiefly contralateral response was found. After surgery, progressively balanced bilateral, rather than contralateral, fMRI response pattern. (From BILECEN et al. 2000)

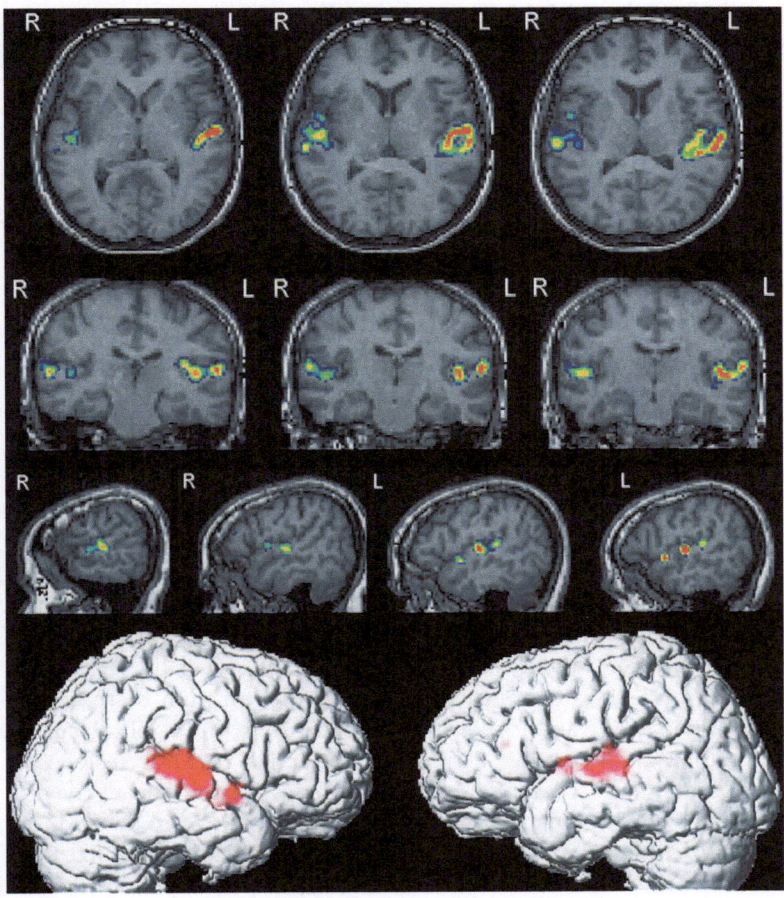

Fig. 16.10. FMRI activity during music listening vs rest ($p<0.05$ corrected for multiple comparisons) overlaid on structural images in transversal, coronal, and sagittal planes, and on a 3D surface reconstruction of the brain of a 34-year-old woman with unilateral left tinnitus. Tinnitus loudness is estimated to be 80 dB and frequency 3–4000 Hz, worsening with exposure to loud high-pitched noise. Note the asymmetry in activation strength and extent of area A1 (L < R), suggestive for cortical reorganization

stimulating intact neurons in the auditory nerve via implanted intracochlear electrodes. Implantees exhibit a wide range of auditory capabilities, e.g., some are conversationally fluent without lip reading, but others are not. As experience with cochlear implantation has increased, the selection criteria have been broadened, and patients with more difficult conditions, such as additional disabilities or special etiologies of deafness, are considered as candidates; therefore, the preoperative diagnostic process becomes more important. In particular, an intact retrocochlear auditory pathway is a basic requirement for a positive outcome with cochlear implantation. Patients could be selected or rejected for implantation, depending on the presence of an intact pathway.

Traditionally, reliable preoperative assessment of the integrity of the central auditory pathway in adult patients is determined by performing the promontory electrical (PT) stimulation test with a needle electrode. This is a subjective test that relies heavily on the patient's sensation and cooperation during stimulation. Especially in congenitally deaf patients, given the fact that these patients have never experienced any auditory sensation, even with an intact retrocochlear auditory pathway and auditory activity, the PT test can be false negative. Furthermore, the PT test cannot be performed in small children or disabled patients because they are unable to cooperate adequately.

Functional MRI could prove to be the objective test that is needed to evaluate those patients. Safe stimulation devices that can be used inside the gauss field of an MR system have recently been developed (OBLER et al. 1999; BERTHEZENE et al. 1997). This MRI-compatible PT test with a needle electrode is used for activation during fMRI. In 1998, MECHLER et al. demonstrated the feasibility of mapping brain activation in response to electrical stimulation of the cochlea in three deaf patients. Using a standard "on"-"off" electrical stimulation, there was clear activation of the contralateral superior temporal lobe, including Heschl's gyrus, in all three subjects. Recently, in a group of 35 profoundly deaf patients, SCHMIDT et al. (2003) reported that 85% of patients who report an auditory sensation during promontory electrical stimulation showed activation of the contralateral auditory cortex. In the group of patients who reported no hearing sensation, 75% did not show activation. The activation in the transverse temporal gyrus (Heschl) was often found in the medial part, an area where high tones should be projected according to the tonotopic organization of the Heschl gyrus. This result could confirm the fact that

the tone heard in PT tests is often described as being very high. Also MECHLER et al. (1998) reported in a patient stimulated with two different electrodes, one located basally in the cochlea (the cochlear region tuned to higher frequencies) and the other located apically (tuned to lower frequencies), that the patterns of activation in auditory cortex for basal vs apical electrical stimulation were in agreement with the normal tonotopic organization (Fig. 16.7).

In conclusion, fMRI examinations with an activated auditory cortex virtually demonstrate an intact auditory pathway, suggesting that these patients are well suited for cochlear implantation; however, a negative examination finding that does not show activation cannot be interpreted as being indicative of a nonfunctioning auditory pathway. Technical problems or a very weak stimulus accounts for false-negative fMRI examinations. Electrical stimulation of the promontory during fMRI can therefore help in making a clinical decision before a cochlear implantation, although a negative result must be considered with great care.

16.4.3
Tinnitus

Tinnitus, the perception of sound when no external sound is present, is a distressing symptom afflicting 15% of the population. Tinnitus can be subdivided into two completely different entities, pulsatile and non-pulsatile tinnitus. Pulsatile tinnitus is the result of a normally functioning auditory system, in which vascular anomalies create a resonance effect in the petrous bone, and can be subdivided into an arterial pulse-synchronized tinnitus and a venous hum. On the contrary, the pathophysiological mechanisms underlying non-pulsatile tinnitus are poorly understood. Recent findings have provided a physiological measure of tinnitus and support the view that non-pulsatile tinnitus is caused by an abnormally functioning and reorganized auditory system (MUHLNICKEL et al. 1998). Any lesion along the auditory tract, influencing its normal function, can generate non-pulsatile tinnitus. Alteration of the normal sensory input, or especially deprivation of input, can lead to reorganization of the entire auditory pathways including the cerebral cortex, e.g., in a frequency-selective cochlear lesion. For example, a high-frequency lesion caused by ototoxic antibiotics, the tonotopic map in the auditory cortex, and brain stem nuclei can reorganize such that cortical neurons deprived of their usual afferent input become supersensitive and now responds to tone frequencies adjacent to the frequency range damaged by the lesion, leading to the symptom of tinnitus.

Recent functional imaging work has contributed to the pathophysiological understanding of tinnitus. MELCHER et al. (2000) studied changes induced by tinnitus at the level of the inferior colliculus. For lateralized tinnitus subjects, they hypothesized that sound-evoked activation would be abnormally asymmetric because of the asymmetry of the tinnitus percept. This was tested using two reference groups for comparison: non-tinnitus subjects and non-lateralized tinnitus subjects. Binaural noise produced abnormally asymmetric inferior colliculus activation in every lateralized tinnitus subject ($n=4$). In reference subjects ($n=9$), activation in the right vs left inferior colliculus did not differ significantly. Compared with reference subjects, lateralized tinnitus subjects showed abnormally low percent signal change in the colliculus inferior contralateral, but not ipsilateral, to the tinnitus percept. Consequently, activation asymmetry (i.e., the ratio of percent signal change in the inferior colliculus ipsilateral vs contralateral to the tinnitus percept) was significantly greater in lateralized tinnitus subjects as compared with normal subjects.

Monaural noise also produced abnormally asymmetric inferior colliculus activation in lateralized tinnitus subjects. MELCHER et al. (2000) proposed two possible models to explain why inferior colliculus activation was abnormally low contralateral to the tinnitus percept in lateralized tinnitus subjects; both assume that the percept is associated with abnormally high ("tinnitus-related") neural activity in the contralateral inferior colliculus. Additionally, they assume that either (a) additional activity evoked by sound was limited by saturation or (b) sound stimulation reduced the level of tinnitus-related activity as it reduced the loudness of (i.e., masked) the tinnitus percept.

Where MELCHER et al. (2000) studied the colliculus inferior only, we recently investigated the primary and secondary auditory cortices in patients with lateralized tinnitus and observed a similar asymmetric activation at the level of the cortex. Functional MRI of the auditory cortex was performed with a stimulation paradigm in which music listening is alternated with no auditory stimulation demonstrating an asymmetrical cortical activity in Heschl's gyrus, with normal activity in the ipsilateral hemisphere and slightly less activity in the contralateral hemisphere (Fig. 16.10).

16.5
Conclusion

The foregoing review demonstrates that fMRI of the auditory system is feasible in both healthy and diseased subjects, and that it is valuable both for basic neuroscience as pathophysiological issues of the auditory system.

The technical difficulties of stimulus delivery in a loud MR scanner environment have been largely dealt with, and future developments in both MR scanner hardware (some manufacturers are announcing completely silent MR scanners in the next decade) and sequences will contribute to a more widespread use of fMRI of the auditory system, eventually also in the clinical setting. The capability of visualizing auditory activity down to the subcortical level, in structures as small as the colliculus inferior, are at present not equaled by any other imaging technique. FMRI thus allows studying early, as well as the later, stages of auditory processing.

As the growing number of studies in healthy volunteers is contributing to the understanding of the normal physiology of the auditory system in humans, clinical applications are emerging (e.g., in patients with hearing loss, cochlear implants, and tinnitus). Clearly, this preliminary clinical work is just the tip of the (future) iceberg, and fMRI should dramatically advance our understanding of human auditory function and dysfunction.

References

Bandettini PA, Wong EC, Hinks RS, Tikofsky RS, Hyde JS (1992) Time course EPI of human brain function during task activation. Magn Reson Med 25:390–397

Bandettini PA, Jesmanowicz A, van Kylen J, Birn RM, Hyde JS (1998) Functional MRI of brain activation induced by scanner acoustic noise. Magn Reson Med 39:410–416

Belin P, Zatorre RJ, Hoge R, Evans AC, Pike B (1999) Event-related fMRI of the auditory cortex. Neuroimage 10: 417–429

Belin P, Zatorre RJ, Lafaille P, Ahad P, Pike B (2000) Voice-selective areas in human auditory cortex. Nature 403:309–312

Berthezene Y, Truy E, Morgon A, Giard MH, Hermier M, Franconi JM, Froment JC (1997) Auditory cortex activation in deaf subjects during cochlear electrical stimulation. Evaluation by functional magnetic resonance imaging. Invest Radiol 32:297–301

Bilecen D, Radu EW, Scheffler K (1998a) The MR tomograph as a sound generator: fMRI tool for the investigation of the auditory cortex. Magn Reson Med 40:934–937

Bilecen D, Scheffler K, Schmid N, Tschopp K, Seelig J (1998b)

Tonotopic organization of the human auditory cortex as detected by BOLD-FMRI. Hear Res 126:19–27

Bilecen D, Seifritz E, Radu EW, Schmid N, Wetzel S, Probst R, Scheffler K (2000) Cortical reorganization after acute unilateral hearing loss traced by fMRI. Neurology 54: 765–767

Binder JR, Rao SM, Hammeke TA, Yetkin FZ, Jesmanowicz A, Bandettini PA, Wong EC, Estkowski LD, Goldstein MD, Haughton VM et al. (1994) Functional magnetic resonance imaging of human auditory cortex. Ann Neurol 35: 662–672. Comment in: Ann Neurol 35:637–638

Binder JR, Frost JA, Hammeke TA, Rao SM, Cox RW (1996) Function of the left planum temporale in auditory and linguistic processing. Brain 119:1239–1247

Brodmann K (1909) Vergleichende Lokalisationslehre der Grosshirnrinde. Johann Ambrosius Barth, pp 130–139

Cho ZH, Chung SC, Lim DW, Wong EK (1998) Effects of the acoustic noise of the gradient systems on fMRI: a study on auditory, motor, and visual cortices. Magn Reson Med 39:331–335

Di Salle F, Formisano E, Seifritz E, Linden DE, Scheffler K, Saulino C, Tedeschi G, Zanella FE, Pepino A, Goebel R, Marciano E (2001) Functional fields in human auditory cortex revealed by time-resolved fMRI without interference of EPI noise. Neuroimage 13:328–338

Eden GF, Joseph JE, Brown HE, Brown CP, Zeffiro TA (1999) Utilizing hemodynamic delay and dispersion to detect fMRI signal change without auditory interference: the behavior interleaved gradients technique. Magn Reson Med 41:13–20

Elliott MR, Bowtell RW, Morris PG (1999) The effect of scanner sound in visual, motor, and auditory functional MRI. Magn Reson Med 41:1230–1235

Frahm J, Bruhn H, Merboldt KD, Hanicke W (1992) Dynamic MR imaging of human brain oxygenation during rest and photic stimulation. J Magn Reson Imaging 2:501–505

Guimaraes AR, Melcher JR, Talavage TM, Baker JR, Ledden P, Rosen BR, Kiang NY, Fullerton BC, Weisskoff RM (1998) Imaging subcortical auditory activity in humans. Hum Brain Mapp 6:33–41

Hall DA, Haggard MP, Akeroyd MA, Palmer AR, Summerfield AQ, Elliott MR, Gurney EM, Bowtell RW (1999) „Sparse" temporal sampling in auditory fMRI. Hum Brain Mapp 7:213–223

Hedeen RA, Edelstein WA (1997) Characterization and prediction of gradient acoustic noise in MR imagers. Magn Reson Med 37:7–10

Hesselmann V, Wedekind C, Kugel H, Schulte O, Krug B, Klug N, Lackner KJ (2001) Functional magnetic resonance imaging of human pontine auditory pathway. Hear Res 158:160–164

Kretschmann HJ, Weinrich W (1998) Neurofunctional systems. 3D reconstructions with correlated Neuroimaging. Thieme, Stuttgart

Kwong KK, Belliveau JW, Chesler DA, Goldberg IE, Weisskoff RM, Poncelet BP, Kennedy DN, Hoppel BE, Cohen MS, Turner R et al. (1992) Dynamic magnetic resonance imaging of human brain activity during primary sensory stimulation. Proc Natl Acad Sci USA 89:5675–5679

Mansfield P, Maudsley AA (1977) Medical imaging by NMR. Br J Radiol 50:188–194

Melcher JR, Eddington DK, Garcia N, Qin M, Sroka J, Weiss-koff RN (1998) Electrically evoked cortical activity in cochlear implant subjects can be mapped using fMRI. Neuroimage 7:S385

Melcher JR, Sigalovsky IS, Guinan JJ Jr, Levine RA (2000) Lateralized tinnitus studied with functional magnetic resonance imaging: abnormal inferior colliculus activation. J Neurophysiol 83:1058–1072

Millen SJ, Haughton VM, Yetkin Z (1995) Functional magnetic resonance imaging of the central auditory pathway following speech and pure-tone stimuli. Laryngoscope 105:1305–1310

Muhlnickel W, Elbert T, Taub E, Flor H (1998) Reorganization of auditory cortex in tinnitus. Proc Natl Acad Sci USA 95: 10340–10343

Muller RA, Rothermel RD, Behen ME, Muzik O, Mangner TJ, Chugani HT (1997) Receptive and expressive language activations for sentences: a PET study. Neuroreport 8: 3767–3770

Obler R, Kostler H, Weber BP, Mack KF, Becker H (1999) Safe electrical stimulation of the cochlear nerve at the promontory during functional magnetic resonance imaging. Magn Reson Med 42:371–378

Ogawa S, Lee TM, Kay AR, Tank DW (1990) Brain magnetic resonance imaging with contrast dependent on blood oxygenation. Proc Natl Acad Sci USA 87:9868–9872

Scheffler K, Bilecen D, Schmid N, Tschopp K, Seelig J (1998) Auditory cortical responses in hearing subjects and unilateral deaf patients as detected by functional magnetic resonance imaging. Cereb Cortex 8:156–163

Schmidt AM, Weber BP, Vahid M, Zacharias R, Neuburger J, Witt M, Lenarz T, Becker H (2003) Functional MR imaging of the auditory cortex with electrical stimulation of the promontory in 35 deaf patients before cochlea implantation. Am J Neuroradiol 24:201–207

Schwaber MK, Garraghty PE, Kaas JH (1993) Neuroplasticity of the adult primate auditory cortex following cochlear hearing loss. Am J Otol 14:252–258

Shah NJ, Jancke L, Grosse-Ruyken ML, Muller-Gartner HW (1999) Influence of acoustic masking noise in fMRI of the auditory cortex during phonetic discrimination. J Magn Reson Imaging 9:19–25

Strainer JC, Ulmer JL, Yetkin FZ, Haughton VM, Daniels DL, Millen SJ (1997) Functional MR of the primary auditory cortex: an analysis of pure tone activation and tone discrimination. Am J Neuroradiol 18:601–610

Talavage TM, Ledden PJ, Benson RR, Rosen BR, Melcher JR (2000) Frequency-dependent responses exhibited by multiple regions in human auditory cortex. Hear Res 150:225–244

Thulborn KR, Waterton JC, Matthews PM, Radda GK (1982) Oxygenation dependence of the transverse relaxation time of water protons in whole blood at high field. Biochim Biophys Acta 714:265–270

Turner R, Howseman A, Rees GE, Josephs O, Friston K (1998) Functional magnetic resonance imaging of the human brain: data acquisition and analysis. Exp Brain Res 123:5–12

Ulmer JL, Biswal BB, Yetkin FZ, Mark LP, Mathews VP, Prost RW, Estkowski LD, McAuliffe TL, Haughton VM, Daniels DL (1998) Cortical activation response to acoustic echo planar scanner noise. J Comput Assist Tomogr 22: 111–119

Vasama JP, Makela JP (1995) Auditory pathway plasticity in

adult humans after unilateral idiopathic sudden sensori-neural hearing loss. Hear Res 87:132–140

Villringer A, Dirnagl U (1995) Coupling of brain activity and cerebral blood flow: basis of functional neuroimaging. Cerebrovasc Brain Metab Rev 7:240–276

Wessinger CM, VanMeter J, Tian B, van Lare J, Pekar J,

Rauschecker JP (2001) Hierarchical organization of the human auditory cortex revealed by functional magnetic resonance imaging. J Cogn Neurosci 13:1–7

Zatorre RJ (1997) Functional neuroimaging in the study of the human auditory cortex. Am J Neuroradiol 18:621–623

Subject Index

List of Contributors

CARLO BARTOLOZZI, MD
Professor and Chairman
Division of Diagnostic and Interventional Radiology
Department of Oncology, Transplants,
and Advanced Technologies in Medicine
University of Pisa
Via Roma 67
56100 Pisa
Italy

A. BEHIN, MD
Department of Neuroradiology Charcot
Group Hospitalier Pitié-Salpêtrière
47 Boulevard de l'Hôpital
75013 Paris
France

STEFANO BERRETTINI, MD
Division of Otolaryngology
Department of Neuroscience
University of Pisa
Via Roma 67
56100 Pisa
Italy

CARLA CAPPELLI, MD
Division of Diagnostic and Interventional Radiology
Department of Oncology, Transplants,
and Advanced Technologies in Medicine
University of Pisa
Via Roma 67
56100 Pisa
Italy

DAVIDE CARAMELLA, MD
Division of Diagnostic and Interventional Radiology
Department of Oncology, Transplants,
and Advanced Technologies in Medicine
University of Pisa
Via Roma 67
56100 Pisa
Italy

J. CHIRAS, MD
Department of Neuroradiology Charcot
Group Hospitalier Pitié-Salpêtrière
47 Boulevard de l'Hôpital
75013 Paris
France

C. CZERNY, MD
MR and Osteology, Leitstelle 8F
Universitäts-Klinik für Radiodiagnostik AKH
Ludwig-Boltzmann-Institut für radiologische
und physikalische Tumordiagnostik
Währinger Gürtel 18-20
1090 Vienna
Austria

BERT DE FOER, MD
Department of Radiology
A.Z. Sint Augustinus
Oosterveldlaan 24
2610 Antwerp (Wilrijk)
Belgium

INGEBORG DHOOGE, MD
Ghent University Hospital
De Pintelaan, 185
9000 Ghent
Belgium

A. DIRISAMER, MD
MR and Osteology, Leitstelle 8F
Universitäts-Klinik für Radiodiagnostik AKH
Ludwig-Boltzmann-Institut für radiologische
und physikalische Tumordiagnostik
Währinger Gürtel 18-20
1090 Vienna
Austria

ROBERT HERMANS, MD, PhD
Professor, Department of Radiology
University Hospitals K.U. Leuven
Herestraat 49
3000 Leuven
Belgium

HERWIG IMHOF, MD
Professor, MR and Osteology, Leitstelle 8F
Universitäts-Klinik für Radiodiagnostik AKH
Ludwig-Boltzmann-Institut für radiologische
und physikalische Tumordiagnostik
Währinger Gürtel 18-20
1090 Vienna
Austria

Spyros S. Kollias, MD
Chief of MRI
Institute of Neuroradiology
University Hospital of Zurich
Frauenklinikstrasse 10
8091 Zurich
Switzerland

Marc Lemmerling, MD, PhD
Medische Beeldvorming
A.Z. St. Lucas
Groenebriel 1
9000 Gent
Belgium

Nadine Martin-Duverneuil, MD
Department of Neuroradiology Charcot
Group Hospitalier Pitié-Salpêtrière
47 Boulevard de l'Hôpital
75013 Paris
France

Emanuele Neri, MD
Division of Diagnostic and Interventional Radiology
Department of Oncology, Transplants,
and Advanced Technologies in Medicine
University of Pisa
Via Roma 67
56100 Pisa
Italy

E. Oschatz, MD
MR and Osteology, Leitstelle 8F
Universitäts-Klinik für Radiodiagnostik AKH
Ludwig-Boltzmann-Institut für radiologische
und physikalische Tumordiagnostik
Währinger Gürtel 18-20
1090 Vienna
Austria

Stefan Sunaert, MD, PhD
Department of Radiology
University Hospitals K.U. Leuven
Herestraat 49
3000 Leuven
Belgium

Hervé Tanghe, MD
Department of Radiology
Section of Neuroradiology
Dijkzigt, Sophia Children & Daniel Den Hoed Hospitals
Erasmus University Medical Centre
Dr. Molenwaterplein 40
3015 GD Rotterdam
The Netherlands

Luc van den Hauwe, MD
Departttment of Radiology
AZ Klina
Augustlijnslei 100
2930 Brasschaat
Belgium

MEDICAL RADIOLOGY Diagnostic Imaging and Radiation Oncology

Titles in the series already published

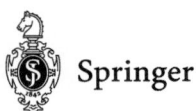

Springer

MEDICAL RADIOLOGY Diagnostic Imaging and Radiation Oncology

Titles in the series already published

RADIATION ONCOLOGY

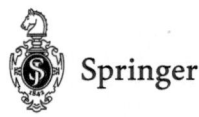
Springer